Julius July • Eka J. Wahjoepramono
Editors

Neurovascular Surgery

Surgical Approaches for Neurovascular Diseases

Editors

Julius July
Department of Neurosurgery
Pelita Harapan University
Tangerang
Indonesia

Eka J. Wahjoepramono
Department of Neurosurgery
Pelita Harapan University
Tangerang
Indonesia

https://doi.org/10.1007/978-981-10-8950-3

Preface

This book is a compilation of the practical details and practices of the key steps in doing a neurosurgery for residents and young neurosurgeons, which provides a variety of illustrations of the intraoperative photographs that will help neurosurgeons gain a better understanding in the neurosurgery field. The chapters are grouped into three parts. The first part, from Chap. 1 through 10, is about an approach-based topic which focuses primarily on the commonly used approach for vascular lesion. The second part, from Chap. 11 through 25, consists of a variety of surgery procedures for specific location of vascular lesion or specific pathology.

The first two groups provide the expert's trick on how to avoid complications during the surgery and some additional expert opinions. The third part, from Chap. 26 through 32, compiles the miscellaneous information that contains some supportive knowledge, technology improvement, and other options of treatment modalities. The detailed and step-by-step approach presented in each chapter with the intraoperative pictures will help provide guidance, especially for many young neurosurgeons who are in the areas with limited resources.

It is a goal to keep this book simple and practical by providing the strength of basic surgical anatomy orientation. Each specific pathology or location requires different approaches that have been addressed in some of the chapters. Every thought and idea shared in the chapters of this book is written by experts who have been in their fields, practicing for many years. Every contributor represents his or her region's best practices that have been proven true based from the neurosurgery results and testimonies they collected and experienced.

We would like to say many thanks to all the contributors who unselfishly shared their expertise and time and to the Springer Publishing Co., which made the publication possible, especially to Dr. Eti Dinesh who encouraged the editors to get this book published. Our gratitude to all the people who are involved in the preparation, from the moment this book was conceptualized. A special thanks to Dr. Megah Indrasari whose support motivated us to believe in what we see for the future of neurosurgery and to never give up on our dreams. And to all our friends who journeyed along with us through this project.

May this book serve as a quick and practical reference for many young neurosurgeons and to those who may need it, in all parts of the world.

Tangerang, Indonesia Julius July
Tangerang, Indonesia Eka J. Wahjoepramono

Contents

Part II Surgery for Specific Location of Vascular Lesion or Specific Pathology

About the Editors

Julius July completed his fellowship in neurovascular surgery at the Department of Neurosurgery, Fujita Health University Hospital, Toyoake, Nagoya, Japan in 2003 and in neuro-oncology and skull-base surgery at the Department of Neurosurgery, Toronto Western Hospital, University of Toronto, Canada in 2007. He is also a certified International Fellow of the American Association of Neurological Surgeons (IFAANS), and a member of the Congress of Neurological Surgeons (CNS), and Asian Congress of Neurological Surgeons (ACNS).

He is a member of the neuro-oncology and neurovascular committee of the Indonesian Society of Neurological Surgeons (PERSPEBSI) and vice treasurer of the Indonesian Society of Neurological Surgeons (PERSPEBSI). He has published numerous journal articles and books and is an editorial board member of Medicinus (Medical Journal of Pelita Harapan University), the Journal of Spine and Neurosurgery, the Indonesian Biomedical Journal, and the Asian Journal of Neurosurgery. He is currently an associate professor at Department of Neurosurgery and director of clinical education at the Medical Faculty of Universitas Pelita Harapan, Tangerang, Indonesia. He is also a staff neurosurgeon at the Neuroscience Center, Siloam Hospital Lippo Village. He is involved in teaching and mentoring neurosurgery residents and medical students. His areas of interest include neurovascular surgery, neuro-oncology, and neuro-endoscopy surgery.

Eka J. Wahjoepramono is currently a professor, chairman, and dean of the Medical Faculty of Universitas Pelita Harapan, Tangerang, Indonesia. He is an active neurosurgeon at the Neuroscience Center, Siloam Hospital Lippo Village. He is an editorial board member of several national and international journals and is a widely published author. He is also a member of AANS (American Association of Neurological Surgeons), vice treasurer of WFNS World Federation of Neurosurgical Societies, chair of the educational committee of AASNS (Asian Australasian Society of Neurological Surgeons), the past president of ACNS (Asian Congress of neurological surgeons), and a member of neurovascular committee of the Indonesian Society of Neurological Surgeons (PERSPEBSI).

Contributors

Jafri Malin Abdullah, MD Department of Neurosciences, Centre for Neurosciences Services and Research, School of Medical Sciences, Universiti Sains Malaysia Health Campus, Kota Bharu, Kelantan, Malaysia

Hugo Andrade-Barazarte, MD Department of Neurosurgery, Helsinki University Central Hospital, Helsinki, Finland

Miguel A. Arraez, MD, PhD Department of Neurosurgery, Carlos Haya University Hospital, Malaga, Spain

Hildo Azevedo-Filho, MD, PhD, MSc, FRCS SN Department of Neurological Surgery, Hospital da Restauracao, Recife, Brazil

Abdul Hafid Bajamal, MD Department of Neurosurgery, Universitas Airlangga, Dr. Soetomo General Hospital, Surabaya Neuroscience Institute, Surabaya, Indonesia

Miguel Dominguez, MD, PhD Department of Neurosurgery, Carlos Haya University Hospital, Malaga, Spain

Rosalia Duarte, MD Department of Neurosurgery, Helsinki University Central Hospital, Helsinki, Finland

Asra Al Fauzi, MD Department of Neurosurgery, Universitas Airlangga, Dr. Soetomo General Hospital, Surabaya Neuroscience Institute, Surabaya, Indonesia

Alberto Feletti, MD, PhD Department of Neurosurgery, Fujita Health University, Banbuntane Hotokukai Hospital, Nagoya city, Aichi, Japan

Department of Neurosurgery, NOCSAE Modena Hospital, Modena, Italy

Antonio López González, MD Department of Neurosurgery, Virgen Macarena and Virgen del Rocío University Hospitals, Seville, Spain

Senanur Gulec Department of Neurosurgery, Faculty of Medicine Universitas Pelita Harapan (UPH), Neuroscience Centre Siloam Hospital Lippo Village, Tangerang, Indonesia

Marmara University School of Medicine, Istanbul, Turkey

Julian Han, MD National Neuroscience Institute (NNI), Singapore, Singapore

Harsan, MD, PhD Department of Neurosurgery, Faculty of Medicine Universitas Pelita Harapan (UPH), Neuroscience Centre Siloam Hospital Lippo Village, Tangerang, Indonesia

Christian Heinen, MD Department of Neurosurgery, Evangelisches Krankenhaus Oldenburg, Oldenburg, Germany

Lutfi Hendriansyah, MD, PhD Gamma Knife Center Indonesia, Siloam Hospitals Lippo Village, Tangerang, Indonesia

Juha Hernesniemi, MD, PhD Department of Neurosurgery, Helsinki University Central Hospital, Helsinki, Finland

Ferzat Hijazy, MD Department of Neurosurgery, Helsinki University Central Hospital, Helsinki, Finland

Jun Hiramoto, MD Department of Neurosurgery, Fuchu Keijinkai Hospital, Tokyo, Japan

Guillermo Ibañez, MD Department of Neurosurgery, Carlos Haya University Hospital, Malaga, Spain

Zamzuri Idris, MD Department of Neurosciences, Centre for Neurosciences Services and Research, School of Medical Sciences, Universiti Sains Malaysia Health Campus, Kota Bharu, Kelantan, Malaysia

Fusao Ikawa, MD Department of Neurosurgery, Shimane Prefectural Central Hospital, Izumo, Japan

Behnam Rezai Jahromi, MB, MD Department of Neurosurgery, Helsinki University Central Hospital, Helsinki, Finland

Julius July, MD, PhD, MHSc, IFAANS Department of Neurosurgery, Faculty of Medicine Universitas Pelita Harapan (UPH), Neuroscience Centre Siloam Hospital Lippo Village, Tangerang, Indonesia

Imad N. Kanaan, MD, FACS, FRCS Department of Neurosciences, King Faisal Specialist Hospital and Research Center, Alfaisal University, College of Medicine, Riyadh, Saudi Arabia

Regunath Kandasamy, MD Department of Neurosciences, Centre for Neurosciences Services and Research, School of Medical Sciences, Universiti Sains Malaysia Health Campus, Kota Bharu, Kelantan, Malaysia

Yoko Kato, MD, PhD Department of Neurosurgery, Fujita Health University, Toyoake, Aichi, Japan

Tsukasa Kawase, MD, PhD Department of Neurosurgery, Fujita Health University, Banbuntane Hotokukai Hospital, Nagoya city, Aichi, Japan

Yong Bae Kim, MD Department of Neurosurgery, Yonsei University College of Medicine, Gangnam Severance Hospital, Seoul, South Korea

Thomas Kretschmer, MD, PhD Department of Neurosurgery, Evangelisches Krankenhaus Oldenburg, Oldenburg, Germany

Naoya Kuwayama, MD, PhD Division of Neuroendovascular Therapy, Department of Neurosurgery, University of Toyama, Toyama, Japan

Aki Laakso, MD, PhD Department of Neurosurgery, Helsinki University Central Hospital, Helsinki, Finland

Kyu Sung Lee, MD Department of Neurosurgery, Yonsei University College of Medicine, Gangnam Severance Hospital, Seoul, South Korea

Martin Lehecka, MD, PhD Department of Neurosurgery, Helsinki University Central Hospital, Helsinki, Finland

Hanna Lehto, MD Department of Neurosurgery, Helsinki University Central Hospital, Helsinki, Finland

Dilshod Mamadaliev, MD Department of Neurosurgery, Fujita Health University, Banbuntane Hotokukai Hospital, Nagoya city, Aichi, Japan

Republican Scientific Center of Neurosurgery, Tashkent, Uzbekistan

Johan Marjamaa, MD, PhD Department of Neurosurgery, Helsinki University Central Hospital, Helsinki, Finland

Tushit Mewada, MCh Department of Neurosurgery, Fujita Health University, Banbuntane Hotokukai Hospital, Nagoya city, Aichi, Japan

G. B. Pant Institute of Post Graduate Medical Education and Research, New Delhi, India

Kentaro Mori, MD, PhD Department of Neurosurgery, National Defense Medical College, Tokorozawa, Saitama, Japan

Ivan Ng, MD National Neuroscience Institute (NNI), Singapore, Singapore

Mohsen Nouri, MD Gundishapour Academy of Neuroscience, Ahvaz, Iran

Andrés Muñoz Nuñez, MD Department of Neurosurgery, Virgen Macarena and Virgen del Rocío University Hospitals, Seville, Spain

Aruma O'shahinan, MD Department of Neurosurgery, Helsinki University Central Hospital, Helsinki, Finland

Naoki Otani, MD Department of Neurosurgery, National Defense Medical College, Tokorozawa, Saitama, Japan

Sophie Peeters, MD Department of Neurosurgery, Faculty of Medicine Universitas Pelita Harapan (UPH), Neuroscience Centre Siloam Hospital Lippo Village, Tangerang, Indonesia,

Department of Neurosurgery, University of California Los Angeles (UCLA), Los Angeles, CA, USA

Anna Piippo, MD, PhD Department of Neurosurgery, Helsinki University Central Hospital, Helsinki, Finland

Francisco Javier Márquez Rivas, MD, PhD Department of Neurosurgery, Virgen Macarena and Virgen del Rocío University Hospitals, Seville, Spain

Bienvenido Ros, MD Department of Neurosurgery, Carlos Haya University Hospital, Malaga, Spain

Ittichai Sakarunchai, MD Division of Neurosurgery, Department of Surgery, Faculty of Medicine, Prince of Songkhla University, Songkhla, Thailand

Tetsuro Sameshima, MD, PhD Department of Neurosurgery, Hamamatsu University School of Medicine, University Hospital, Hamamatsu city, Japan

Cristina Sanchez-Viguera, MD Department of Neurosurgery, Carlos Haya University Hospital, Malaga, Spain

Ferry Senjaya, MD Department of Neurosurgery, Faculty of Medicine Universitas Pelita Harapan (UPH), Neuroscience Centre Siloam Hospital Lippo Village, Tangerang, Indonesia

Thomas Schmidt, MD Department of Neurosurgery, Evangelisches Krankenhaus Oldenburg, Oldenburg, Germany

Joseph C. Serrone, MD Department of Neurosurgery, Virginia Mason Medical Center, Seattle, WA, USA

Guowei Shu, MD Department of Neurosurgery, Shuguang Hospital, Shanghai University of Traditional Chinese Medicine, Shanghai, China

Francesca Spedicato, MD Department of Neurosurgery, Faculty of Medicine Universitas Pelita Harapan (UPH), Neuroscience Centre Siloam Hospital Lippo Village, Tangerang, Indonesia

Universita Degli Studi. "A.Moro" School of Medicine, Bari, Italy

Nur Setiawan Suroto, MD Department of Neurosurgery, Universitas Airlangga, Dr. Soetomo General Hospital, Surabaya Neuroscience Institute, Surabaya, Indonesia

Daisuke Suyama, MD Department of Neurosurgery, Fuchu Keijinkai Hospital, Tokyo, Japan

Department of Neurosurgery, Fujita Health University, Banbuntane Hotokukai Hospital, Nagoya city, Aichi, Japan

Ryan D. Tackla, MD Department of Neurosurgery, Virginia Mason Medical Center, Seattle, WA, USA

Mardjono Tjahjadi, MD Department of Neurosurgery, Helsinki University Central Hospital, Helsinki, Finland

Terushige Toyooka, MD Department of Neurosurgery, National Defense Medical College, Tokorozawa, Saitama, Japan

Eduardo Vieira, MD Department of Neurological Surgery, Hospital da Restauracao, Recife, Brazil

Eka J. Wahjoepramono, MD, PhD Department of Neurosurgery, Faculty of Medicine Universitas Pelita Harapan (UPH), Neuroscience Centre Siloam Hospital Lippo Village, Tangerang, Indonesia

Petra Wahjoepramono, MD Department of Neurosurgery, Medical Faculty of Universitas Padjadjaran, Hasan Sadikin Hospital, Bandung, West Java, Indonesia

Department of Neurosurgery, Faculty of Medicine Universitas Pelita Harapan (UPH), Neuroscience Centre Siloam Hospital Lippo Village, Tangerang, Indonesia

Xiangdong Wang, MD Department of Neurosurgery, Fujita Health University, Banbuntane Hotokukai Hospital, Nagoya city, Aichi, Japan

Yasuhiro Yamada, MD, PhD Department of Neurosurgery, Fujita Health University, Banbuntane Hotokukai Hospital, Nagoya city, Aichi, Japan

Kei Yamashiro, MD Department of Neurosurgery, Fujita Health University, Banbuntane Hotokukai Hospital, Nagoya city, Aichi, Japan

Mario Zuccarello, MD Department of Neurosurgery, University of Cincinnati, Cincinnati, OH, USA

Part I

Surgical Approaches

1 Pterional Approach

Sophie Peeters and Julius July

1.1 Introduction

For years, surgeons have been developing surgical approaches attempting to achieve maximal surgical exposure with minimal brain retraction, advantages found within the frontotemporal or pterional approach, first described by Yasargil, four decades ago [1–3]. Compared to its predecessors, this approach allowed for wider frontobasal exposure, secondary to more significant drilling away sphenoid wing; in addition to that surgeon could dissect and split Sylvian fissure wider [1]. Consequently, it was applicable for clipping of both basilar tip and anterior circulation aneurysms, with an excellent safety-efficacy profile [1]. Later on, the approach will be modified and combined with others, and its indications are only growing in number.

S. Peeters
Department of Neurosurgery,
Faculty of Medicine Universitas Pelita Harapan (UPH), Neuroscience Centre Siloam Hospital Lippo Village, Tangerang, Indonesia

Department of Neurosurgery, University of California Los Angeles (UCLA), Los Angeles, CA, USA

J. July (✉)
Department of Neurosurgery, Faculty of Medicine Universitas Pelita Harapan (UPH), Neuroscience Centre Siloam Hospital Lippo Village, Tangerang, Indonesia

1.2 Steps of the Approach

1.2.1 Positioning and Preparation

Position the patient supine, head fixated with a Sugita or Mayfield head holder. Two pins need to be contralateral at superior temporal line right above the temporal muscle, and lastly, the third pin is placed at the ipsilateral mastoid (Fig. 1.1).

When positioning the head, pay attention to five movements: (1) traction when moving the head toward the surgeon; (2) lifting the surgical area to a level above the atrium, to avoid impeding venous return; (3) deflection and (4)

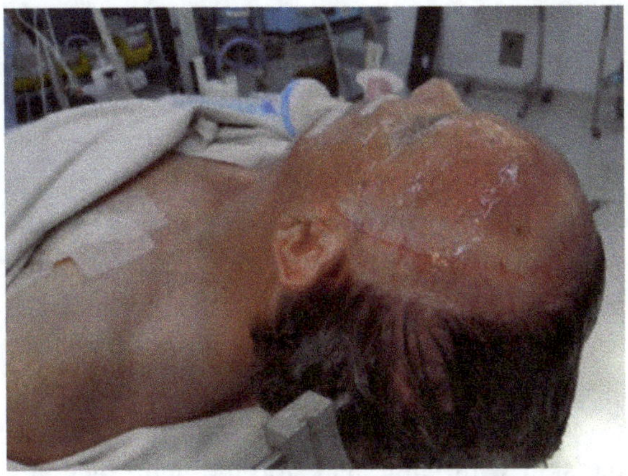

Fig. 1.1 Supine position, head is fixed with Sugita head holder with three pins fixed. The angle of head rotation can be tailored according to tip of exposure that we want to achieve. Usual angle for pterional approach would be around 30–60° head rotation to the contralateral side

J. July, E. J. Wahjoepramono (eds.), *Neurovascular Surgery*,
https://doi.org/10.1007/978-981-10-8950-3_1

rotation, both related to the surgical indication; and (5) torsion, with the angle between the head, neck, and shoulder, large enough to give the surgeon a satisfying lateral operating position [4]. Conditions needing slight deflection with rotation 45–60° from vertical line to the floor include cavernous sinus pathologies and basal lesions, for example, internal carotid (IC)-ophthalmic aneurysm, IC-posterior communicating aneurysm, and IC-choroidal segment aneurysm. Contrarily, conditions requiring increased deflection with rotation 30–45° from vertical line to the floor include carotid bifurcation aneurysm, middle cerebral artery (MCA) aneurysm, anterior communicating aneurysms, and anterior cerebral artery aneurysm, as well as suprasellar tumors.

The hair is combed with chlorhexidine solution (Microshield®) or any detergent solution and subsequently shaved about 2 cm from incision line. The shaved skin is then treated with alcohol, getting rid of scalp fat and facilitating sticking of the sterile fields. The incision is marked with methylene blue or marked with transofix (Fig. 1.1) after injection of local anesthetic with lidocaine 10 mg/mL mixed with adrenaline 6.25 µg solution. The injection at pin site and the incision site provides additional protection to pain, and the adrenaline would help to keep the drape clean from the blood loss during incision.

An arcuate semicoronal frontotemporal skin cut is performed starting from the upper edge zygomatic arch, anterior to tragal cartilage. The skin cut should preserve the superficial temporal artery and frontal branch of facial nerve. The incision extends to the midline of the frontal skull, ideally concealed behind the hairline. The arch of Sugita head holder should be placed for suspension and traction of myocutaneous flaps to avoid compression of the eyeball. Finally, incise the skin with knife, and stop the scalp bleeding with bipolar, and apply the Raney clips. Proceed with subgaleal dissection until the line between the superior border of orbital rim and tragus dissects until leaving anterior one fourth of the temporal fascia [5]. Retract the skin flap to anterior, and hold it with fish hooks.

1.2.2 Dissection and Mobilize Temporal Muscle

Interfascial splitting at temporal region was first introduce by Yasargil [6]. The challenge of this step is preserving the frontalis nerve and reducing unwanted cosmetic results after the surgery. The temporal muscle can be divided into two portions: one originating along the superior temporal line and then inserting to mandibular coronoid process and the second portion originating on the temporal squama and inserting onto the mandibular temporal crest [7]. There are also two layers of fascia that cover this muscle (superficial and deep). Deep layer protects the vessel supplying the muscle which consists of anterior, intermediate, and posterior deep temporal arteries, all originating from the maxillary artery. It also protects the innervations that are coming from trigeminal nerve (temporal and mandible branches) [7]. The splitting plane through laminae of the temporal fascia is created, protecting the frontotemporal branch of the frontal nerve [6]. The temporal muscle is retracted away from temporal fossa, thus improving exposure and limiting unnecessary retraction of the cortex while doing surgery. Dissect the superficial fascia vertically with a scalpel of Metzenbaum scissors starting about 2 cm at superior orbital rim to the zygomatic root, along superior temporal line [7]. Avoid monopolar cauterization to limit the risk of temporal muscle atrophy. Placing a hook in the center may aid the separation by scalpel of the superficial fascia with the underlying fat plane, obtaining best identification of the deeper muscle part that contains nerves and vessels. Both the superficial and fat layers are reflected anterolaterally over the skin flap. To detach the temporalis muscle, first use the monopolar (on coagulation to avoid any extra bleeding), and transversally cut the temporal muscle at its insertion, medially to zygoma and frontal zygomatic process. Then, use a scalpel to cut the muscle in an anterior to posterior motion slightly below the superior temporal line. A small portion of the myofascial cuff is intentionally left at superior temporal line on the bone flap for future muscle reconstruction in order to prevent atrophy of the muscle [8, 9].

Secondarily, detach the deep fascia from the skull using a Cushing's elevator. To avoid bleeding, start detaching the muscle flap inferiorly where the muscle is least attached to the bone [9]. These maneuvers release the fascia temporalis, aponeurosis, temporal muscle, and temporal periosteum from the temporal muscle's origin. Once detached, the temporal muscle is retracted inferiorly leaving its tendinous attachment intact, exposing the pterional region. Finally, reflect the periosteum cranial to superior temporal line to the anterior direction. Remember to keep all the tissue moisture by covering it with wet gauge.

1.2.3 Craniotomy

The craniotomy for this will vary based on surgical aim; typically, one or two burr holes are sufficient, though many surgeons will use three. The aim of this craniotomy is more basal exposure as well as generous visibility of the Sylvian fissure. Thus, the goal is to attempt exposure of the inferior frontal, part of the middle frontal, gyrus superior temporal, and superior part of gyrus middle temporal. The burr holes are performed with common drilling system aiming posteriorly and inferiorly to avoid penetrating the orbit [9]. The first and most important burr hole, also called "keyhole," is placed at the meeting point between zygomatic bone, the superior temporal line, and supraorbital edge [9]. Second trepanation is located inferiorly in the temporal bone's squamous portion, near the pterion. Lastly, the third hole, optional but recommended in older patients due to their dura sticking to the skull, is made on the most posterior end of superior temporal line. Use dissectors to detach the dura from the skull. The Sylvian fissure lies beneath the pterion; thus, the inferior frontal gyrus lies between the pterion and the superior temporal line. Use either a Gigli saw or a craniotome for the craniotomy, as long as the cut is made along the outer edge of the trepanations and extended frontally, taking care not to open the frontal sinus. Use a bipolar forceps for hemostasis at low power to prevent more dural shrinking. Greater sphenoid wing lies deep between first and second burr holes and, if too prominent, may require some rongeuring prior to elevate the bone flap; the alternative is fracturing the bone when elevating the flap.

1.2.4 Basal Drilling

Extradural gentle drilling of greater sphenoid wing process, projections of orbital roof, and the rest of temporal squama until exposing the superior orbital fissure may be necessary for better access to the basal structures with limited brain retraction and flatter bone ridges [8]. The exposure will be magnified even more with opening of the cisterns and subsequent drainage of the cerebrospinal fluid. Some even recommend performing lumbar spinal CSF drainage and ventriculostomy to get more relax brain for a skull base approach. Use dissectors to detach the dura from orbital roof and part that left on lesser sphenoid wing bone without extending past the limits of the drilling, to avoid forming extradural dead spaces. Place a spatula, attached to an orthostatic retractor, to serve a shield to protect the dural surface. A cylindrical or round drill is used to remove remaining bony prominences from the outside inward on the orbital roof and the remaining temporal squama. Next, protect the underlying dura with a spatula, and drill the lesser sphenoid until dural cuff containing the meningo-orbital artery located at the superolateral border of the superior orbital fissure is visible. Isolate, coagulate, and section this artery using a scalpel. The best drill for delicate drilling is diamond drill. To relax tension on the dura, if necessary, a small incision at the projection of the lateral fissure level can allow for cerebrospinal fluid drainage. After drilling, anchor the dura by stitching it (3.0 round silk) at bone edge to avoid collection of epidural blood during or after the operation.

1.2.5 Opening the Dura and Exposing the Brain

The purpose of incising and retracting the dura is to keep it smooth when folded back over the bony surface; dural folds can sometimes hinder visibility.

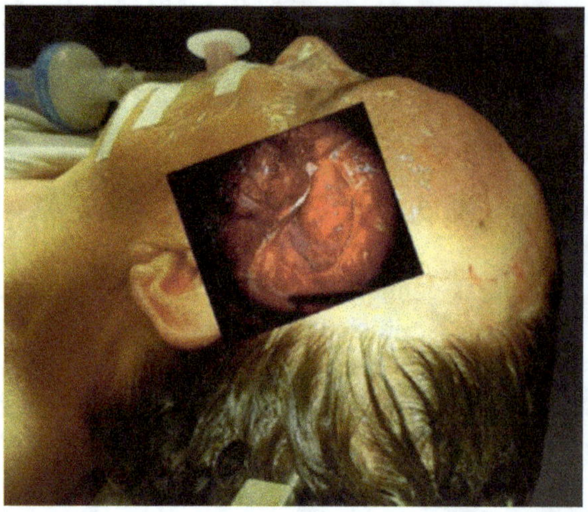

Fig. 1.2 The inserted picture shows the opening flap is retracted toward anterior inferior using fish hook and the C-shape opening of dura with its concave facing the skull base. The brain is slightly tense and red, which is common for aneurysmal subarachnoid bleed. This is the case with left M1 bifurcation aneurysm bleed

Use Metzenbaum scissors to incise the dura in a "C"-shaped manner creating a flap pedunculated toward the previously roungered greater sphenoidal wing, improving parasellar visibility.

The concavity of the incision should be toward the orbit and sphenoid that were previously roungered or flattened using high-speed drill; the pedunculated flap is then retracted over the greater sphenoidal wing remains (Fig. 1.2). This maneuver will exposes the inferior frontal gyrus, the superior temporal gyrus, the middle temporal gyrus, and most importantly the Sylvian fissure.

1.2.6 Splitting Sylvian Fissure

Sylvian fissure can be divided into superficial and a deep part [4]. The stem of the superficial part extends medial to the semilunar gyrus of the uncus between inferior frontal lobe and pole of temporal lobe until lateral portion of sphenoid wing. The stem then split into anterior ascending branches, anterior horizontal branches, and posterior branches. The deeper part of the lateral fissure divides into an anterior part (sphenoidal) and posterior part (operculoinsular). Anterior part is the narrow space between frontal and temporal, located behind sphenoid ridge; it communicates directly cistern around the carotid. The posterior part is made up of two clefts—opercula and insular. Insula becomes visible once the Sylvian fissure's lateral walls are separated. It links the temporal lobe with posterior orbital gyrus through limen insula, a threshold between the fissure laterally and the carotid cistern medially. The insula covers up a set of valuable structures such as internal capsules, external capsule, extreme capsule, the claustrum, the basal ganglia, and the thalamus. Typically, the basal cisterns are opened, prior to the transsylvian dissection, in order to relax the brain through cerebrospinal fluid drainage. This allows for a cisternal approach to aneurysms, first presented by Yasargil [1]. The opening of the Sylvian fissure is started near the pars triangularis of the parasylvian inferior frontal gyrus, where there is the most room between frontal and temporal lobes [4, 9] (Fig. 1.3).

Using microscissors and either a scalpel blade number 11, 25G needle, or diamond knife, the superficial portion of Sylvian fissure is cut and dissected starting from the frontal part of superficial Sylvian vein. The latter typically runs laterally toward the distal end of the temporal lobe and then drains into the sphenoparietal sinus. However, in some cases, the superficial Sylvian vein may drain toward the frontal Sylvian vein and finally into the superior sagittal sinus, justifying a dissection lateral of the superficial Sylvian vein. Relevant anatomical structures identifiable at this stage are ICA, MCA, ACA, and the optic nerve. It is very important to have a good dissec-

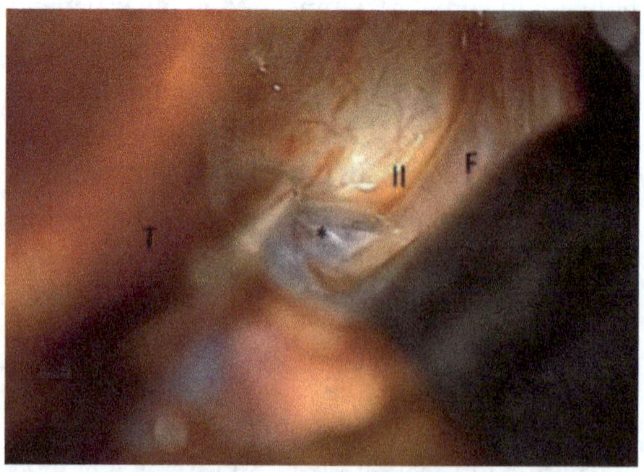

Fig. 1.3 The pars triangularis of the parasylvian inferior frontal gyrus (*), *F* frontal, *T* temporal, *II* optic nerve

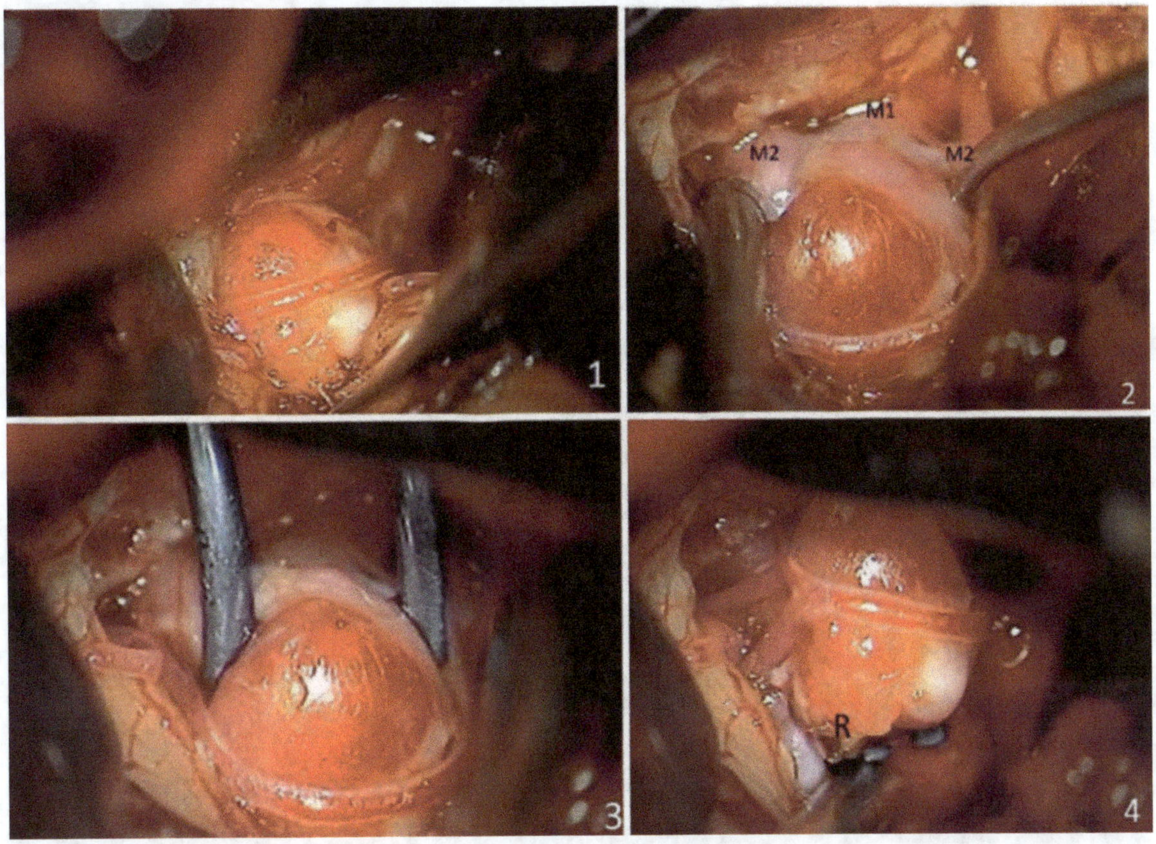

Fig. 1.4 The case of M1 bifurcation aneurysm. (1) The aneurysm was identified, but it's not well exposed yet, and it's necessary to continue dissection to identify all the surrounding, especially to find the parent artery in case the surgeon needs temporary occlusion. (2) Sylvian fissure dissection allows surgeon to expose the M1, M2, and branches. (3) Avoiding the branches and putting the clip on the aneurysm neck. (4) Expose the legs of the clip, and confirm the aneurysm is well clipped (*R* rupture site)

tion of Sylvian fissure for certain cases, such as MCA aneurysm (Fig. 1.4).

Though the gyrus rectus sometimes obscures the view of the AcomA complex, its resection is rarely indicated (Fig. 1.5). This approach grants access to cistern around olfactory, cistern around carotid artery, chiasmatic cistern, sphenoid part of lateral fissure, cistern in front of lamina terminalis, interpeduncular cistern, ambient cistern, and crural cistern, which can be attained by resection of anteromedial segment of uncus.

1.2.7 Closing

When closing, focus on preventing any potential epidural blood collections and attempt to avoid any major surgical cosmetic defects. Hemostasis must be attained prior to fascial closure, with electrocautery and sponge tamponade methods. After closing the dura until watertight, the bone flap is repositioned and secured with miniplates. The burr hole area could be covered with a titanium clamp, or the other options are to fill the hole with bone dust and make sure that it's covered well with periosteum. The periosteum is very important for bone healing and remodeling to the normal appearance. The temporal muscle flap is placed where it belongs, and the temporal muscle is re-sutured to the remaining myofascial cuff on the skull, while the reflected fascia is sutured to the fascia-periosteum complex. Finally, the fascial incision and the scalp incision are closed in the usual manner. The choice of an extradural subgaleal closed suction drain should enhance the healing and reduce fluid collections under the flap [10].

The classical pterional approach is attractive and widely used for many reasons, including smaller size craniotomy yet still allowing a wide

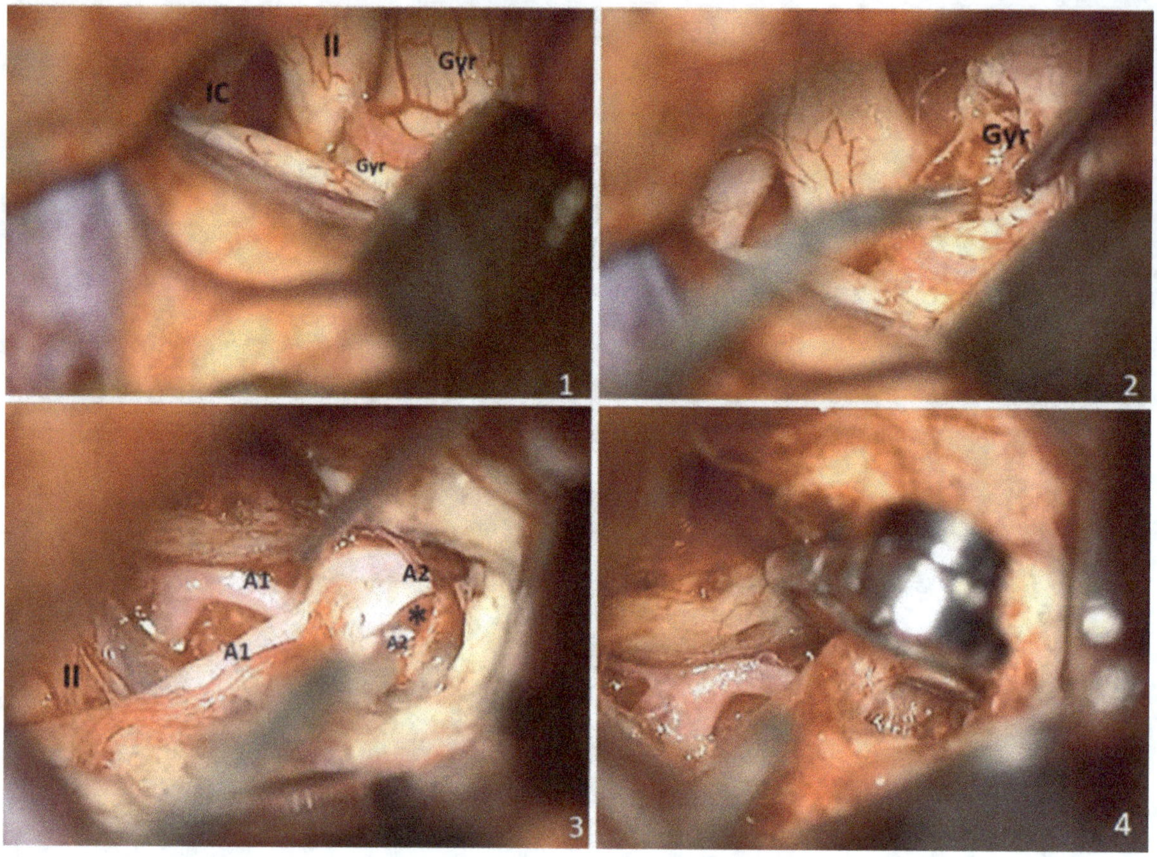

Fig. 1.5 The case of Acom aneurysm rupture, with left pterional approach. (1) The gyrus rectus obscures the AcomA complex. (2) Partial resection of gyrus rectus (Gyr). (3) Exposing the AcomA complex with the aneurysm between the both A2. (4) Clipping with ring clip to spare the A2 on the ipsilateral side

frontobasal exposure and rapid access to basal cisterns and the circle of Willis, without requiring extensive brain retraction. The approach limits unnecessary frontal and temporal lobes exposure. It also prevents risk of injury to the optic radiations or uncinate fasciculus, thus avoiding postoperative visual field deficits and aphasia, in the context of temporal lesion removal [11]. On a cosmetic level, the pterional approach was favorable for its good skin incision behind the hairline, appropriate size bone flap, and the osteoplastic craniotomy preventing some of the postoperative temporalis atrophy.

1.3 Indications of the Approach

Initially, the approach was suggested for most of microsurgical approach for cerebral aneurysms in the whole circle of Willis, particularly in the anterior circulation. Later, the pterional approach was also used for the removal of tumors and other vascular malformations found in cavernous sinus area but also sella, parasellar, temporal, subfrontal, and anterior and anterolateral midbrain regions. Examples of lesions successfully treated through this approach include aneurysms, olfactory groove meningiomas, cavernomas of the anterior mesiotemporal region, temporal horn tumors, and a clival chordoma. It's still one of the most commonly used approaches in neurosurgery practice.

1.4 Limitations of the Approach

The main factors to be considered when selecting the right extent of exposure required are compartment that need to be exposed and of course the location and size of aneurysm. The main issues regarding the pterional approach are obstruction of the operator's visualization by the basal structures, such as orbital roof, sphenoidal ridge, frontal and temporal lobes, and ICA, and temporal muscle. Sometimes surgeon need to work at a deep and narrow naturally available space between the carotid artery and optic or oculomotor nerves [1]. Hence, though the indications for a pterional approach are numerous and it is a widely applicable technique, it is not without limitations, typically exposure-related. The pterional approach is now often modified by or combined with the following approaches, temporopolar, pretemporal, cranioorbitozygomatic (middle cranial fossa lesions or upper clivus, upper basilar complex), and lateral supraorbital, in order to obtain the optimal diameter and angle of exposure for the pathology being treated. For example, if clipping an aneurysm of the posterior circulation (i.e., basilar tip aneurysm), the surgery may have to include removal of the anterior plus or minus the posterior clinoid processes for better visibility; or in order to have better access to the parasellar region, reshaping of the zygomatic complex may be helpful [7]. Additionally, ipsilateral vessels and the gyrus rectus can sometimes hinder ideal exposure of the AcomA complex and the contralateral vessels in a pterional approach; the orbitopterional approach is a great alternative. If a more inferior temporal view is required, removal of the zygomatic arch may be considered.

1.5 Complications and How to Avoid

The main complications that can be expected from this approach are aneurysmal intraoperative rupture, epidural or subdural hematoma, infection, ischemic events, early or late rebleeding, temporal muscle atrophy and/or dysfunction, and lastly, cosmetic cranial defects.

The interfascial flap dieresis technique from the original pterional approach, as described by Yasargil, was found to be associated with more prevalent, worse, and longer-lasting palsy of frontotemporal facial nerve branches, temporalis muscle atrophy, and temporomandibularis joint dysfunction [12]. The aim of this two-layer flap is maximizing visibility at the expense of severe retraction of the temporalis muscle. On the other hand, the myocutaneous flap has considerably less risk for facial nerve injury since temporal muscle is lifted up with scalp in a one-layer flap [5, 13]. However, this myocutaneous flap is at the detriment of worse exposure secondary to the bulkiness of the temporalis muscle [6]. Kim and Delashaw propose an osteomyoplastic monobloc technique in order to prevent both cosmetic and functional undesirable outcomes [14]. The procedure spares the temporalis muscle and the basal bone. It involves dissecting a subperiosteal detachment below the temporal separating it from the underlying bone while maintaining the muscle's attachment to superior temporal line and temporal squama. This is followed by the creation of a keyhole 2 cm posterior to pterion at the Sylvian fissure line. Final step consists of roungering part of the sphenoid wing allowing its removal with the pterion in one piece, along with the bone flap.

Even though most concerns of scalp deformities (temporal depression, skin indentation) linked to craniotomies have decreased since the introduction of miniplating systems and burr hole covers, the pterional approach remains prone to it, especially surrounding the keyhole, due to the complex curvature of the circumferential bone. Moscovici et al. suggested that a craniotomy without the classical MacCarty keyhole leads to superior aesthetic outcomes with minimal bone loss [15]. Their approach involves delicate sphenoid ridge drilling in a plane parallel to the skull base, thus no longer requiring expansion of the bony window basally.

References

1. Yasargil MG, et al. Microsurgical pterional approach to aneurysms of the basilar bifurcation. Surg. Neurology. 1976;6:83–91.
2. Weil AG, Robert T, Alsaiari S, Obaid S, Bojanowski MW. Using the trans-lamina terminalis route via a pterional approach to resect a retrochiasmatic craniopharyngioma involving the third ventricle. Neurosurg Focus. 2016;40 Video Suppl 1, 1.

3. Tayebi Meybodi A, Benet A, Lawton MT. Microsurgical clipping of bilateral superior hypophyseal artery aneurysms through unilateral pterional craniotomy: 3-dimensional operative video. Neurosurgery. 2016;12(2):193.
4. Chaddad-Neto F, et al. The pterional craniotomy: tips and tricks. Arq Neuropsiquiatr. 2012;70:727–32.
5. Miyazawa T. Less invasive reconstruction of the temporalis muscle for pterional craniotomy: modified procedures. Surg Neurol. 1998;50:347–51; discussion 351.
6. Yaşargil MG, Reichman MV, Kubik S. Preservation of the frontotemporal branch of the facial nerve using the interfascial temporalis flap for pterional craniotomy. Technical article. J Neurosurg. 1987;67:463–6.
7. Altay T, Couldwell WT. The frontotemporal (pterional) approach: an historical perspective. Neurosurgery. 2012;71:481–91; discussion 491–492
8. Andaluz N, Van Loveren HR, Keller JT, Zuccarello M. Anatomic and clinical study of the orbitopterional approach to anterior communicating artery aneurysms. Neurosurgery. 2003;52:1140–8; discussion 1148–1149.
9. Olivas A, Garcia L. 3D neurosurgical approaches. 2011:1.
10. Choi SY, et al. Necessity of surgical site closed suction drain for pterional craniotomy. J Cerebrovasc Endovasc Neurosurg. 2015;17:194–202.
11. Campero A, et al. Pterional transsylvian-transinsular approach in three cavernomas of the left anterior mesiotemporal region. Clin Neurol Neurosurg. 2015;130:14–9.
12. de Andrade Júnior FC, de Andrade FC, de Araujo Filho CM, Carcagnolo Filho J. Dysfunction of the temporalis muscle after pterional craniotomy for intracranial aneurysms. Comparative, prospective and randomized study of one flap versus two flaps dieresis. Arq Neuropsiquiatr. 1998;56:200–5.
13. Spetzler RF, Lee KS. Reconstruction of the temporalis muscle for the pterional craniotomy. Technical note. J Neurosurg. 1990;73:636–7.
14. Kim E, Delashaw JB. Osteoplastic pterional craniotomy revisited. Neurosurgery. 2011;68:125–9; discussion 129.
15. Moscovici S, Mizrahi CJ, Margolin E, Spektor S. Modified pterional craniotomy without 'MacCarty keyhole'. J Clin Neurosci. 2016;24:135–7.

2 Eyebrow Keyhole Approach in Aneurysm Surgery

Asra Al Fauzi, Nur Setiawan Suroto, and Abdul Hafid Bajamal

2.1 Basic Consept

The concept of keyhole neurosurgery is not only to perform small incision and reduce the craniotomy size for the sake of a small opening as we called "keyhole," but it is rather to make "minimum craniotomy" required to access deep intracranial lesions at the end of the route. Standard craniotomy forms a "funnel-shaped surgical corridor" to reach deeper area of the brain. In contrast, keyhole mini craniotomy forms a "reverse funnel-shaped surgical corridor" that provides adequate working space through a small incision and bone window to reach the target. The concept of this approach is that the deep area of the brain can be accessed through smaller craniotomy since the superficial optical field is widened if the size of craniotomy is bigger (Fig. 2.1).

Intracranial aneurysm surgery using eyebrow keyhole approach has been reported by Van Lindert and Perneczky in 1998, and since then, this approach has been accepted as minimally invasive approach for aneurysm clipping surgery in addition to the existing standard approach.

2.2 Preoperative Planning

The planning and execution of the approach play a critical role in performing this keyhole surgery. The smaller the craniotomy, the greater the need for precise planning and self-made completion of the approach because the corridor of surgical dissection cannot be changed during the procedure.

It is necessary to have preoperative consideration about the size and aneurysm dome projection, aneurysm location, perforating arteries, surrounding important structures, and how to plan the bone flap. Using excellent diagnostic facilities of CT, MRI, and digital subtraction angiography (DSA), one has today the possibility to demonstrate small details and specific anatomical orientation of the lesion related with surgical planning. In our experience, preoperative planning for eyebrow keyhole surgery is could be mainly by using and rely on 3D CT angiography (3D-CTA). The 3D reconstruction images maybe able to shows from the skin, then skull, cerebral arteries and veins, including size and shape of the aneurysm. The preoperative planning of the keyhole craniotomy can be simulated with 3D-CTA (Fig. 2.2).

A. Al Fauzi (✉) · N. S. Suroto · A. H. Bajamal
Department of Neurosurgery,
Universitas Airlangga, Dr. Soetomo General Hospital,
Surabaya Neuroscience Institute, Surabaya, Indonesia

J. July, E. J. Wahjoepramono (eds.), *Neurovascular Surgery*,
https://doi.org/10.1007/978-981-10-8950-3_2

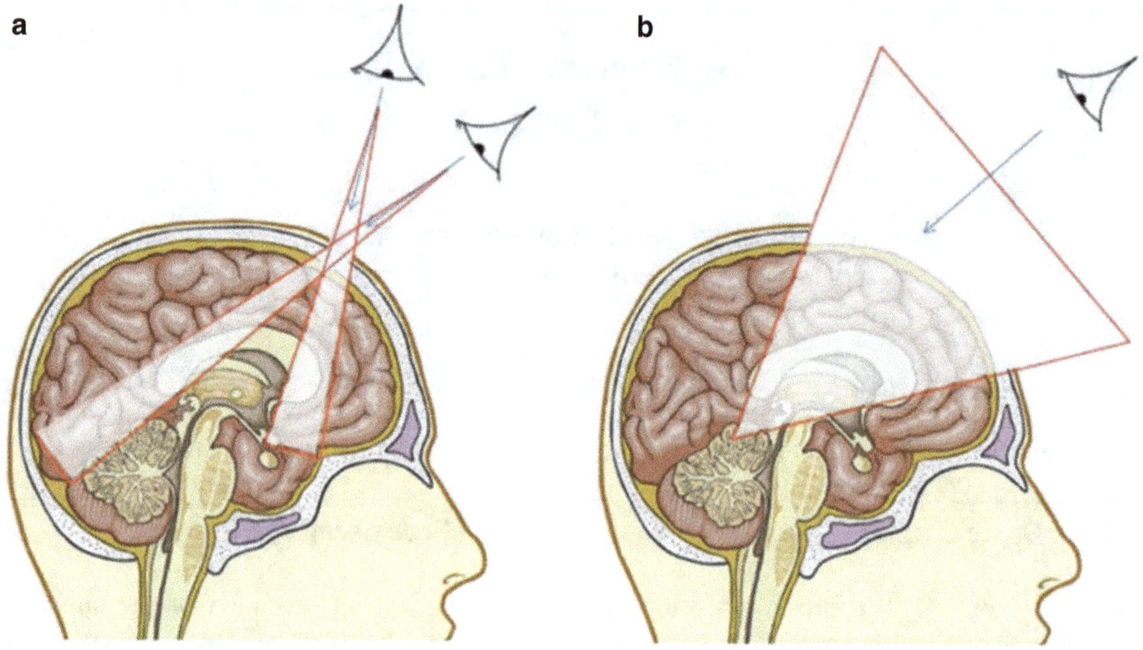

Fig. 2.1 Concept of surgical corridors in keyhole craniotomy. (**a**) Keyhole craniotomy with "reverse funnel-shaped" corridor, (**b**) macrocraniotomy with "funnel-shaped" corridor

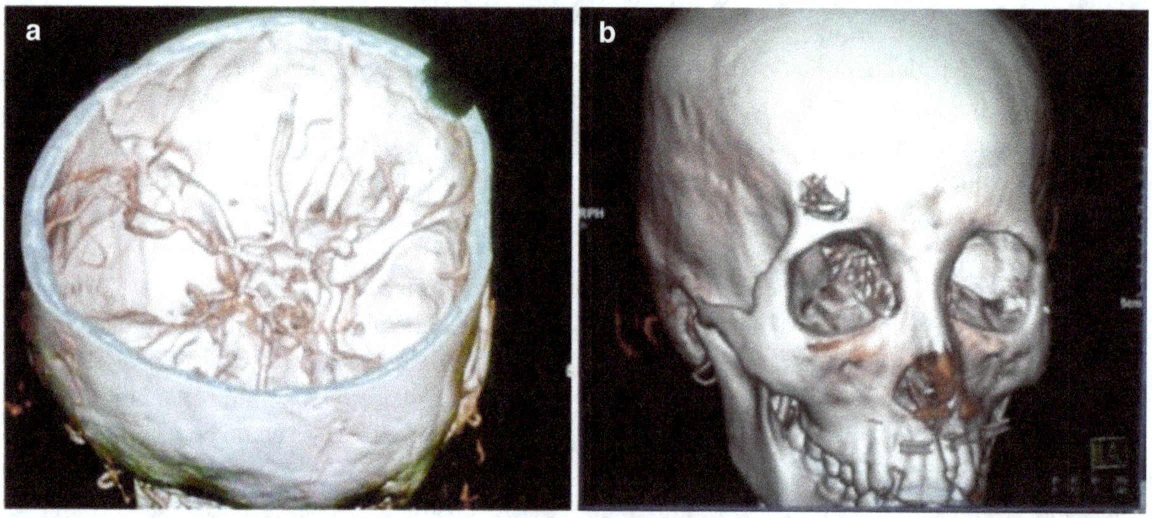

Fig. 2.2 Preoperative planning with 3D CTA images showing the skull, cerebral arteries, and aneurysm pathology. (**a**) The supraorbital keyhole craniotomy and its relationship to the aneurysm are well visualized. (**b**) The supraorbital craniotomy with the lesion is prepared at various angles to have an optimal microsurgical visualization

2.3 Step of the Approach

2.3.1 Positioning and Preparation

The surgeon must plan and perform the proper positioning of the patient by himself. Self-made preparation and positioning are essential for creating keyhole craniotomies. After the patient is anesthetized, the patient head is positioned in supine with head holder, and the head is higher up approximately 15° to facilitate venous drainage. A slightly chin-up position is preferable to support the frontal lobe that will slightly fall down according to the gravity force. The degree of head rotation should be determined by preoperative 3D simulation, but generally the head is

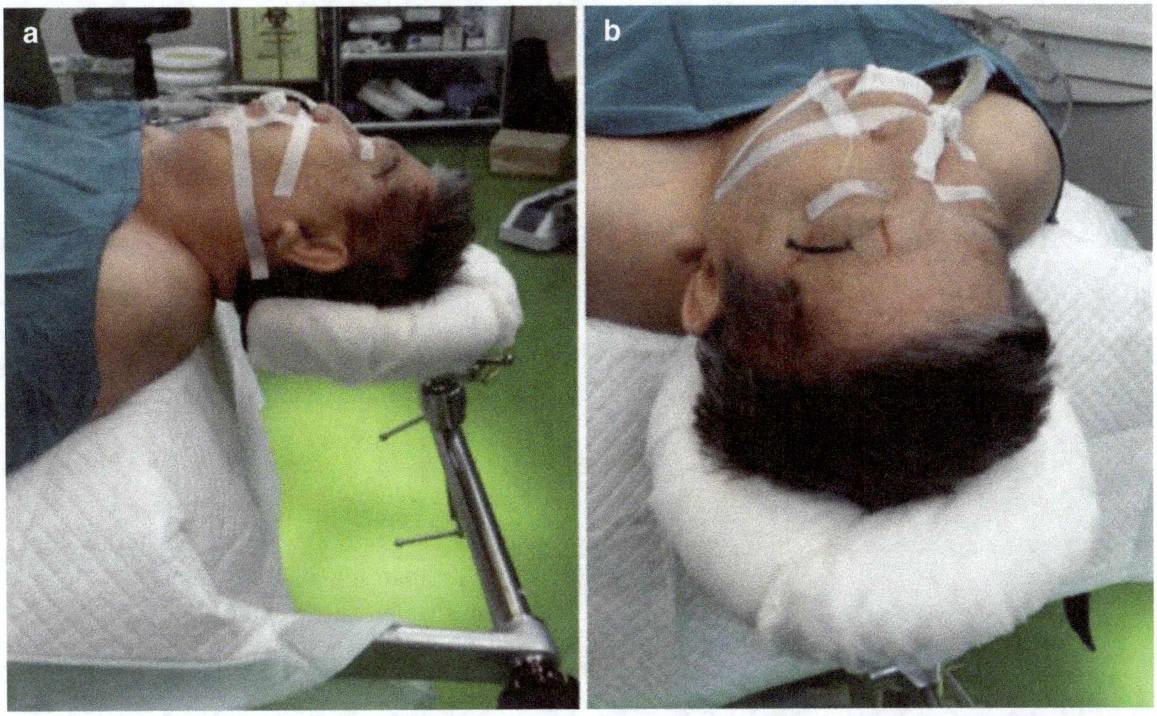

Fig. 2.3 Supine positioning of the patient, slightly extended and the head is turned to contralateral, and depend on aneurysm location. In most cases, the headrest with soft cushion is used for a brief preparation; the use of head fixation clamp is not necessary

rotated between 15° and 45° toward the contralateral side, determined by the location and dome projection of aneurysm. The placement of lumbar drain or extraventricular drainage also allows for brain relaxation specially in ruptured aneurysm case with brain edema.

Frontal anatomic landmarks should be precisely identified, including the foramen supraorbital, superior temporal line, orbital rim, and zygomatic arch, then drawing the skin incision plan on the skin (Fig. 2.3).

2.3.2 Skin Cut

The skin is cut according to the preoperative planning and anatomical orientation. The skin is cut at lateral two-thirds of the eyebrow, from supraorbital notch to the lateral part, sometimes extending few millimeters to the temporal line. To achieve a good cosmetic appearance, the incision should follow the orbital rim, in the hair line. It is advisable not to overuse bipolar coagulation to avoid damaging hair follicles and surrounding tissues. After skin incision, skin flap is dissected subcutaneously to obtain optimal exposure to surrounding muscles. We could clearly identify the frontal, orbicularis oculi and temporal muscles. After dividing the muscular layers gently, we have to identify pericranium at supraorbital edge, and it is cut perpendicularly following superior temporal line to get good bone exposure.

Skin flaps should be gently retracted with three or four temporary stiches at each upper and lower side of the flaps. The frontal muscle should be retracted upward, and the temporal muscle is detached gently from the attachment and retracted laterally to expose ipsilateral temporal line, and then keyhole area is exposed. Gentle detachment and pulling of the muscle are important to prevent local postoperative hematoma (Fig. 2.4).

2.3.3 Mini Craniotomy and Dural Incision

Making a single frontobasal burr hole at the frontozygomatic point just behind the temporal line by using high-speed drill. The placement and direction of the drilling procedure should be in correct man-

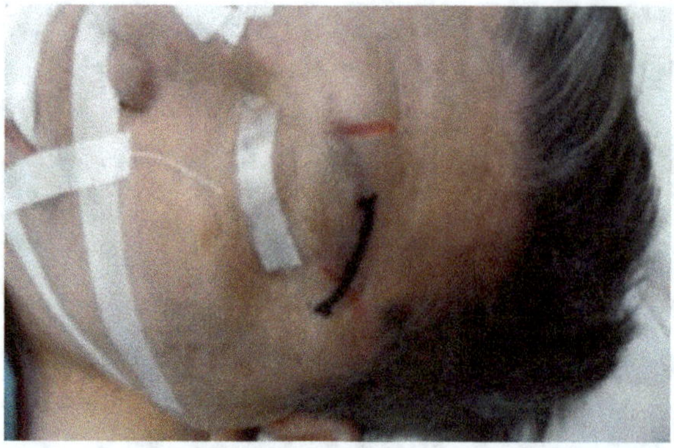

Fig. 2.4 Skin cut from the lateral border of supraorbital notch and extending a few millimeters from the eyebrow line to reach the temporal line

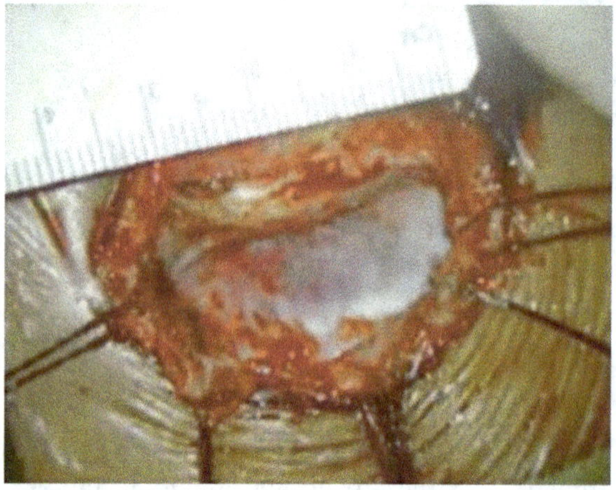

Fig. 2.5 Supraorbital keyhole craniotomy with a width of 25–30 mm and a height of 15–25 mm

ner. Wrong direction during drilling can cause the drill going into the orbit, while we actually want it to go to the anterior frontal floor. The craniotomy flap is then performed with high-speed craniotomy, starting from lateral orbital rim and following the orbital rim to medial, as long as 25–30 mm, then curving cranially about 15–25 mm, and cutting back to the burr hole site, thus creating a small bone flap. An important point is the bone cut should be very close and approaching orbital roof and if necessary additional drilling to make any prominence at the frontal floor totally flat. This may provide a few millimeters more exposure and avoid the bony prominence to obstruct surgical visualization and facilitate optimal microsurgical maneuvers using microscope and microinstruments (Fig. 2.5).

Opening the dura with semicircular shape and the base parallel along the orbital rim. The dura flap is reflected basally and fixed downward with three or four sutures so that dural window is formed in optimal opening following craniotomy corridor (Fig. 2.6).

2.3.4 Intradural Dissection

After opening the dura, the first-step maneuver is to gently remove sufficient cerebrospinal fluid by opening the arachnoid membrane through the chiasmatic and carotid cistern or furthermore to Sylvian fissure. Ventricular puncture and drainage sometimes may be needed in case of brain edema; the authors only use the lumbar spinal drain for very selective cases. With adequate drainage of CSF (cerebrospinal fluid), the brain becomes relaxed, then a brain spatula is put in the frontal lobe, and the purpose is to protect the cortex and *not* to retract the cortex. With this efficient and adequate surgical corridor, we can get to the aneurysm precisely and avoid extensive cortical retraction (Fig. 2.7).

2.3.5 Closure and Bone Flap Replacement

After the intracranial procedure is performed, the next step is filling the intradural space with warm normal saline. Close the dura with watertight and interrupted sutures, and then make sure that any defects are well repaired. If the frontal sinus opened during the surgery, it is a must to seal off the frontal sinus to avoid postoperative infection. Bone flap is placed back, and hold it with mini plates and be careful not to penetrate frontal sinus by the screws. Authors prefer using three mini plate fixations at medial, lateral, and upper part of craniotomy to make sure a strong fixation to prevent postoperative deformity. Reapproximate the temporal muscle to zygoma by one or two sutures. After final hemostasis control, reapproximate the subcutaneous layer by interrupted sutures; then the skin is also closed by interrupted sutures in the eyebrow (Fig. 2.8).

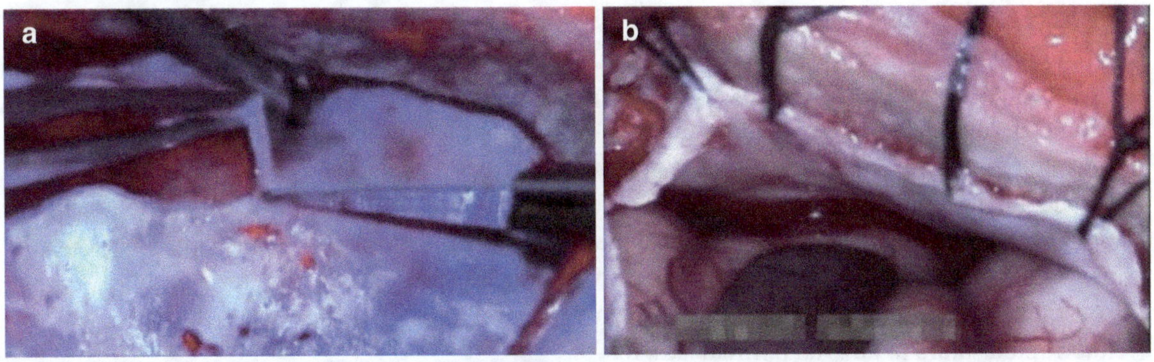

Fig. 2.6 (a) Opening the dura in a curved fashion toward the frontal base, (b) optimal surgical corridor to the skull base after dural opening

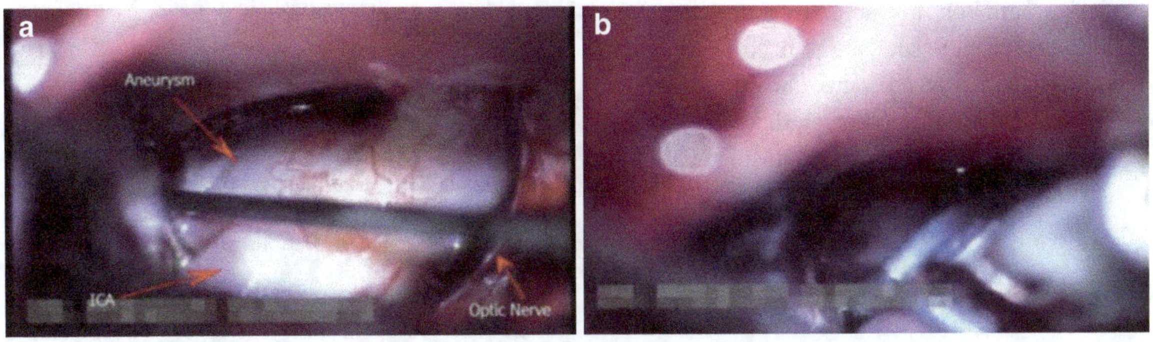

Fig. 2.7 (a) Intradural dissection and securing the aneurysm using microinstruments, (b) clipping procedure

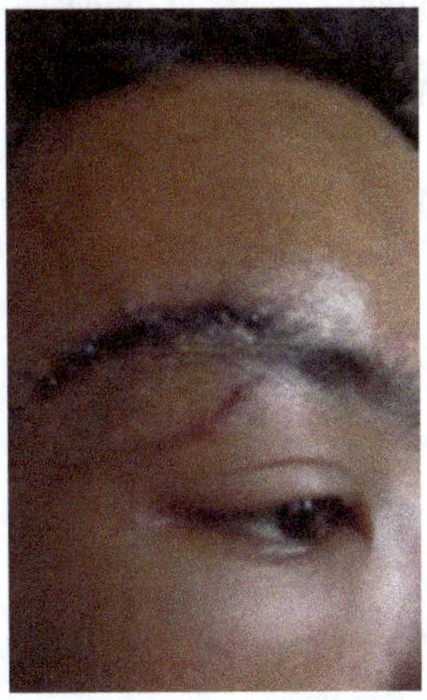

Fig. 2.8 The skin is closed with interrupted suture to control the skin tension for a good cosmetic result

2.4 Complications and How to Avoid

There are some complications that could be occurred associated with surgical technique in eyebrow keyhole approach.

1. Temporary or permanent supraorbital hypesthesia. In eyebrow keyhole craniotomy, the surgical field is very narrow, and medially the surgical field is limited by supraorbital notch that contains supraorbital nerve. Perioperative anatomical landmark should be prepared precisely to avoid damaging these structures. Certainly, keeping a distance of the craniotomy site at least 5–10 mm lateral to the orbital notch can reduce the risk of supraorbital nerve injury. Sometimes stretching the nerve during surgery is unavoidable, but preserving the nerve continuity will provide good chance to have functional recovery after surgery.
2. Frontal deformity. The frontobasal burr hole needs to be placed behind the temporal line after retracting the temporal muscle laterally. The burr hole site will be covered with the muscle to prevent deformity in this area. Proper repositioning of the bone flap is also an important step to prevent frontal deformity for a better cosmetic result. Bone flap should be fixed frontally and medially without any bony

distance; make sure the mini plate tightly fixed the bone in proper position.
3. Suboptimal cosmetic result. Skin incision should be made within the eyebrow and follow the orbital rim. Retraction of the skin flap should be in gentle manner to prevent soft tissue necrosis, and it is better to minimize the use of bipolar cauterization during skin and soft tissue procedures. The skin is closed with interrupted suture to have an optimal skin tension with good approximation.
4. Infection. If the frontal sinus opened during procedure, careful repair is mandatory. The periosteum or fascia flap, bone wax, or abdominal fat tissue can be used to repair the injured sinus. Make sure the dura is closed watertightly with interrupted suture; if still dehiscence occurred, a small muscle patch should be used for this purpose.

2.5 Limitations

1. This approach is contraindicated in patient with massive brain swelling after subarachnoid hemorrhage.
2. This approach could not be a standard for all of aneurysm surgery; the indication should be strict and rely on the surgeon's experience.
3. The keyhole craniotomy may limit the microsurgery working angles, so it is mandatory to use a high magnification microscope and specific keyhole microsurgery instruments.
4. It is preferred not to use this approach for patient with large frontal sinus, because the greater risk of infection may occur.

Bibliography

1. Jallo GI, Bognar L. Eyebrow surgery: the supraciliary craniotomy: technical note. Neurosurgery. 2006;59:ONSE157–8.
2. Mori K. Keyhole concept in cerebral aneurysm clipping and tumor removal by the supraciliary lateral supraorbital approach. Asian J Neurosurg. 2014;9:14–20.
3. Ormond DR, Hadjipanayis CG. The supraorbital keyhole craniotomy through an eyebrow incision: its origins and evolution. Minim Invasive Surg. 2013;2013:1–11.
4. Paladino J, Mrak G, Miklic JH, Mihaljevic D. The keyhole concept in aneurysm surgery—a comparative study: keyhole versus standard craniotomy. Minim Invas Neurosurg. 2005;48:251–8.
5. Perneczky A, Reisch R. Keyhole approaches in neurosurgery, vol. 1. Concept and surgical technique. Wien: Springer; 2008.
6. Reisch R, Perneczky A. Ten-year experience with the supraorbital subfrontal approach through an eyebrow skin incision. Neurosurgery. 2005;57:ONS242–55.

3 Fronto-orbito-zygomatic (FOZ) Approach

Imad N. Kanaan

3.1 Introduction

Surgical management of skull base pathologies remains one of the most challenging tasks for neurosurgeons. Advances in neuroimaging and evolution of modern technologies have paved the way for a more precise diagnosis and better selection of the surgical approach.

The fronto-orbito-zygomatic (FOZ) approach welds several surgical avenues and satisfies the philosophy of skull base surgery by removing bone obstacles in favor of better exposure with minimal brain retraction. Historically, this approach evolved from the pioneering work of avant-garde neurosurgeons. Removal of the supraorbital ridge as part of the frontal craniotomy was first described by McArthur [11] in 1912 and Frazier [5] in 1913 to remove a pituitary tumor. Jane et al. [8] revived this approach to include the anterior orbital roof osteotomy in a single flap to approach vascular lesions and remove orbital tumors. The original description of pterional approach was credited to Heuer [6] in 1918, modified by Dandy [3] to clip an anterior communicating artery aneurysm in 1941, and later was refined and popularized by Yasargil [14] in 1969. Pellerin [13] and Hakuba [7] first described the orbito-zygomatic-malar approach to central skull base lesions in the early 1980s. FOZ approach was eventually adopted and modified by Al Mefty [1] and others [9, 12, 15] to include several variations that match the patient's clinical condition, the pathology dealt with, and the neurosurgeon's preference.

The FOZ approach provides an excellent neurosurgical avenue for safe removal of skull base tumors and management of complex vascular lesions around the central skull base, cavernous sinus, and upper clivus [1, 4, 7, 15]. Several publications quantified this approach and highlighted its advantages in the contemporary practice of skull base surgery [2].

3.2 Steps of the Approach

3.2.1 Position and Preparation

The patient is placed in supine position with elevation of the trunk 25° and ipsilateral shoulder (gravity-supported venous drainage). The head is elevated, extended, tilted slightly away from the ipsilateral shoulder, and rotated 25° to the contralateral side (Fig. 3.1). The leg is prepped should a graft of fascia lata, fat, or saphenous vein be needed for reconstruction. Lumbar drain may be considered, and the patient receives antibiotics, steroids, H1-receptor antagonists, as well as anticonvulsant and mannitol if needed.

I. N. Kanaan
Department of Neurosciences,
King Faisal Specialist Hospital and Research Center,
Alfaisal University, College of Medicine, Riyadh,
Saudi Arabia

J. July, E. J. Wahjoepramono (eds.), *Neurovascular Surgery*,
https://doi.org/10.1007/978-981-10-8950-3_3

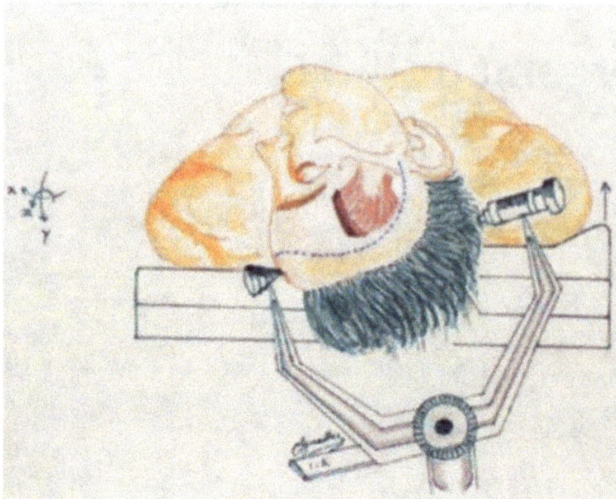

Fig. 3.1 Supine position with the head fixed in the Mayfield head clamp. The head and upper body is elevated up 25° with elevation of the ipsilateral shoulder, hyperextended, and rotated to the opposite side by 25°. Additional rotation or manipulation of the position can be adjusted by the table's control buttons. The blue dotted line represents the skin incision. *X*, *Y*, *Z* curved arrows represent the three axes of the head for orientation

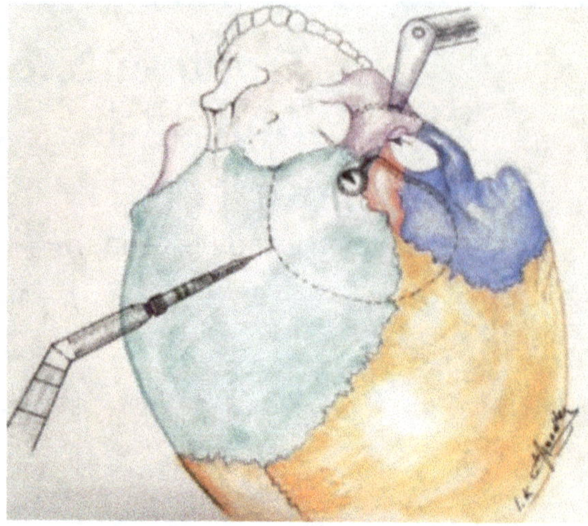

Fig. 3.2 Artistic illustration of the right fronto-orbito-zygomatic approach (FOZ). Arrowhead, McArthur's burr-hole; arrow, to inferior orbital fissure; dashed line, frontotemporal craniotomy including the orbital rim and part of the zygoma

3.2.2 Skin Incision and Soft Tissue Dissection

Elevate a frontal skin flap, starting within 1 cm anterior to the tragus at the level of the zygomatic arch, extending behind the hairline, and just passing the midline in a slightly curved fashion. Pay special attention not to injure the frontal branch of the facial nerve or damage the superficial temporal artery for its potential use in EC-IC bypass.

Incise and dissect sharply a large vascularized frontal pericranial flap and reflect it over the skin flap to be in continuity with the periorbita at the level of the orbital roof. Mobilize the temporal muscle basely and laterally under the arch of the zygoma, but leave a muscle cuff attached to the superior temporal line on the frontal bone for reattachment.

3.2.3 Craniotomy and Orbito-zygomatic Osteotomy

Perform two burr holes: one at McArthur's point (keyhole) and the second at the bottom of the temporal squama. Complete a frontotemporal craniotomy, and include the superior and lateral orbital rim (zygoma) medial to the supraorbital notch and down to the malar eminence (Fig. 3.2). This flap will include the anterior part of the orbital roof and the lateral wall of the orbit; hence, it negates the need for later reconstruction. We have used the oscillating saw and Midas Rex B1bone cutter or pediatric osteotome to perform this step. The cut of the orbital roof is placed lateral to the ethmoid sinuses, and the one at the lateral orbit is made between the outer edge of the superior and inferior orbital fissures. These cuts are best judged from an intraorbital perspective. Special attention is paid to dissect and protect both the frontobasal dura and the periorbita over the lacrimal gland using cotton patties or narrow brain spatula. This step can be performed as a single or two-piece bone flap. The latter is advocated in elderly patients with very thin dura or in patients with thick orbital roof. The elevation of this flap will facilitate the extradural resection of the sphenoid wing and drilling of the anterior clinoid process, as well as the decompression of the superior orbital fissure, the optic canal, and the posterior orbit using a high-speed diamond-tipped burr and small rongeurs. The need for the double cut of the zygomatic arc does not warrant total skeletonization of the bone and is limited to the extended subtemporal approach for surgical management of cavernous sinus lesions, complex basilar tip aneurysm, or upper clivus tumors. These cuts of the zygoma are now performed with pre-platting concept for best cosmetic results. For access to the cavernous sinus, petrous apex, and upper clivus, the lateral temporal fossa will be flattened using a high-speed drill; the foramen spinosum will be obliterated in order to proceed with extradural access to these areas as described by Dolenc [4] and Kawase [10], with special attention to maintain the integrity of the greater and lesser superficial petrosal nerves (GSPN and LSPN) during the exposure of the petrous carotid for proximal control (Fig. 3.3).

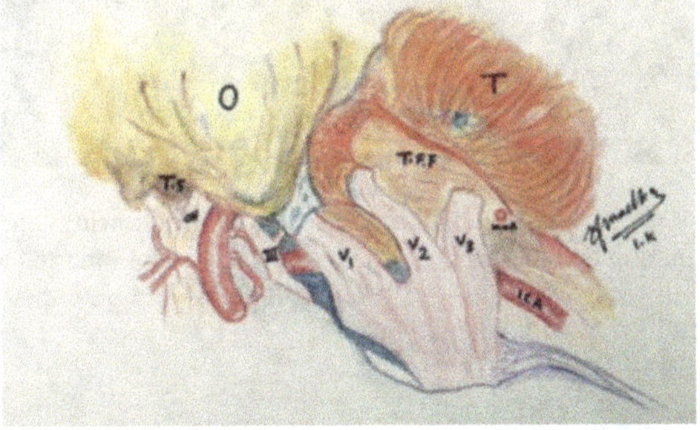

Fig. 3.3 Artistic illustration of a right front-orbito-zygomatic (FOZ) approach. The wide exposure demonstrates access to the orbit, frontal fossa, central skull base, and suprasellar area, as well as to the cavernous sinus, middle fossa, and upper petroclival region. The following anatomical structures are shown: *T* temporal muscle, *O* orbit, *TFF* temporal fossa floor, *TS* tuberculum sellae, *ON* optic nerve, *ICA* internal carotid artery, *MMA* middle meningeal artery, *III* oculomotor nerve, and *V1, V2, V3* represent the three branches of the trigeminal nerve

3.2.4 Surgical Closure

Upon conclusion of the planned intradural intervention, the dura is closed in a watertight fashion using dura substitutes in order to guarantee brain relaxation and tent the dura to prevent postoperative epidural collection. The fronto-orbito-zygomatic bone flap is replaced and fixed in position with miniplates. The preservation of the roof and lateral wall of the orbit does not warrant additional bone reconstruction; however, if the osteotomy defect is large, then this can be reconstructed by using low-profile craniofacial miniplates that can be fixed to the FOZ flap and measured to the size and shape of the bone defect. The temporal muscle and fascia flap are sutured to the myofascial cuff left on the frontal bone. The skin incision is closed in a multilayer fashion leaving a small subgaleal closed drainage system.

3.3 Indications of the Approach

Fronto-orbito-zygomatic approach provides multiple short, wide, and direct corridors giving access for safe surgical management of complex skull base tumors and vascular pathologies located in the posterior orbit or at the central skull base, interpeduncular fossa, cavernous sinus, and upper clivus.

Variations of FOZ approach [1, 7–9, 12, 15] are tailored to the nature of the pathology being dealt with and its anatomical location and extent and governed by meticulous evaluation of the patient's clinical condition and imaging studies. The FOZ approach or its variants (Figs. 3.4, 3.5, and 3.6) are to be considered in surgical management of suprasellar, perisellar, and anterior clinoid meningiomas, craniopharyngiomas, giant pituitary tumors, trigeminal schwannomas, chordomas, cavernous sinus lesions, and complex anterior circulation, or basilar bifurcation aneurysms. A trans-eyebrow mini-FOZ approach was described in the literature and may suffice adequately in some selected indications [9].

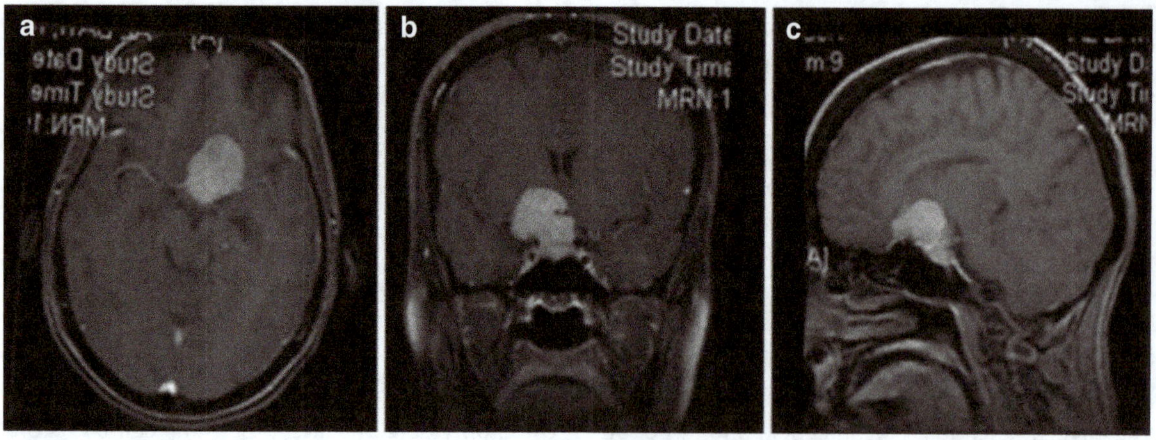

Fig. 3.4 Preoperative MRI T1 with gadolinium of a 42-year-old female patient who presented with 8 months' history of headache and progressive visual impairment, more pronounced on the right side. Her neurological examination confirmed the presence of right optic nerve atrophy, decreased visual acuity to 20/100, and temporal visual field defect; (**a**) axial; (**b**) coronal; (**c**) sagittal projection showing homogenous enhancement of the lesion

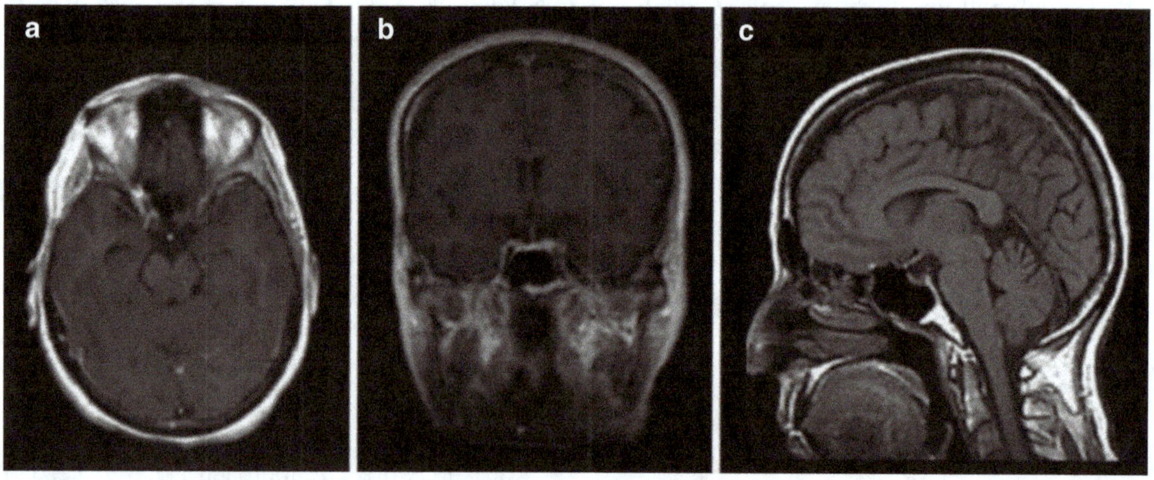

Fig. 3.5 Postoperative MRI with gadolinium; (**a**) axial; (**b**) coronal; (**c**) sagittal views. It demonstrates complete resection of the diaphragma sellae meningioma. The patient underwent a modified FOZ approach with opening of the optic canal and resection of the sphenoid wings and sparing the cut of the zygoma arc. The patient reported a full recovery of her vision and symptoms at the 9-month follow-up with no complications

3.4 Limitation and Complication and How to Avoid

The FOZ approach may appear to be a complex intervention, but it is worth the effort whenever it is indicated. It provides excellent working channels and maneuverability to handle intraoperative complications. Risks of facial nerve injury and temporal muscle atrophy can be avoided by the subperiosteal elevation of the temporal muscle and minimal use of cautery. The approach as described above negates the need for major reconstruction; however, enophthalmos may occur in some cases as the result of greater bone loss due to excessive drilling or damage to the periorbital area during dissection. Therefore, proper placement of the osteotomy at the orbital roof and lateral wall under protection of the periorbita and repair of any ensuing defect in the periorbita by using a small pericranial patch are very important measures. It is recommended to reconstruct a larger bone defect in the orbita by

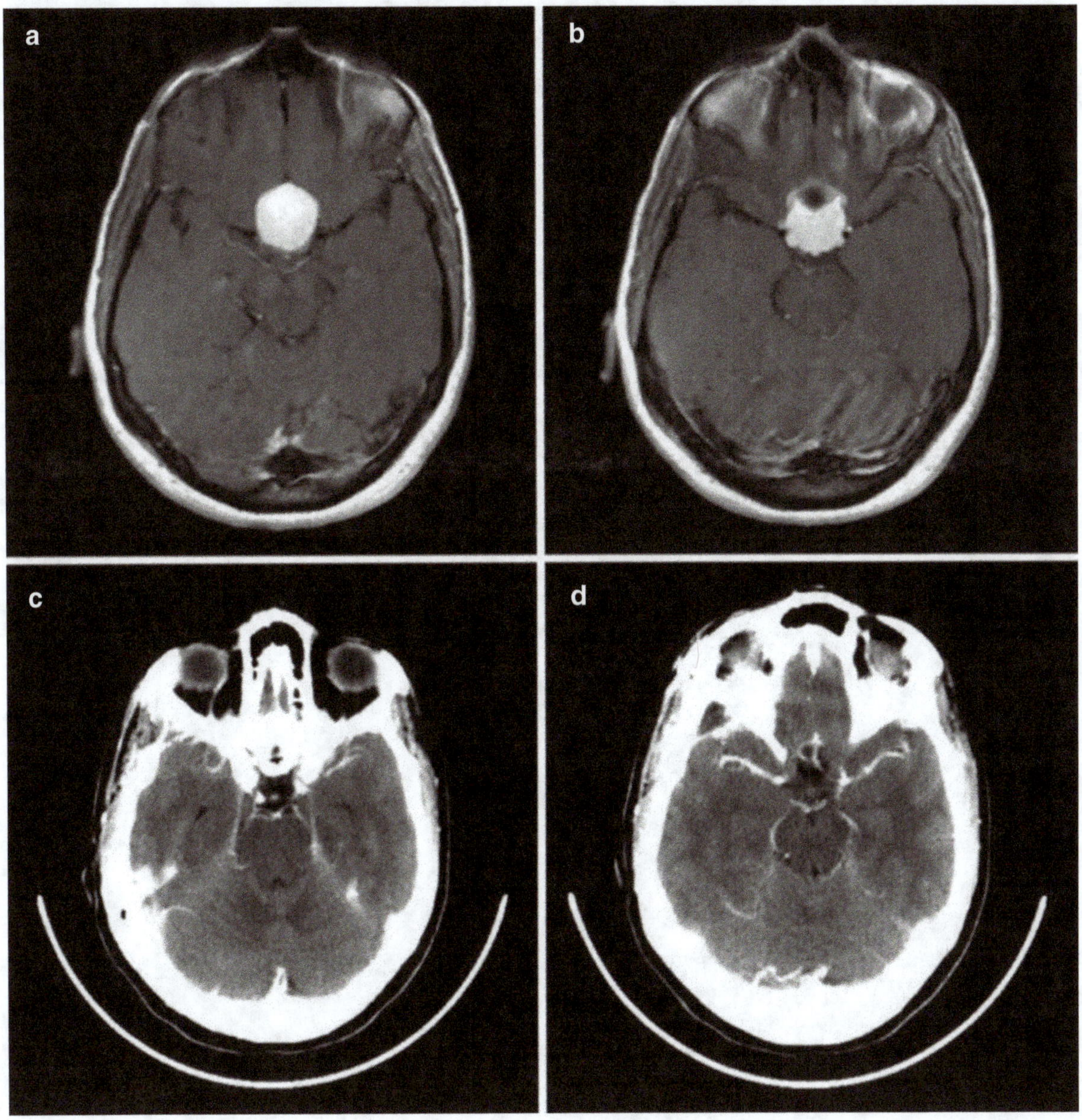

Fig. 3.6 Preoperative MRI, T1 with gadolinium (**a** and **b**) of a middle-age female patient, who presented with 1-year history of progressive visual loss and recent episode of generalized seizure. These images revealed a planum sphenoidale lesion with hyperostosis, which was compatible with the diagnosis of meningioma. The patient underwent trans-eyebrow modified mini-FOZ for gross total resection of the planum sphenoidale meningioma as shown on the postoperative CT scan with contrast (**c** and **d**) resulting an excellent clinical recovery

using miniplates that can be fixed to the bone flap. Careful repair and obliteration of any opened air cells or air sinuses should handle the potential risk of CSF leakage resulting from drilling of the anterior clinoid process or the wall of the sinuses. The relatively common problem of transient periorbital swelling can be managed by early ambulation, head elevation, and application of cold compress.

References

1. Al-Mefty O. Supraorbital-pterional approach to skull base lesions. Neurosurgery. 1987;21:474–7.
2. Andaluz N, Keller JT, van Loveren HR, Zuccarello M. Anatomical and clinical study of the orbitopterional approach to anterior communicating artery aneurysms. Neurosurgery. 2003;52(5):1140–9.
3. Dandy WE. Intracranial arterial aneurysms. New York: Hafner; 1944 Reprinted 1969.

4. Dolenc VV. Extradural approach to intracavernous ICA aneurysms. Acta Neurochir Suppl. 1999;72:99–106.
5. Frazer CH. An approach to the hypophysis through the anterior cranial fossa. Ann Surg. 1913;57(2):145–50.
6. Heuer GJ, Dandy WE. A new hypophysis operation. Johns Hopkins Hosp Bull. 1918;29:154.
7. Hakuba A, Liu SS, Shuro N. The orbitozygomatic infratemporal approach: a new surgical technique. Surg Neurol. 1986;26(3):271–6.
8. Jane JA, Park TS, Pobereskin LH, et al. The supraorbital approach: technical note. Neurosurgery. 1982;11(4):537–42.
9. Kanaan IN. Trans-eyebrow mini-orbitozygomatic pterional approach for minimally invasive skull base surgery. Minim Invas Neurosurg. 2005;48(1):34–8.
10. Kawase T, Toya S, Shiobara R, et al. Transpetrosal approach for aneurysms of the lower basilar artery. J Neurosurg. 1985;63:857–61.
11. McArthur LL. An aseptic surgical access to the pituitary body and its neighborhood. JAMA. 1912;58:2009–11.
12. McDermott MW, Durity FA, Rootman J, et al. Combined frontotemporal-orbitozygomatic approach for tumors of the sphenoid wing and orbit. Neurosurgery. 1990;26(1):107–16.
13. Pellerin P, Lesoin F, Dhellemmes P, et al. Usefulness of the orbitofrontomalar approach associated with bone reconstruction for frontotemporosphenoid meningiomas. Neurosurgery. 1984;15(5):715–8.
14. Yasargil MG, Antic J, Laciga R, Jain KK, Hodosh RM, Smith RD. Microsurgical pterional approach to aneurysm of the basilar bifurcation. Surg Neurol. 1976;6(2):83–91.
15. Zabramski JM, Kiris T, Sankhla SK, Cabiol J, Spetzler RF. Orbitozygomatic craniotomy: Technical note. J Neurosurg. 1998;89(2):336–41.

4 Lateral Supraorbital Approach

Juha Hernesniemi, Hugo Andrade-Barazarte, Rosalia Duarte, Joseph Serrone, and Ferzat Hijazy

4.1 Introduction

The lateral supraorbital (LSO) approach is the most common craniotomy used in Helsinki by Professor Juha Hernesniemi. He has used the LSO approach for more than 30 years and in more than 6000 surgeries. This approach is a simpler, faster, and less invasive modification of the classically established pterional approach described by Yasargil. It provides excellent exposure of anterior fossa lesions, suprasellar lesions, and most anterior circulation aneurysms.

Like the pterional craniotomy, the skin incision is just behind the hairline. However, the incision for this approach is kept short and does not reach the zygoma inferiorly. In the LSO approach, the skin-muscle flap is opened as a single-layer flap, sparing the meticulous and laborious subfascial dissection of the pterional approach that puts the frontotemporal branches of the facial nerve at risk of injury. The temporalis muscle is split only in its superior aspect, decreasing postoperative pain and masticatory dysfunction. Additionally, it provides better cosmetic results due to less dissection of the temporalis muscle, which preserves its neurovascular supply.

J. Hernesniemi (✉) · H. Andrade-Barazarte
R. Duarte · F. Hijazy
Department of Neurosurgery,
Helsinki University Central Hospital,
Helsinki, Finland
e-mail: juha.hernesniemi@hus.fi

J. Serrone
Department of Neurosurgery, Virginia Mason
Medical Center, Seattle, WA, USA

4.2 Steps of the Approach

4.2.1 Positioning

The patient is positioned supine with the head and shoulders elevated above the cardiac level (Fig. 4.1) to reduce the bleeding by facilitating cerebral venous drainage. This in turn creates a "slack brain." The head is fixed with three or four pins to the head frame (Mayfield or Sugita) and is rotated 15–30° toward the opposite side, flexed slightly laterally (Fig. 4.2), and either flexed or extended according to the location of the lesion to be approached. If the head is rotated too much toward the opposite side, the temporal lobe obstructs access into the Sylvian fissure. The degree of head flexion and extension depends on the craniocaudal distance between the pathology and the base of the anterior cranial fossa. Higher lesions require more extension of the head, whereas lesions located nearer to the skull base require slight flexion of the head. We use the Sugita's head frame because it provides a strong retraction force by the spring hooks and also allows the surgeon to rotate the head during the surgery. When this feature is not possible, the operating table can be rotated according to the surgeon needs.

J. July, E. J. Wahjoepramono (eds.), *Neurovascular Surgery*,
https://doi.org/10.1007/978-981-10-8950-3_4

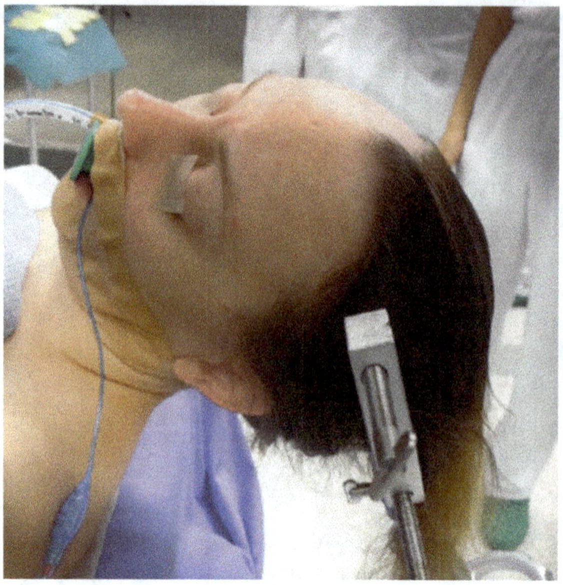

Fig. 4.1 Lateral view. The patient is positioned supine with the head and shoulders elevated above the cardiac level to reduce the bleeding

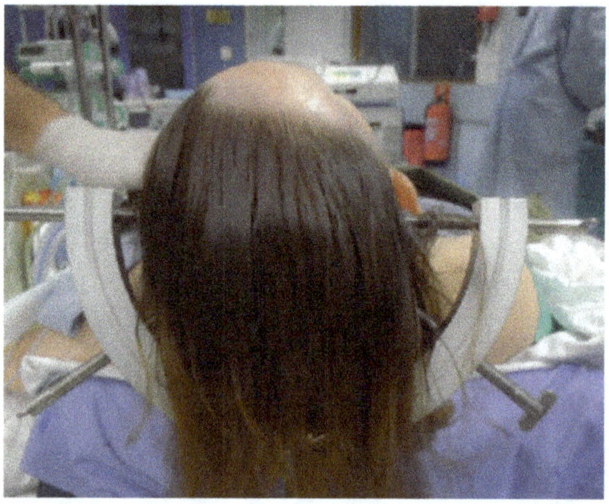

Fig. 4.2 The head is fixed with three or four pins to the Sugita's head frame and is rotated 15–30° toward the opposite side and flexed slightly laterally

4.2.2 Incision

After minimal shaving, an oblique frontotemporal skin incision is made behind the hairline. The incision starts 3 centimeters (cm) above the root of the zygoma and extends 2 cm medial to the ipsilateral midpupillary line (Fig. 4.3). In balding patients, the medial part of the incision can be placed in a skin wrinkle to provide better cosmetic results. The skin-galea-muscle flap is elevated in a single layer and retracted anteriorly with spring hooks until exposure of the superior orbital rim and frontal root of the zygoma. Raney clips are placed on the posterior margin of the skin incision for hemostasis (Fig. 4.4). The temporalis muscle is split only in its most superior and anterior part (only 3 cm of temporalis muscle is detached), and a spring hook is used to retract the muscle toward the zygomatic arc (Fig. 4.5).

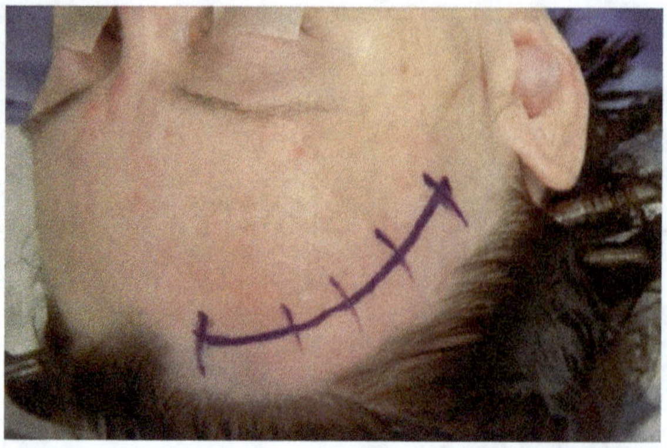

Fig. 4.3 Superior view. Oblique frontotemporal skin incision, behind the hairline

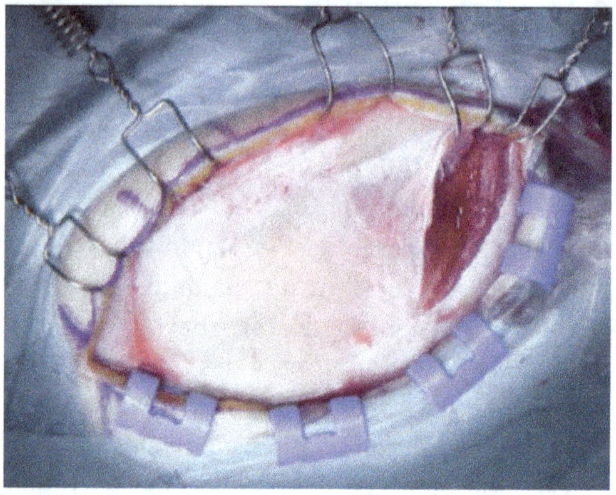

Fig. 4.4 The skin-galea-muscle flap elevated as a single layer and retracted anteriorly with spring hooks

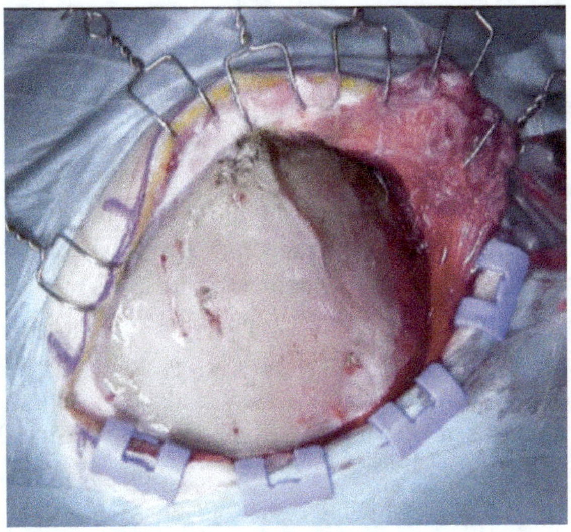

Fig. 4.5 Exposure of the superior orbital rim and frontal root of the zygoma. The temporalis muscle is detached only in its superior portion

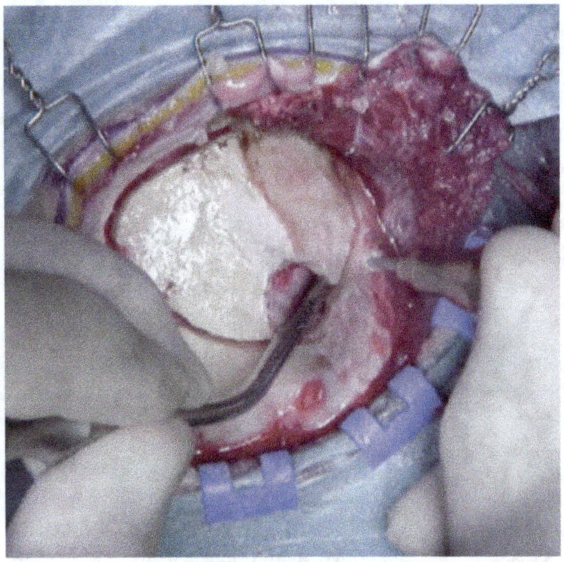

Fig. 4.6 A single burr hole is placed under the superior temporal line, and two cuts are made with the craniotome until obtaining a bone flap of 4 × 4 cm approximately

4.2.3 Craniotomy

A single burr hole is placed under the most posteriorly exposed insertion line of the temporalis muscle. If necessary, another burr hole may be placed over the pterion, depending on the size of the flap, thickness of the bone, and adherence of the dura to the inner skull surface. A curved and stout dissector is used to detach the dura from the bone. Next, a side-cutting craniotome with a footplate is used to obtain an approximately 4 cm × 4 cm bone flap with the Sylvian fissure located at the inferior limit of the craniotomy. The first cut starts from the burr hole and curves superiorly and then anteriorly toward the zygomatic process of the frontal bone. The second cut again starts in the burr hole and proceeds inferiorly toward the temporal bone, leaving the sphenoid ridge between these two cuts. The side-cutting craniotome without footplate is used to drill small holes around the craniotomy edges for future placement of dural tack-up sutures (Fig. 4.6). The thick frontal bone and lateral sphenoid ridge is thinned using the side-cutting craniotome. The bone flap is elevated posteriorly and cracked along the drilled line over the frontal and sphenoid bones.

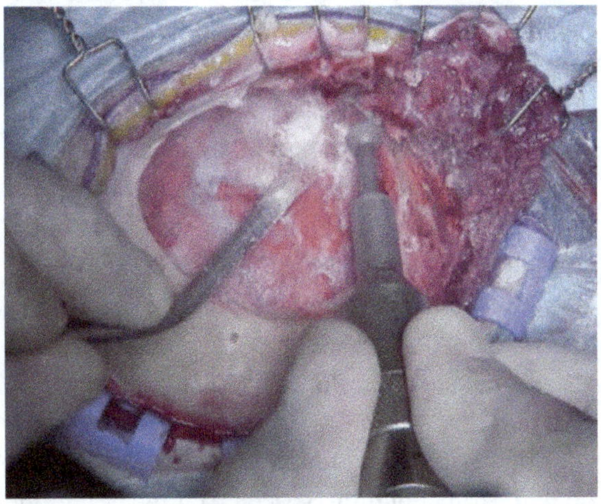

Fig. 4.7 Hot drilling technique of the sphenoid ridge and lateral and superior orbital wall

After the removal of the bone flap, the lateral sphenoid ridge is drilled off using first a high-speed drill with a rounded bit, starting at the lateral wall of the orbit toward the lesser sphenoid wing. Further drilling is continued with diamond-tipped drill bit without irrigation to smooth the surface and stop oozing of blood from the bone (Fig. 4.7). This so-called hot drilling technique (diamond-tipped drill

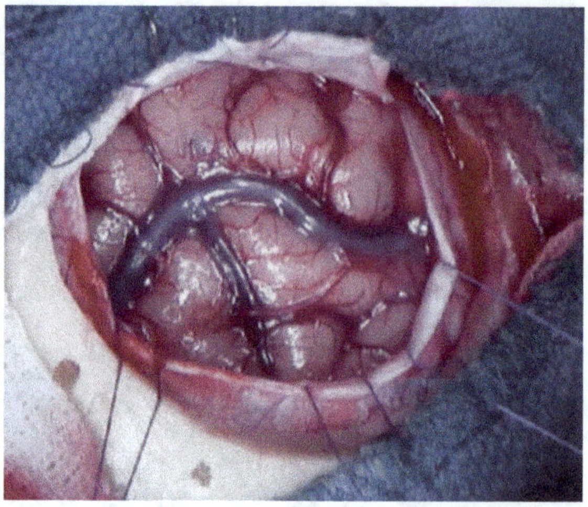

Fig. 4.8 The dura is opened in a curvilinear fashion and reflected anterolaterally. Multiple tack-up sutures are placed to retract the dural edges toward the craniotomy margins. White arrow and line demonstrated the place of the Sylvian Fissure

without saline irrigation heating the bone and sealing the bleeding) finishes the bone removal and offers excellent hemostasis. Before opening the dura, the area surrounding the craniotomy is covered with three hydrogen peroxide-soaked towels for antimicrobial effect. A green cloth is attached with staples at the anterior and inferior limit of the craniotomy to decrease the color balance in the operative field and improve visualization.

The dura is opened in a curvilinear fashion and reflected anterolaterally. Multiple tack-up sutures (Fig. 4.8) are placed to retract the dural edges toward the craniotomy margins preventing oozing from epidural space. At this point, the operating microscope is brought in place.

Before beginning the intracranial dissection, fibrin glue and small pieces of Surgicel® are used to achieve hemostasis and obtain a clear surgical field. Usually, the main goal of the initial subarachnoid dissection is to reach the basal cisterns to release cerebrospinal fluid (CSF) for brain relaxation. The dissection proceeds along the frontobasal surface of the frontal lobe slightly medial to the proximal Sylvian fissure until the entrance of the ipsilateral optic nerve into the optic canal. The arachnoid membranes limiting the optic cistern are opened and CSF is released. Furthermore, CSF can be released through the carotid cistern lateral to the ipsilateral optic nerve. Once a slack brain is achieved, the dissection proceeds according to the pathology being treated. In cases of a very tight brain, CSF can also be released from the ventricles by opening of the lamina terminalis. To reach the lamina terminalis, the dissection continues from the ipsilateral optic nerve to the optic chiasm. The frontal lobe is retracted gently using tandem work of the suction and bipolar until the lamina terminalis is visualized, just posterior to the optic chiasm. The lamina terminalis is punctured with a sharp bipolar forceps or with microscissors allowing further drainage of CSF directly from the third ventricle.

In the LSO approach, the Sylvian fissure is located on the temporal edge of the craniotomy, and all the work to open the fissure is performed from the frontal side. An 18-guage sharp needle is used to open a small gap into the arachnoid membrane of the fissure. This small opening is filled with water (water dissection technique by Toth) to expand the subarachnoid space and facilitate a bloodless subarachnoid dissection. Then the dissection continues according to the pathology to be treated.

4.2.4 Closure

The complete closure is performed under high magnification of the operative microscope. The dura is closed tightly as much as possible, in a continuous fashion with a resorbable filament (Safil 4-0). Dural defects are sealed using hemostatic agents like TachoSil®, fibrin glue, and Surgicel®. Careful and meticulous hemostasis is performed with bipolar coagulation. Additional tack-up sutures can be placed between the dura and the previously drilled holes around the craniotomy edges to elevate the dura and decrease the risk of postoperative epidural hematoma. At the final stage of the dural suturing, a blunt needle is inserted through a small gap between the dural margins, to fill the subdural space with saline and remove the air. After this, the gap is covered with TachoSil®, fibrin glue, and/or Surgicel®.

The bone flap is replaced and fixed using two CranioFix® clamps. The temporalis muscle is sutured using interrupted resorbable take-off filaments (Vicryl 2-0 or 1-0). The galea and subcutaneous layer are sutured simultaneously using a running suture with resorbable filament (Vicryl 3-0) without placing any drain. The skin is closed using surgical staples. However, in small children or young patients, the skin is closed with running resorbable intracutaneous suture (Monocryl 4-0). In some reoperations, the distance between the staples is less than 4–5 mm to ensure an uneventful wound healing.

4.3 Indications of the Approach

The LSO approach provides access to all anterior circulation aneurysms, except those located at the distal anterior cerebral artery. In addition, this approach can be used for high-positioned basilar bifurcation and basilar-superior cerebellar artery aneurysms. The trajectory of the approach provides an excellent view of the anterior fossa, the sellar and suprasellar regions, and the anterior part of the Sylvian fissure. Moreover, the LSO approach can be tailored more frontally or temporally depending of the location of a specific lesion.

4.4 Limitation of the Approach

This approach has certain limitations. It is not feasible for lesions requiring significant lateral (temporal) exposure. Examples of these cases include large posterior communicating artery aneurysms projecting posteriorly, large or giant middle cerebral artery aneurysms projecting laterally against the sphenoid wing, middle cerebral artery aneurysms associated with large temporoparietal intracerebral hematomas, or basilar tip aneurysms lying below the posterior clinoid process. In those cases, different approaches such as pterional, subtemporal, or a combination of both is necessary to treat the pathology.

4.5 Complication and How to Avoid

During the drilling of the sphenoid ridge, it is common to open the lateral and superior orbital wall causing extrusion of the periorbital fat into the surgical field. To solve this problem, we place a piece of TachoSil® over the defect. This keeps the periorbital fat contained while the bony work is completed. During the dural opening, we place two stiches at the inferior and anterior limit of the dural flap and retract this segment anteriorly using high tension. This maneuver keeps the periorbital fat away from the surgical field and provides 2–3 mm of extra space.

Since the LSO approach is a simple and less invasive approach, the rate of complications is less. CSF leakage represents a minor complication related to the approach. To decrease the risk of postoperative CSF leakage, we take special care during the dural closure placing small pieces of TachoSil®, Surgicel®, and fibrin glue in the dural defect to obtain a complete closed surface. Due to the small size of the bone flap, the risk of an epidural hematoma is low. To further decrease this risk, we place multiple tack-up sutures between the dura and the small holes drilled around the craniotomy edges.

The LSO approach represents a fast and simple approach to treat a multitude of vascular lesions and tumors. This approach follows the basic principles described by the senior author (J.H): "Simple, clean, while preserving the normal anatomy."

Bibliography

1. Hernesniemi J, Ishii K, Karatas A, et al. Surgical technique to retract the tentorial edge during subtemporal approach: technical note. Neurosurgery. 2005;57(4 Suppl):E408; discussion E408.
2. Kivelev J, Hernesniemi J. Four-fold benefit of wound closure under high magnification. Surg Neurol Int. 2013;4:115.
3. Lehecka M, Laakso A, Hernesniemi J. Helsinki microneurosurgery basics and tricks. Germany: Aesculap AG; 2011.
4. Romani R, Elsharkawy A, Laakso A, Kangasniemi M, Hernesniemi J. Complications of anterior clinoidectomy through lateral supraorbital approach. World Neurosurg. 2012;77(5–6):698–703.
5. Romani R, Laakso A, Kangasniemi M, Niemela M, Hernesniemi J. Lateral supraorbital approach applied to tuberculum sellae meningiomas: experience with 52 consecutive patients. Neurosurgery. 2012;70(6):1504–18; discussion 1518–1509.

5 Interhemispheric Approach

Alberto Feletti, Dilshod Mamadaliev, Tushit Mewada, Kei Yamashiro, Yasuhiro Yamada, Tsukasa Kawase, and Yoko Kato

5.1 Introduction

The interhemispheric (IH) approach is the best access to lesions located in the midline along the corpus callosum and can be used also for lesions in the lateral and third ventricles and in the pineal region.

Depending on the position of the target along the anteroposterior direction, the skin incision and craniotomy can vary. However, as the majority of distal anterior cerebral artery (DACA) aneurysms located along the corpus callosum especially the rostrum part, the anterior approach represents the most common way to reach them. The approach may minimally displace the frontal lobe to get enough space to expose the falx, the anterior cerebral arteries, and the corpus callosum.

Unilateral low anterior IH approach is a variation, which allows reaching the anterior communicating artery (ACoA) aneurysms.

5.2 Steps of the Approach

5.2.1 Positioning

As for other approaches, patient position is supine with the head and shoulders slightly higher than the heart to reduce bleeding by facilitating cerebral venous drainage. The head is fixed with either Mayfield (three pins) or Sugita (four pins) head holder, in straight position, and either with slight extension or flexion to get the best projection to the lesion. The degree of head flexion and extension depends on the relative position of the pathology compared to rostral part of

A. Feletti (✉)
Department of Neurosurgery, Fujita Health University, Banbuntane Hotokukai Hospital, Nagoya city, Aichi, Japan

Department of Neurosurgery, NOCSAE Modena Hospital, Modena, Italy

D. Mamadaliev
Department of Neurosurgery, Fujita Health University, Banbuntane Hotokukai Hospital, Nagoya city, Aichi, Japan

Republican Scientific Center of Neurosurgery, Tashkent, Uzbekistan

T. Mewada
Department of Neurosurgery, Fujita Health University, Banbuntane Hotokukai Hospital, Nagoya city, Aichi, Japan

G. B. Pant Institute of Post Graduate Medical Education and Research, New Delhi, India

K. Yamashiro · Y. Yamada · T. Kawase
Department of Neurosurgery, Fujita Health University, Banbuntane Hotokukai Hospital, Nagoya city, Aichi, Japan
e-mail: kawasemi@hm8.aitai.ne.jp

Y. Kato
Department of Neurosurgery, Fujita Health University, Toyoake, Aichi, Japan
e-mail: kyoko@fujita-hu.ac.jp

J. July, E. J. Wahjoepramono (eds.), *Neurovascular Surgery*,
https://doi.org/10.1007/978-981-10-8950-3_5

corpus callosum. More distal lesions require more flexion of the head, whereas lesions located close to the rostral part may just be approached with head in neutral position.

In the unilateral anterior IH approach, the patient's head is rotated to orient the midline horizontally and tilted 45° superiorly.

5.2.2 Incision

After minimal or no shaving, a frontal scalp incision is made starting just behind the hairline, 1 cm beyond the midline. The incision extends backwards parallel to the midline for 4–5 cm, bends laterally to cross the midline, and prolongs for 4–5 cm. The skin-galea flap is elevated and retracted anterolaterally with skin hooks. At the edge of skin incision, we may apply Raney clips for hemostasis.

Alternatively, a bicoronal skin incision can be performed just behind the hairline from one side to the other, starting 2 cm above the zygomatic arc. The temporalis muscle must be preserved.

5.2.3 Craniotomy

Start with two burr holes at the anterior and posterior margin of the bone flap, preferable exactly to expose the midline. If necessary, additional lateral burr holes can be placed if the dura adheres very tight to the inner table of the bone (Fig. 5.1). The dura is released from the inner table of the bone, using curved and blunt dissector. Craniotomy is then performed using a side-cutting craniotome with a footplate to obtain an approximately 4 cm × 4 cm bone flap encompassing the median line. In case of unilateral craniotomy, it is advisable to leave the median side of the craniotomy as the last step, as it has the highest risk for dural damage and consequent superior sagittal sinus opening. Actually, if that happens, less time would be required to elevate the bone flap and compress the sagittal sinus to reduce blood loss.

In the unilateral anterior (basal) IH approach, the bone flap is placed more frontally, as the skin is retracted anteriorly to a wider extent in order to obtain a more favorable direction toward the ACoA under the rostrum of the corpus callosum. Efforts should be made to preserve the frontal sinus. The bone flap is then elevated using a blunt dissector (Fig. 5.2).

Before opening the dura, the margins of the skin incision are covered with povidone-iodine-soaked towels, which can be secured to the skin using Raney clips.

Surgeon open the dura with a "U" shape, and the base of the flap lying along the superior sagittal sinus (Fig. 5.3). The two branches of the dural incision extend to the limit of the sagittal sinus, avoiding its violation. If the sagittal sinus is inadvertently opened at this stage, a dural clip can be placed to stop the bleeding. Two or three tack-up sutures are placed to retract the dural edge toward

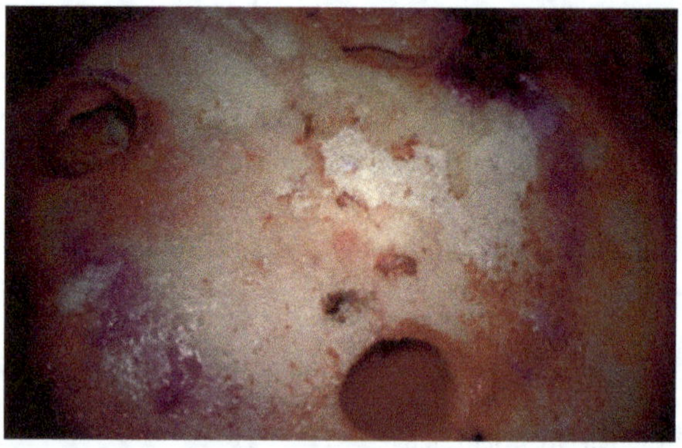

Fig. 5.1 Two burr holes are placed at the most anterior and posterior portion of the exposed midline. Occasionally, a third lateral burr hole can be placed when the dura is not easily detachable from the inner theca of the skull

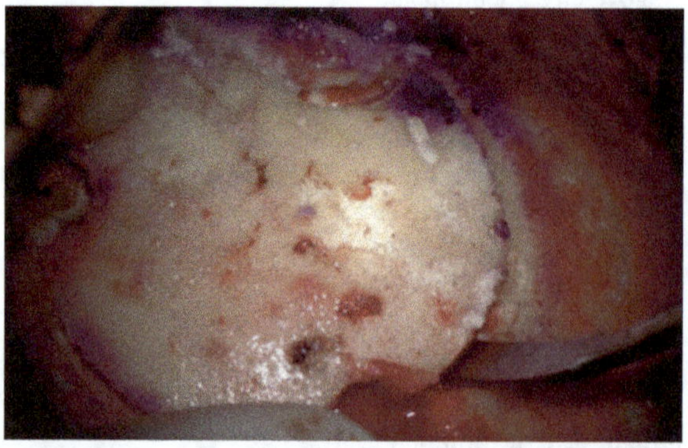

Fig. 5.2 The bone flap is elevated using a blunt dissector

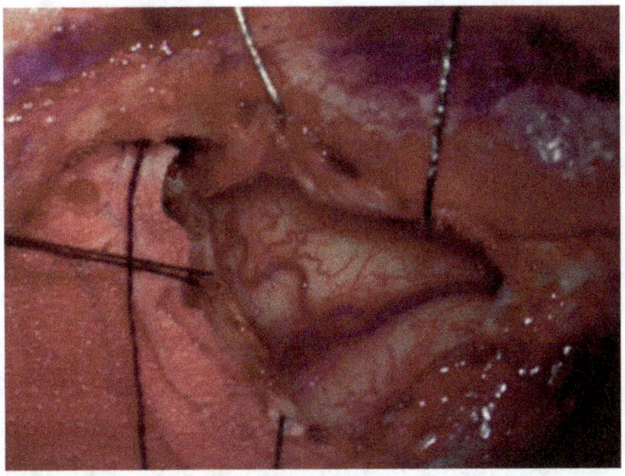

Fig. 5.3 The dura is opened and elevated toward the median line (on the left)

the median craniotomy margin. When approaching an ACoA aneurysm, sometimes a wider exposure is needed depending on the anatomical characteristics of aneurysm and vessels. In this case, the superior sagittal sinus can be closed using stiches placed at its most anterior part in the proximity of crista galli, and then cut. The dura and the falx can be therefore retracted posteriorly. The surgical microscope is placed so the surgeon may have all the flexibility for surgical maneuver.

Before beginning dissection of interhemispheric fissure, it is necessary to identify the best entry point and direction. Usually, the entry point is chosen in the space between the eventual bridging veins, to minimize vascular traction and damage. Neuronavigation systems provide a valuable tool to detect the appropriate direction of dissection. As the brain is progressively detached from the falx, a retractor can be placed to mildly retract the frontal lobe obtaining wider space and better vision along the falx. In the unilateral anterior IH approach, there is no need for active retraction as gravity itself pushes the frontal lobe downward. In any case, the cerebrospinal fluid (CSF) release obtained with subarachnoid dissection allows gradual brain relaxation and wider surgical exposure.

The dissection proceeds along the falx until either the ACAs or the ACoA are visualized (Fig. 5.4). In case of ACoA aneurysms, crista galli must be removed to obtain a wide operative field and full control of vessels.

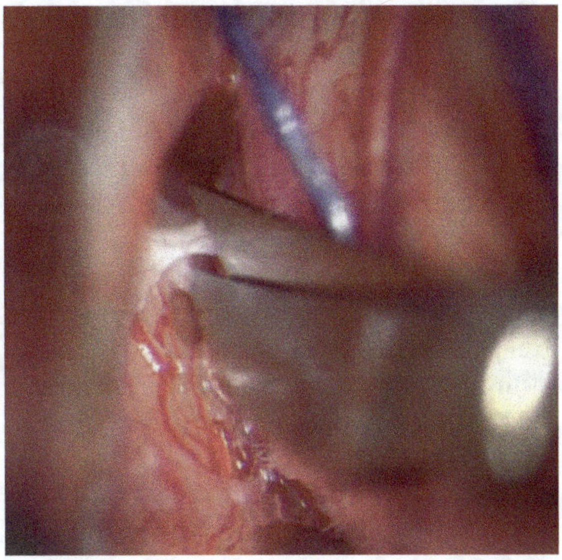

Fig. 5.4 Following the direction of the falx (on the left), subarachnoid dissection is performed

5.2.4 Closure

Before closure, any retractor must be removed and the underlying brain must be visualized in order to detect and block eventual bleedings. The dura is tightly closed in a waterproof manner with a resorbable filament (Safil 3-0 or 4-0), eventually adding fibrin glue along the dural suture. Suture should begin from the lower end of the dural opening and proceed to the upper end. In this way, just before the very last sutures, a blunt needle can be inserted intradurally to fill the subdural space with saline and remove the air. Additional tack-up sutures can be placed at the dura to the craniotomy edge, to minimize the risk of postoperative epidural hematoma. It is advisable to avoid placing these sutures along the median side of the craniotomy to prevent any puncture of the superior sagittal sinus.

The bone flap is replaced and fixed using either microplates and microscrews or sutures placed between the previously drilled holes around the craniotomy edges and along the bone flap margins. The galea and subcutaneous layer are sutured simultaneously using separate sutures with resorbable filament (Vicryl 3-0) with or without drain. The skin is closed using surgical staples or running resorbable intracutaneous suture (Monocryl 4-0).

5.3 Indication of the Approach

The IH approach provides access to aneurysms of DACA (usually for segment A2, A3), as those originating at the origin of callosomarginal artery from the pericallosal artery. This approach is also adequate for highly positioned ACoA aneurysms with superoposterior projection of the dome. The unilateral anterior IH approach has been proposed to clip unruptured small and medium sized ACoA aneurysms, as it requires minimal brain retraction and carries less risk on olfactory nerves.

5.4 Limitation of the Approach

The unilateral anterior IH approach has some limitations. Compared to the more frequently used pterional approach, it provides less clear proximal control on A1 portions of ACAs, especially when the ACoA aneurysm is large or it is projecting anteriorly. This is the reason why it has been proposed for unruptured small- and medium-sized ACoA aneurysms.

5.5 Complication and How to Avoid

When placing the burr holes along the median line, or during the craniotomy between the two burr holes, it is possible to injure superior sagittal sinus and cause copious venous bleeding. But such complication is very rare. In this case, bipolar coagulation is useless and sometimes harmful. The best way to stop the bleeding is the addition of hemostatic material such as Spongostan® or Surgicel® overlaid by a cottonoid and mechanical compression over it.

The damage of bridging veins is another potential complication of IH approach. It can be minimized by selecting the wider space between two bridging veins as the entry point to the interhemispheric fissure. If a bridging vein is fissured, placing small pieces of Surgicel® and fibrin glue can stop the bleeding. Coagulation of the vein is the last choice in case of failure of conservative attempts.

Brain contusions due to retractors must be taken into account and can be avoided applying only gentle retraction. Appropriate subarachnoid dissection and CSF release usually give significant help.

CSF leakage represents a minor complication related to this approach and can be minimized by careful waterproof dural closure. The risk of epidural hematoma is also low and can be further reduced placing multiple tack-up sutures of dura and craniotomy edges. A central suture can be also placed between the dura and two small holes at the center of the bone flap.

Bibliography

1. El-Noamany H, Nakagawa F, Hongo K, Kakizawa Y, Kobayashi S. Low anterior interhemispheric approach—a narrow corridor to aneurysms of the anterior communicating artery. Acta Neurochir (Wien). 2001;143(9):885–91.
2. Hayashi N, Sato H, Akioka N, Kurosaki K, Hori S, Endo S. Unilateral anterior interhemispheric approach for anterior communicating artery aneurysms with horizontal head position - technical note. Neurol Med Chir (Tokyo). 2011;51(2):160–3.
3. Hernesniemi J, Dashti R, Lehecka M, Niemela M, Rinne J, Lehto H, et al. Microneurosurgical management of anterior communicating artery aneurysms. Surg Neurol. 2008;70(3):8–29.
4. Hori T, Kawamata T, Amano K, Aihara Y, Ono M, Miki N. Anterior interhemispheric approach for 100 tumors in and around the anterior third ventricle. Neurosurgery. 2010;66(ONS Suppl 1):ons65–74.
5. Lehecka M, Dashti R, Hernesniemi J, Niemela M, Koivisto T, Ronkainen A, et al. Microneurosurgical management of aneurysms at the A2 segment of anterior cerebral artery (proximal pericallosal artery) and its frontobasal branches. Surg Neurol. 2008;70(3):232–46.
6. Levy ML, Berto S. Interhemispheric transcallosal transchoroidal approach to the third ventricle. In: Nader R, Gragnaniello C, Berta SC, Sabbagh AJ, Levy ML, editors. Neurosurgery tricks of the trade. 1st ed. New York: Thieme; 2013. p. 19.
7. Oda J, Kato Y, Chen SF, Sodhiya P, Watabe T, Imizu S, et al. Intraoperative near-infrared indocyanine green-videoangiography (ICG-VA) and graphic analysis of fluorescence intensity in cerebral aneurysm surgery. J Clin Neurosci. 2011;18:1097–100.

6 Subtemporal Approach

Yong Bae Kim and Kyu Sung Lee

6.1 Introduction

Historically, the first form of subtemporal approach had been described for the treatment of trigeminal neuralgia early in the twentieth century. Temporal craniotomies had offered surgical corridor to the various lesions situated in middle cranial fossa. By the 1960s, subtemporal approach entered in flourishing period by Drake's pioneering work of surgical treatment for more than 1700 basilar and posterior circulation aneurysms. Subsequently, modifications of subtemporal route, such as subtemporal key hole approach, extended exposure with zygomatic resection, or removal of petrous apex, were developed to reach peri-mesencephalic and mid-clival regions.

Here, in this chapter, the subtemporal approach will be illustrated mainly focusing on Drake's original description, while modifications for extended exposure are included for relevant occasions.

Y. B. Kim · K. S. Lee (✉)
Department of Neurosurgery,
Yonsei University College of Medicine,
Gangnam Severance Hospital, Seoul, South Korea
e-mail: ybkim69@yuhs.ac;
KYUSUNG@yuhs.ac; kyusung@yumc.yonsei.ac.kr

6.2 Steps of the Approach

After induction of general anesthesia, a lumbar drain is inserted to achieve adequate intraoperative brain relaxation. Albeit Drake and some others prefer to place patient in lateral decubitus position, supine position with the ipsilateral shoulder elevated is usually satisfactory for routine practice. Mostly right-sided (non-dominant-sided) approach is selected unless the location and/or direction of the lesion, left third nerve palsy, compromised left vision, or right hemiparesis mandate left-sided approach.

The head is rotated to the contralateral side, aligning anterior-posterior axis parallel with the floor. The vertex is slightly tilted down toward the floor for efficient intraoperative viewing trajectory as the base of the middle cranial fossa inclines upward steeply. The aim of subtemporal approach is to operate as close to the base of middle cranial fossa of the skull as possible. Therefore, the skin incision should be designed to expose temporal squama at least to the extent of root of the zygomatic arch. Usually, an inverted U-shaped skin incision is made, beginning at the level of the root of the zygomatic arch, within 1–2 cm anterior to the tragus. The incision is curved anteriorly and upwardly and then backward over the pinna around the ear. Alternately, a linear skin incision originating from the inferior rim of the zygomatic arch, approximately one finger's width, anterior to the external auditory

J. July, E. J. Wahjoepramono (eds.), *Neurovascular Surgery*,
https://doi.org/10.1007/978-981-10-8950-3_6

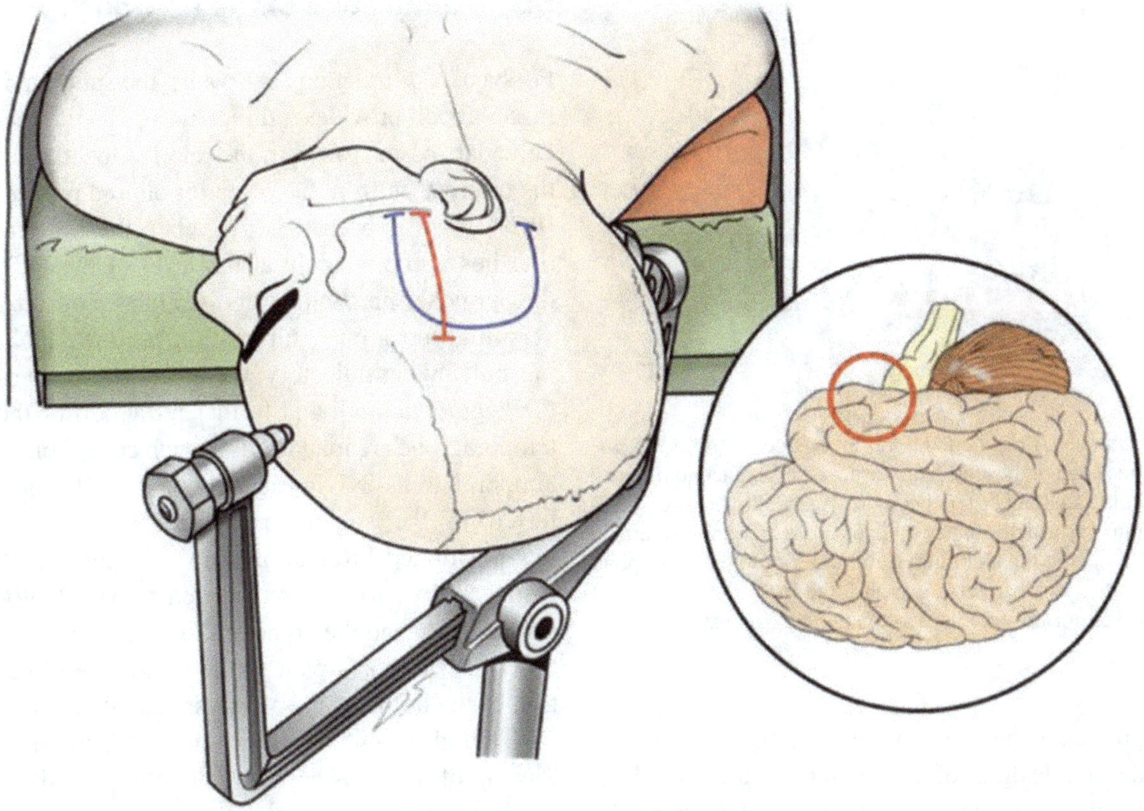

Fig. 6.1 The patient is usually positioned in supine with ipsilateral shoulder elevated. The head is rotated to the contralateral side and slightly tilted down toward the floor. An inverted U-shaped incision or linear incision can be used to expose the temporal squama just above the zygomatic tubercle

canal can be adopted for minimized temporal bone flap (Fig. 6.1).

The skin flap is then reflected inferiorly, and the temporalis muscle is divided and reflected as well, exposing the zygomatic process of the temporal bone and the root of the zygomatic arch. A 4–5 cm-sized craniotomy at exposed temporal squama is performed, placing inferior border of the bone flap as lower as possible. If mastoid air cells are inadvertently opened, careful closure by bone waxing or temporal muscle flap should be completed. It is critical to drill down the inferior overhanging edge of the temporal bone to flush with the base of the middle cranial fossa.

The dura is opened and reflected with several tack-up sutures. At this point, the lumbar drain is opened until sufficient brain relaxation is gained. Gentle retraction of the temporal lobe should progress in stepwise manner as the floor of the middle cranial fossa shapes convex. Small bridging veins from undersurface of the temporal lobe to the tent can be divided when necessary. However, care must be taken never to violate the vein of Labbe, which is usually running just beyond the posterior border of the temporal craniotomy. As the temporal lobe is being retracted further, the free edge of the tentorial incisura and the arachnoid sheath of the ambient cistern become visualized. Opening of the ambient cistern will provide further cerebrospinal fluid drainage and clear view of cisternal contents. The trochlear nerve can be identified usually underneath of the tentorium, when the free edge is lifted up only few millimeters. More anteriorly, the interpeduncular cistern comes into view by elevating the uncus. A thick arachnoid membrane, so-called Liliequist's membrane, is extending from the anterior edge of the mammillary bodies to the superior border of the dorsum sellae, separating interpeduncular cistern from the carotid and chiasmatic cisterns. Laterally, this membrane is perforated by the posterior communicating artery and the oculomotor nerve. A vertical incision at the tentorium just behind the entry point of the trochlear nerve will

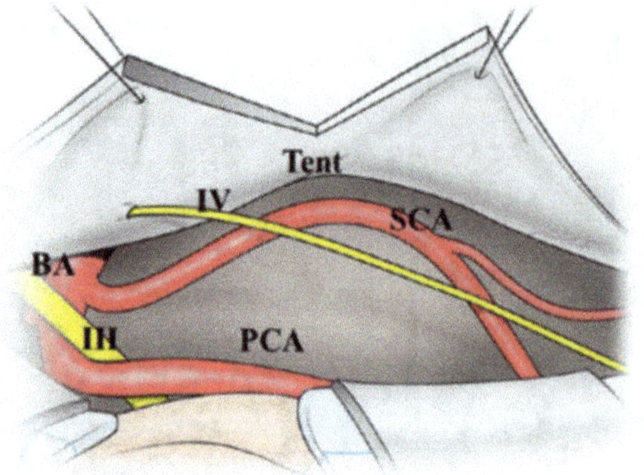

Fig. 6.2 After the temporal lobe is gently retracted, the free edge of the tentorial incisura and the arachnoid sheath of the ambient cistern become visualized. The trochlear is running usually underneath of the tentorium. A vertical incision at the tentorium right posterior to the entry point of the trochlear nerve is made, and the incised leaflets of the tentorium are raised up bilaterally using stay sutures

provide wider opening of the ambient cistern. The incised leaflets of the tentorium are raised up bilaterally using stay sutures. At this stage, the ambient segment of the superior cerebellar artery (SCA) is firstly seen on the anterolateral side of the pontomesencephalic junction. Anteriorly, the oculomotor nerve arises from the medial surface of the cerebral peduncle and traverses between the posterior cerebral artery (PCA) and the SCA (Fig. 6.2). After opening the Liliequist's membrane, the bifurcation of the basilar artery (BA) is found within interpeduncular cistern (Fig. 6.4). The PCA is joined by the posterior communicating artery at the lateral margin of the interpeduncular cistern and passes over the oculomotor nerve along crural and ambient cisterns. The direct perforators to the brain stem and thalamus usually arise from the superior surface of the PCA; therefore, it should be safer to follow the PCA along the inferior surface medially to the basilar apex. If the posterior communicating artery is hypoplastic, and obscuring surgical view around the basilar apex, then the artery may be divided only when perforators are not compromised. The origin of SCA is usually located inferior to the trochlear nerve. When temporary clip of the BA trunk is necessary, a few millimeters segment of the BA below the origin of the SCA is ideal because there is seldom existence of the BA perforators.

6.3 Indication of the Approach

For basilar bifurcation aneurysms, the subtemporal approach provides a direct avenue to interpeduncular fossa. However, the relative location of the bifurcation from the posterior clinoid process (PCP) is an important issue. When the bifurcation lies approximately at the level of the PCP, the surgical approach can be straightforward. A very high-positioned bifurcation requires looking-up viewing trajectory; therefore, resection of the zygomatic arch and further retraction of the temporal lobe are mandated. In such case, frontotemporal trans-Sylvian approach could be preferred to the subtemporal approach. A very low-positioned bifurcation may be significantly hampered by narrow corridor even with the tentorial incision, and the dome of the aneurysm often obscures surgeon's path to the neck. The direction of the dome of the aneurysm should also be considered when selecting surgical approach. Placing of the clips becomes straightforward for BA aneurysms projecting anteriorly, as the dome is exposed directly into view while the neck of the aneurysm tends to be free of the PCA and its perforators. On the contrary, posterior-projecting aneurysms may pose difficulties in direct clipping. The dome can be buried high up in the interpeduncular fossa, and numerous perforators from basilar terminus are usually adhered with the back of the aneurysm. It is critical to separate those perforators form the site where the final clip is to be deployed. The neck of the aneurysm is often hidden underneath the ipsilateral oculomotor nerve and the PCA. Such configurations may possess blind spots around the neck of the aneurysm, resulting in incomplete or mispositioned final clip.

For aneurysms arisen at the origin of the SCA, the subtemporal approach provides excellent visualization of the neck and fundus of the aneurysms. They are usually projecting laterally toward the approach side, and no perforators emanate from the BA segment between the PCA and SCA, making clipping simple and straightforward. Only concerns should be given not to compromise or kink the BA and the SCA orifice.

The aneurysms arisen at the P1 (from the origin of the PCA to the junction with the posterior communicating artery) and P2 (within peduncular and ambient cisterns) segment of the PCA can best be dealt with subtemporal approach. One may require resecting some parts of the parahippocampal gyri when the aneurysm is hidden under them.

Because the subtemporal approach exposes mesial temporal lobe, and the lateral aspect of mesencephalon, vascular malformations such as the arteriovenous malformations and cavernous malformations situated around these structures are good candidates for the subtemporal approach. Cavernous malformations or other vascular lesions developed at the level of upper pons can be removed when the subtemporal approach is combined with removal of petrous apex (extended subtemporal exposure, or anterior transpetrosal approach) (Figs. 6.3, 6.4, 6.5, 6.6, 6.7, 6.8, and 6.9). Open surgical treatment for the

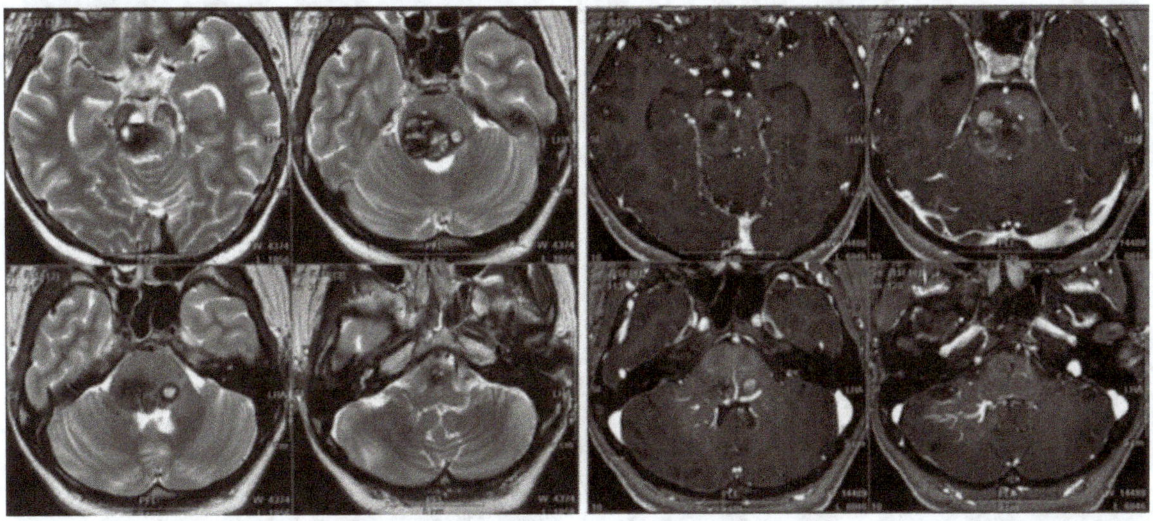

Fig. 6.3 Axial T2-weighted (left) and gadolinium-enhanced T1-weighted (right) magnetic resonance images reveal cavernous malformation residing in upper pons. Note fluid-fluid layer inside the lesion, implying previous episodes of intralesional rupture. Dorsal surface of the lesion is engulfed by network of the venous malformation; therefore approaches from the midline of the posterior fossa are impossible. Instead, extended subtemporal transtentorial approach is selected to approach from the right posterolateral aspect of the brain stem

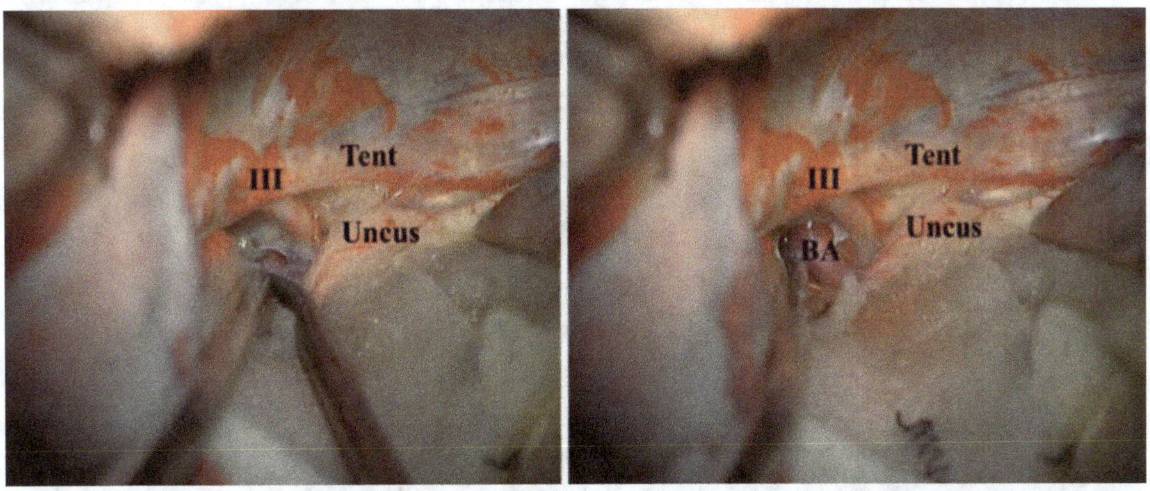

Fig. 6.4 For extended subtemporal exposure, the patient is placed in lateral decubitus position. A curvilinear incision is made extending from the inferior border of the root of the zygomatic arch, curving anteriorly to the midline behind the hairline. By using interfascial technique to avoid facial nerve injury, the zygomatic arch is exposed and resected. After gentle retraction of the temporal lobe, the free edge of the tentorium becomes visualized. The uncus is the landmark to identify the oculomotor nerve (III). Note that the thick arachnoid membrane over the interpeduncular fossa (Liliequist's membrane) is adherent laterally to the oculomotor nerve (left). After the membrane is opened, the terminus of the basilar artery is then exposed (right)

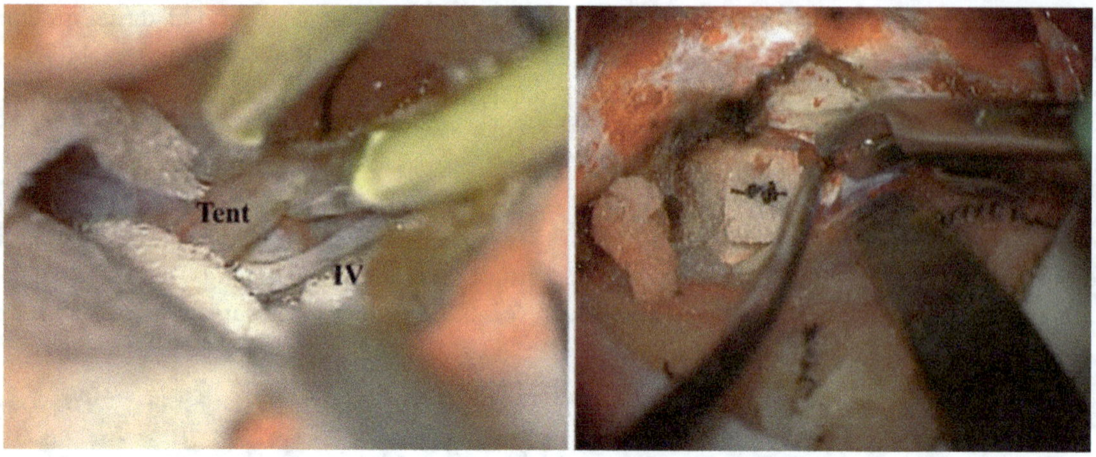

Fig. 6.5 Posteriorly to the oculomotor nerve, the crural and ambient cistern is opened. The tentorium is incised posterior to the entry point of the trochlear nerve to gain wider surgical window (left). The extension of the tentorial incision is performed toward the superior petrosal sinus to remove dural cover at the area of the petrous apex. The superior petrosal sinus is ligated using hemoclip (right)

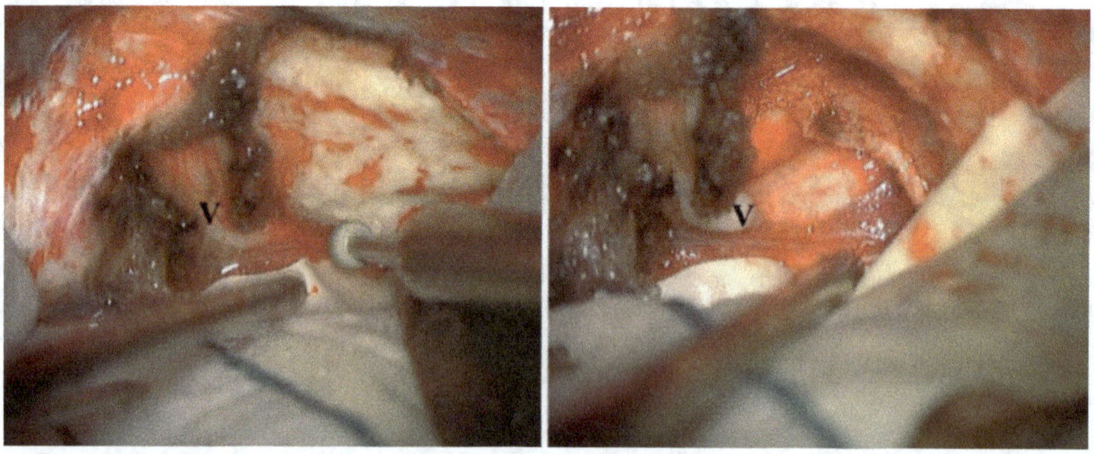

Fig. 6.6 The dura over the Meckel cave and the petrous apex is uncovered (left). With gentle mobilization and protection of the trigeminal nerve, the petrous apex is removed using diamond drill (right)

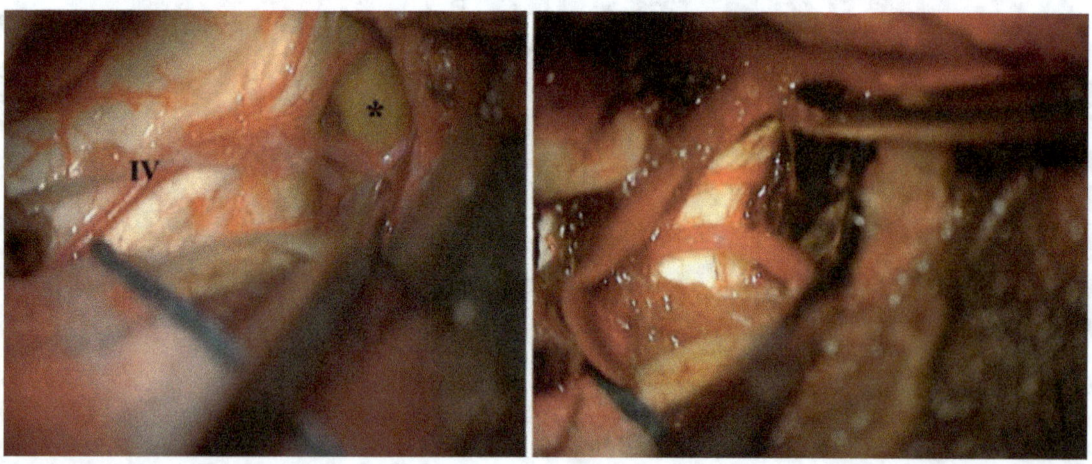

Fig. 6.7 By removal of the petrous apex, upper half of the retroclival region is exposed. Note the yellowish discoloration on the surface of the pons (left, asterisk). A small incision at the discolored surface of the pons is made, and the cavernous malformation is being removed (right)

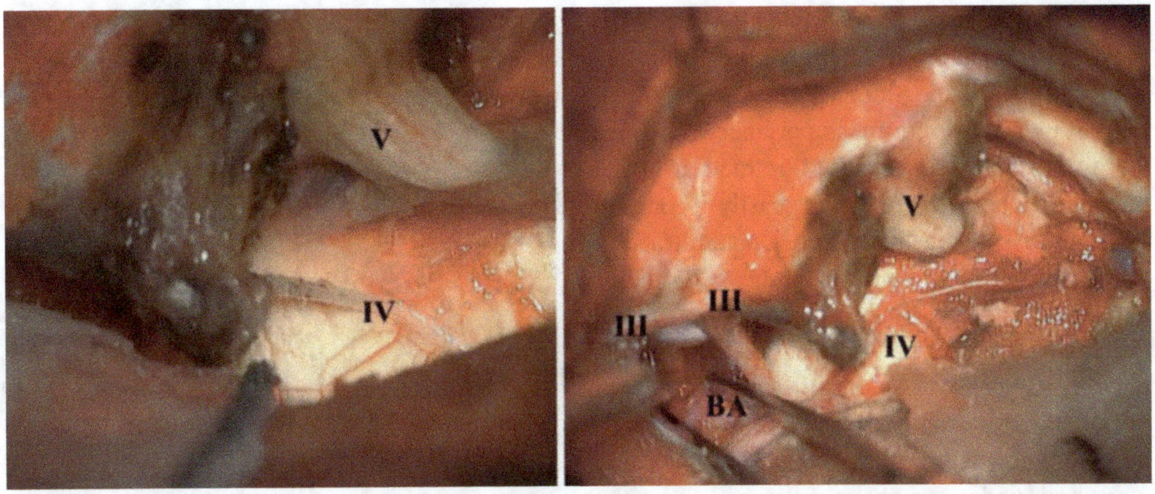

Fig. 6.8 The overall extent of intraoperative view from extended subtemporal transtentorial approach utilizing resection of the zygomatic arch and the petrous apex. The retroclival and anterolateral mesencephalo-pontine area are fully exposed. Note the bilateral oculomotor nerves, the trochlear nerve, the trigeminal nerve, and the BA (right)

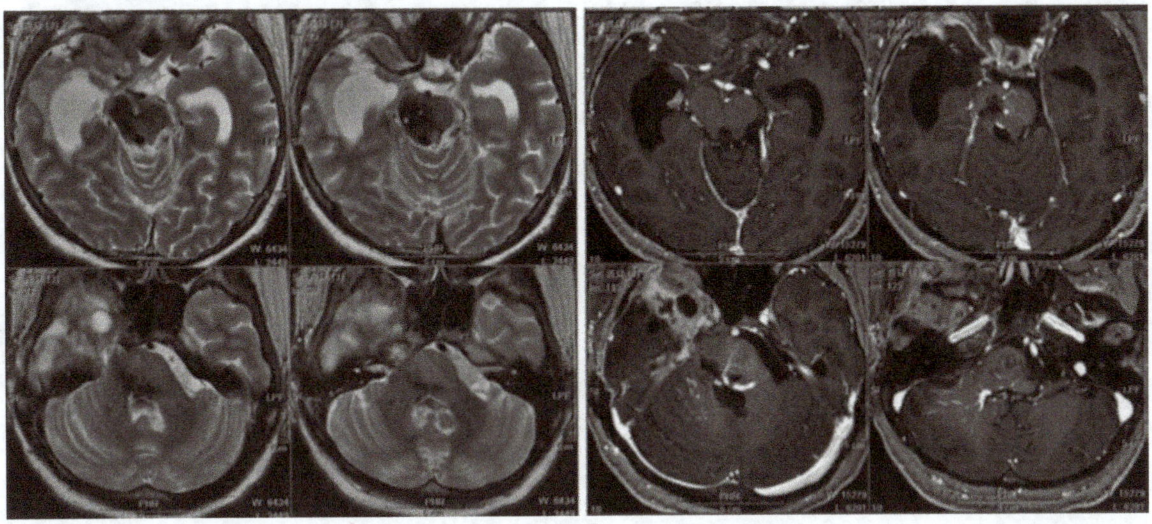

Fig. 6.9 Axial T2-weighted (left) and gadolinium-enhanced T1-weighted (right) magnetic resonance images reveal complete removal of the cavernous malformation. The venous channels at the dorsum of the lesion are well preserved

dural arteriovenous fistulae in the tentorial incisura can also be considered in suitable condition via subtemporal approach.

6.4 Limitation, Complication, and How to Avoid

Although the subtemporal approach may provide relatively straightforward exposure of anatomy and an adequate visualization of the terminal basilar complex, the narrow working window of lateral surgical trajectories often permit only limited maneuverability. Therefore, reflecting the tentorial edge is the key step to increase working space around the cerebral peduncle. When making incision at the tentorium, the entrance of the trochlear nerve to its dural canal should be identified first to avoid the trochlear nerve injury.

Nevertheless, the essential part of this approach is assured only by retracting temporal lobe in certain degree. The injury to the temporal lobe by pressuring retraction must be one of the most disadvantageous consequences in this approach. Adequate drainage of cerebrospinal fluid is, therefore, of prime importance. When the draining vein is compromised, retraction of the temporal lobe will be more easily prone to postoperative venous infarction. Uncal retraction may cause tethering injury to the oculomotor nerve. Ordinarily, it is advocated to leave the oculomotor nerve attached and ensheathed within thick arachnoid without manipulation to avoid postoperative palsies. In selected cases, it may be necessary to dissect the oculomotor nerve and work both under and above the nerve. Once the integrity of the oculomotor nerve is well preserved, postoperative palsies should be transient. Due to the relatively lateral to medial direction of line of sight, the contralateral PCA and perforating vessels are often difficult to identify so that retraction or indentation of the aneurysm itself may be necessary to visualize the hind aspect of the aneurysm. Selecting appropriate length of clips is also important not to blindly bite the vessels and nerves embedded in deep opposite side. Fenestrated clips are very useful for passing the ipsilateral PCA through the aperture.

Bibliography

1. Drake CG. Surgical treatment of ruptured aneurysms of the basilar artery. Experience with 14 cases. J Neurosurg. 1965;23(5):457–73.
2. Yasargil MG, Antic J, Laciga R, Jain KK, Hodosh RM, Smith RD. Microsurgical pterional approach to aneurysms of the basilar bifurcation. Surg Neurol. 1976;6(2):83–91.
3. Kawase T, Shiobara R, Toya S. Anterior transpetrosal-transtentorial approach for sphenopetroclival meningiomas: surgical methods and results in 10 patients. Neurosurgery. 1991;28:869–76.
4. Hernesniemi J, Ishii K, Niemelä M, Kivipelto L, Fujiki M, Shen H. Subtemporal approach to basilar bifurcation aneurysms: advanced technique and clinical experience. Acta Neurochir Suppl. 2005;94:31–8.
5. McLaughlin N, Martin NA. Extended subtemporal transtentorial approach to the anterior incisural space and upper clival region: experience with posterior circulation aneurysms. Neurosurgery. 2014;10(Suppl 1):15–24.

7 Lateral Suboccipital Approach (Retrosigmoid)

Senanur Gulec, Francesca Spedicato, Ferry Senjaya, and Julius July

7.1 Introduction

After first description by Fedor Krause in 1903 [1], the unilateral approach to the cerebellopontine angle (CPA) have been developed and modified further by many surgeons. These include the transmastoid-translabyrinthine approach, the transtemporal extradural approach, and the lateral suboccipital (retrosigmoid) approach.

Many good achievements by surgeon from various different operative approaches, which more determined by the familiarity and experience of individual surgeon rather than the approaches themselves. Still, an ever-growing amount of evidence suggests that the goals of CPA surgery are best achieved with the retrosigmoid approach [2]. One of the advantages of retrosigmoid approach is that it provides a good exposure to the cranial nerve, brainstem, lateral cerebellum, and the vessels; also it can be extended inferiorly by combining with the far-lateral transcondylar approach [3] or far-lateral retrocondylar approach. The retrosigmoid approach also can be extended superiorly and combined with the intradural suprameatal approach [1].

Vascular lesions and other pathology at this area can be exposed adequately by doing the classical retrosigmoid approach or its modifications [4]. This approach enables the surgery to be performed under visual control, due to wide panoramic view, and it is essential to have a clear exposure while doing dissection near brainstem. Additional to that, the retrosigmoid approach is the best technique for patients with big vestibular schwannoma (VS).

When the intraoperative neurophysiological monitoring becomes available, it provides a basis for a much safer surgery [5]. Nowadays this monitoring is done starting from the very beginning of the surgery until the very end of surgery. Various monitoring systems are available nowadays; in some cases the monitoring system is absolutely important, such as the somatosensory evoked potentials to detect spinal cord compression while doing semi-sitting position [4].

S. Gulec
Department of Neurosurgery,
Faculty of Medicine Universitas Pelita Harapan (UPH), Neuroscience Centre Siloam Hospital Lippo Village, Tangerang, Indonesia

Marmara University School of Medicine, Istanbul, Turkey

F. Spedicato
Department of Neurosurgery,
Faculty of Medicine Universitas Pelita Harapan (UPH), Neuroscience Centre Siloam Hospital Lippo Village, Tangerang, Indonesia

Universita Degli Studi. "A.Moro" School of Medicine, Bari, Italy

F. Senjaya · J. July (✉)
Department of Neurosurgery,
Faculty of Medicine Universitas Pelita Harapan (UPH), Neuroscience Centre Siloam Hospital Lippo Village, Tangerang, Indonesia

J. July, E. J. Wahjoepramono (eds.), *Neurovascular Surgery*,
https://doi.org/10.1007/978-981-10-8950-3_7

7.2 Steps of the Approach

7.2.1 Positioning of the Head

Patient can be positioned in semi-sitting, lateral, or ¾ lateral position (park bench), or even some surgeon prefers supine position and the head rotated to contralateral side [5–7]. Each of these positions has its advantages and disadvantages from the points of providing sufficient access and avoiding complications. However, the surgeon preference and familiarity is the most important part while deciding the patient position. We prefer to use the park bench position for many reasons and arguments that we think safer for the patient and easy for anesthesia monitoring. Head and neck position is almost neutral if we consider the cervical stenosis in to the risk factor if we turn and flex the neck. The disadvantage part is requiring slightly longer time to put the patient in to such position. We do not describe sitting position in this chapter, simply because it requires specific monitoring system to detect air embolism such as trans-esophageal echocardiography, end-tidal carbon dioxide, and precordial Doppler echocardiography [8]. All those monitoring systems might not be always available.

The positioning has to start with the body in the lateral position, and we like to put it slightly prone to push the shoulder away from the surgical field. The front and back of the patient body were held with body holders. The contralateral arm is positioned lower than the body, sitting on the arm rest. The contralateral armpit is supported with silicon bolster, just at the edge of the table. We can use Mayfield or Sugita head pin fixation system, but *do not* fix the head until the body is in good position and well held (Fig. 7.1). The head is fixed with three pin fixations and slightly flexed. Remember to avoid any occlusion of venous jugular outflow. The ipsilateral arm is kept aligned with the body, and the contralateral arm is always wrapped with waterproof and soft pad to avoid skin burn.

7.2.2 Skin Incision: Craniotomy

Shave the hair behind the ear just enough to identify the anatomical landmark. The incision is planned according to the need, but usually the skin incision is tailored according to the bone opening. Surgical landmark on the skin projection is important. At the level of acoustic meatus should be the vestibular-facial nerve region, and 1 cm (one finger) superior to it would be the projection of transverse sigmoid junction. If we draw a line from this junction to the protuberantia occipitalis externa, the line would represent the transverse sinus (Fig. 7.2).

We prefer to use the lazy "S" incision, because it's simple and sufficient. The underlying neck muscles are incised in line with the skin. The skin

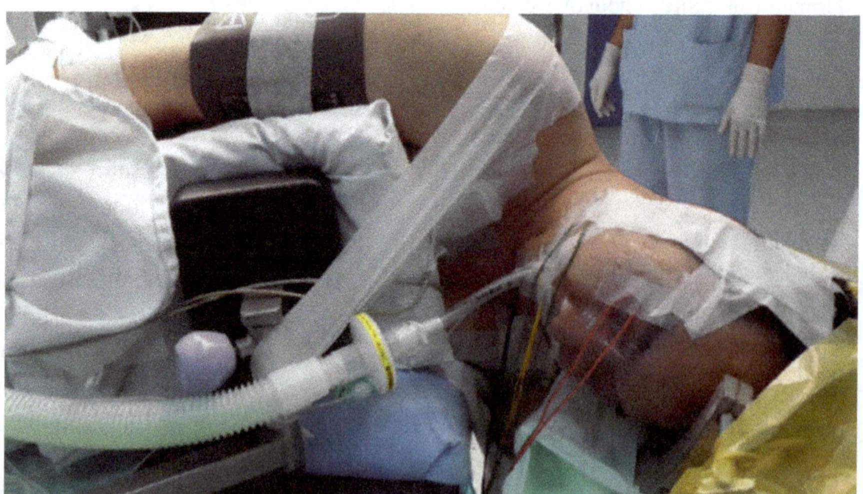

Fig. 7.1 The patient position. Right side (park bench), the chest and back are held with body holder and locked. The ipsilateral shoulder is tapped gently to the anterior and inferior of the patient to bring the shoulder away from the surgical field. The contralateral armpit is supported with silicon bolster at the edge of the surgical table. Then the head is fixed with Sugita pin fixation with the head slightly flexed

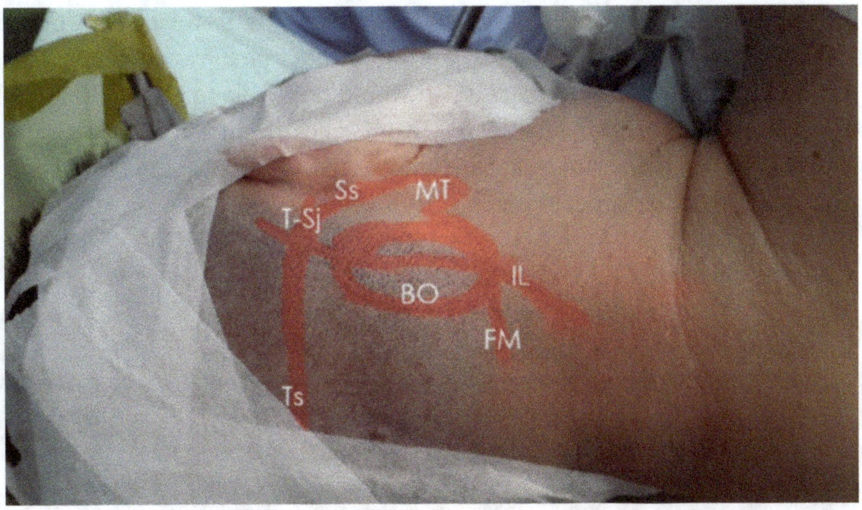

Fig. 7.2 The incision planning to expose the right CN VIII/VII complex and LCN (lower cranial nerve). *Ts* transverse sinus, *T-Sj* transverse sigmoid junction, *Ss* sigmoid sinus, *MT* mastoid tip, *BO* bone opening, *FM* foramen magnum, *IL* incision line

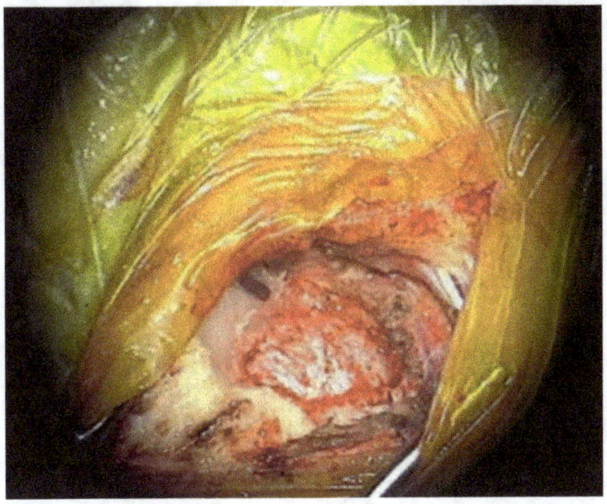

Fig. 7.3 The right side. The skin flap and muscles are retracted with self-retaining retractor. The bone opening is ellipsoid

flap and the muscles are split and held using a self-retaining retractor (Fig. 7.3).

Performing whether craniectomy or craniotomy is a matter of surgeon's choice, and they both have advantage and disadvantage. The size of the bone opening is according to how much the surgeon needs the exposure. The surgeon may expose the borders of transverse and sigmoid sinuses if necessary, but it is unnecessary to expose it routinely because it may lead to laceration and subsequent thrombosis [4].

The burr hole is placed half centimeter inferomedial to the asterion, and remember that the asterion may serve as a landmark where transverse sinus curves and turns to be sigmoid sinus [5]. The transverse sinus and sigmoid sinus generally curve around the asterion. However, recent studies have proven that asterion is not an entirely consistent anatomical point; it may vary in cranio-caudal direction or in anterior-posterior direction [9].

Doing the opening of the dura with a curvilinear shape approximately 2 mm medial away from sigmoid sinus and 2 mm inferior away from transverse sinus. For protection of the cerebellum, leave the dural flap over the cerebellum. If necessary, additional dural incisions should be made laterally toward the curve between the transverse sinus and sigmoid sinus. The resulting curvilinear-shaped dural leave is sutured to the surrounding tissue (Fig. 7.4).

To relax the cerebellum, the inferior cerebellum is retracted gently, and the arachnoid that cover the cistern is opened to release CSF. The surgeon should be aware that excessive cerebellar relaxation may cause a venous tear near the tentorium or in the area of petrosal sinus, even some remote areas in the supratentorial area. Complications of remote bleeding such as subdural hemorrhage or even epidural hemorrhage have been incidentally reported.

The later steps of surgery depend on the underlying pathology. It is very important to be familiar with all the cranial nerves, vessels, and anatomical landmark in this area. The best is to use the microvascular decompression case as a role case for normal anatomy. If we direct the microscope toward inferior lateral, we would be able to see the lower cranial nerve (IX, X, and XI); if we change the microscope slightly superior, we would be able to see the subarcuate artery, VIII and VII complex going to meatus acusticus internus (MAI), and the labyrinthine artery as a branch of anterior inferior cerebellar artery (AICA). If we dissect the prepontine arachnoid, we could see the VI nerve going in to the Dorello's canal (Fig. 7.5).

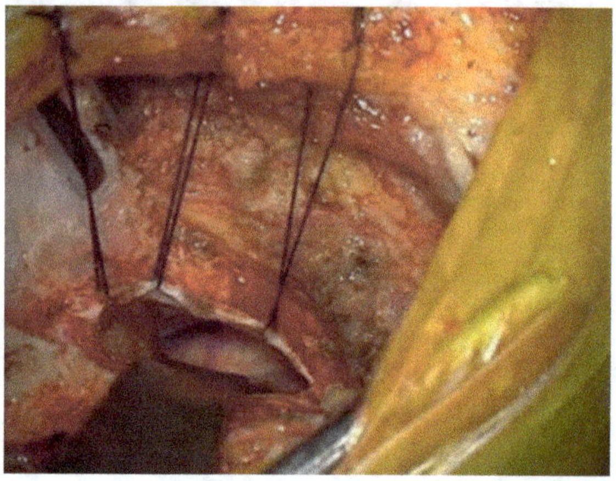

Fig. 7.4 The right side. The curvilinear shape dural leave is sutured to the muscle, providing 2–3 mm more visual field. The retractor is used gently just to hold the cerebellum to avoid jigging movement to the brain

If we change the microscope more superior after viewing the VIII/VII complex, we should be able to see the V, sometimes IV, superior petrosal vein and the superior cerebellar artery (SCA) and of course the tentorium (Fig. 7.6).

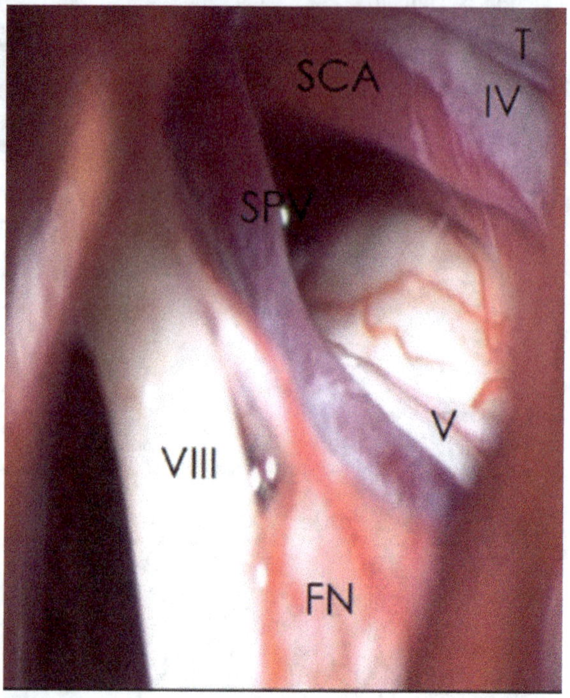

Fig. 7.6 Left retrosigmoid approach, exposing the upper part of the CP angle. *VIII* vestibular nerve, *V* trigeminal nerve, *SPV* superior petrosal vein, *IV* trochlear nerve, *T* tentorium, *SCA* superior cerebellar artery

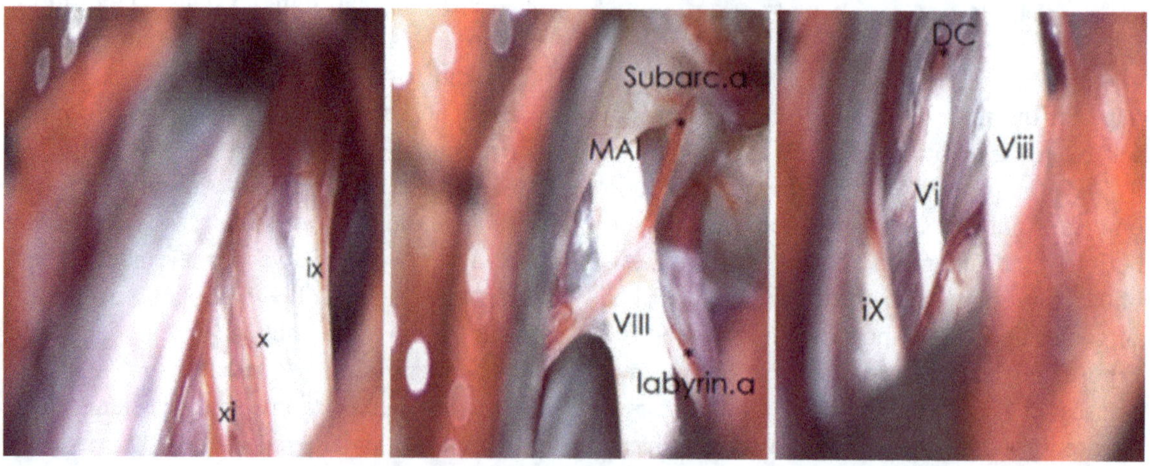

Fig. 7.5 Left retrosigmoid approach is exposing the left cerebellopontine angle anatomy. *Left*, inferiorly we expose lower cranial nerve (IX, X, XI); *middle*, more superior we could see the VIII/VII complex, MAI (meatus acusticus internus), labyrinthine artery and subarcuate artery; *right*, after dissection of the prepontine arachnoid, we could expose VI nerve going into the DC (Dorello's canal)

7.2.3 Closure

When the mastoid air cells are opened during drilling of the bone, it is important to make sure they are occluded with muscle, fat, and fibrin glue. The dura should be closed with watertight suture and has to be done under the microscope, and if needed, the fat harvested from subcutaneous layer or muscle is necessary if watertight suture cannot be achieved. The fat or the muscle should be sutured to the suture line, and it will seal the leak. If there is significant bleeding from the edges of the bone, bone wax may be used to control the bleeding.

7.3 Indication of the Approach

This retrosigmoid approach is good to approach several vascular lesions such as resection of the pontine cavernoma, posterior inferior cerebellar artery (PICA) aneurysm, vertebral artery aneurysm, anterior inferior cerebellar artery (AICA) aneurysm, and cortical segment aneurysm of superior cerebellar artery (SCA). Of course this approach is more common to take out CPA tumor and for microvascular decompression of fifth and seventh nerve. If we extend to inferiorly in combination with far lateral approach, we may take out the lower brainstem cavernoma or prepare the proximal control for aneurysm surgery.

Lesion that is located in lateral or anterior part of foramen magnum area can be successfully approached by lateral suboccipital (retrosigmoid) approach, combined with C1 hemilaminectomy/laminectomy [10]. The foramen magnum needs to be opened widely, and additional C1 laminectomy will provide enough space for dissection. The vertebral artery can be identified and can be mobilized if necessary.

7.4 Limitation of the Approach

Limitation of the approach is defined by the limitations to viewing angles imposed on the surgeon by the operating microscope and several factors that could contribute to it such as the lesion itself (tumor or vessel) and the working space in the CPA. Intraoperative use of endoscope may extend the view to the corner looking at the perforator that could not be provided by microscopic view.

7.5 Complication and How to Avoid

If craniectomy is performed, methyl methacrylate is used to reconstruct the posterior skull base. Complication such as pseudomeningocele should be avoidable by doing meticulous watertight closure of dura. The reconstruction of the posterior fossa with bone dust and held with fibrin glue is useful for small opening. But bigger bone opening needs substitute of methyl methacrylate to prevent adhesion between the dura and the neck muscles that may cause suboccipital headache [4] and also to have a better cosmetic result. In such case, subcutaneous infiltration with local anesthetic generally cures the headache. If the pain remains disturbing the patient and resistant to medication, a surgery to release the scar can be performed due to immediate beneficial effect [6].

References

1. Tatagiba M, Acioly MA. Retrosigmoid approach to the posterior and middle fossae. In: Ramina R, Aguiar PHP, Tatagiba M, editors. Samii's essentials in neurosurgery. Berlin: Springer; 2008. p. 136–47.
2. Samii M, Gerganov V. Cerebellopontine angle tumors. In: Ellenbogen R, Abdulrauf S, editors, Sekhar L, ass editor. Principles of neurological surgery, 3rd ed. Philadelphia: Saunders;2012. p. 585–90.
3. Fisch U. Chirurgie im inneren Gehörgang und an benachbarten Strukturen. In: Naumann HH, editor. Kopfund Hals-Chirurgie, vol. 3. Stuttgart: Thieme; 1976. p. 457–543.
4. Samii M, Gerganov VM. Suboccipital lateral approaches (retrosigmoid). In: Cappabianca P, et al., editors. Cranial, craniopharyngeal and skull base surgery, vol. 2010. Milan: Springer; 2010. p. 143–9.
5. Ciric I, Zhao JC, Rosenblatt S, et al. Suboccipital retrosigmoid approach for vestibular schwannomas: facial nerve function and hearing preservation. Neurosurgery. 2005;56:560–70.
6. Samii M, Gerganov V, Samii A. Improved preservation of hearing and facial nerve function in vestibular schwannoma surgery via the retrosigmoid approach in a series of 200 patients. J Neurosurg. 2006;105:527–35.

7. Yasargil MG, Smith RD, Gasser JC. The microsurgical approach to acoustic neuromas. Adv Tech Stand Neurosurg. 1977;4:93–128.
8. Von Goesseln HH, Samii M, Sur D, et al. The lounging position for posterior fossa surgery: anesthesiological considerations regarding air embolism. Childs Nerv Syst. 1991;7:368–74.
9. Bozbuga M, Boran BO, Sahinoglu K. Surface anatomy of the posterolateral cranium regarding the localization of the initial burr-hole for a retrosigmoid approach. Neurosurg Rev. 2006;29:61–3.
10. Samii M, Klekamp J, Carvalho G. Surgical results for meningiomas of the craniocervical junction. Neurosurgery. 1996;39:1086–95.

8 Transmastoid Approach for Retrolabyrinthine and Translabyrinthine

Tetsuro Sameshima

8.1 Introduction

It is very important to understand the anatomical landmark of this approach (Fig. 8.1). There are some well-known triangle and skin incisions related to retrolabyrinthine and translabyrinthine approaches (Fig. 8.1a, b).

The retrolabyrinthine approach exposes the posterior fossa dura between sigmoid sinus, posterior semicircular canal, jugular bulb, and superior petrosal sinus. Retrolabyrinthine access to the cerebellopontine angle (CPA) with hearing preservation can be accomplished; however, exposure is generally limited. The most frequent indication for an isolated retrolabyrinthine approach is selective vestibular nerve section. More frequently the retrolabyrinthine approach is combined with cutting temporal bone and splitting tentorium to expose lateral pons and basilar artery from the confluence of the vertebral arteries to the dorsum sellae (the combined petrosal approach).

When hearing that preservation is not a consideration, the CPA can be more widely exposed by removing the vestibular labyrinth and skeletonizing the internal auditory canal through the translabyrinthine approach. Advocates of this approach cite early identification of the facial nerve in the IAC and minimal brain retraction as factors for improved results in acoustic tumor surgery. Either the retro- or translabyrinthine approaches can be combined with other lateral skull base procedures to enhance exposure, depending on size and location of lesion being exposed and the patient's hearing status such as the total petrosectomy approach with facial nerve translocation.

T. Sameshima
Department of Neurosurgery,
Hamamatsu University School of Medicine,
University Hospital,
Hamamatsu city, Japan

8.2 Steps of the Surgery

8.2.1 Positioning, Incision, and Bony Landmarks

The head is held with lateral position, facing away from the surgeon. A postauricular incision through the galea is made, one inch behind the postauricular crease. The incision extends from the mastoid tip and curves forward to end just above the pinna (or midpoint of supramastoid crest) (Fig. 8.1d left).

The scalp is elevated by sharply dissecting the subgaleal connective tissue which spans the galea and the underlying pericranium. The pericranium is contiguous with the temporalis fascia above and the fascia overlying the sternocleidomastoid muscle below. A second incision is made in this deep layer composed of temporalis fascia and

J. July, E. J. Wahjoepramono (eds.), *Neurovascular Surgery*,
https://doi.org/10.1007/978-981-10-8950-3_8

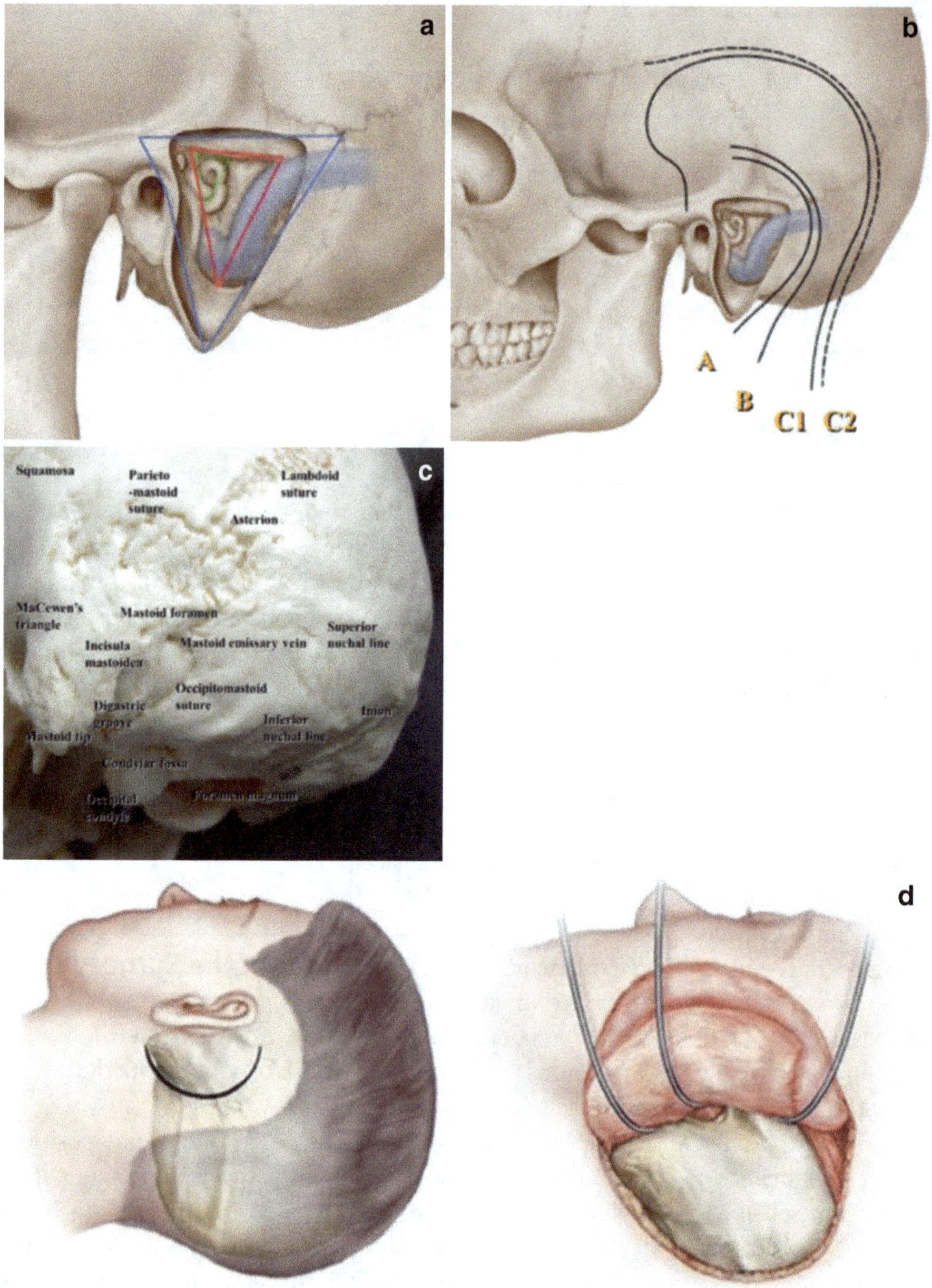

Fig. 8.1 (**a**) Surface anatomy of the temporal bone and mastoid triangles. Blue, Fukushima's outer mastoid triangle (asterion-root of zygoma posterior point-mastoid tip) [1, 2]; red, Fukushima's inner mastoid triangle (sinodural angle-aditus-digastric ridge) [1, 2]; Trautman's triangle (sinodural angle-superior aspect of posterior semicircular canal-jugular bulb) [3]; green, MacEwen's triangle or suprameatal triangle (mastoid antrum) which is a flat or depressive area [4]. (**b**) Skin incision. (A) Small C-shaped transmastoid incision represents standard transmastoid, retrolabyrinthine, or translabyrinthine incision used by neuro-otologists; (B) extended transmastoid incision represents a combined transmastoid and suboccipital (retrosigmoid) approach frequently used for the preservation of hearing function in acoustic neuroma surgery; (C) combined transpetrosal incision represents a question mark (C1) or L-shaped incision (C2) used in this skull base dissection for combined petrosal approach. (**c**) Bony landmark. (**d**) *Left*, skin incision; *right*, after the skin and muscle elevated and exposing the bony landmarks

muscle, periosteum, and sternocleidomastoid fascia to fashion a musculofascial flap that is important in obtaining a water tight, cosmetic closure. The two flaps are elevated anteriorly to reveal posterior edge of external auditory canal, spine of Henle, and root of zygoma posterior point. Large blunt scalp hooks are used to reflect these flaps. The bony landmarks which should be visualized at this point are the root of zygoma posterior point, the spine of Henle, the squamosal suture, the asterion, the supramastoid or temporal crest, the mastoid tip, and the digastric groove (Fig. 8.1c, d right).

8.2.2 Mastoidectomy and Retrolabyrinthine Exposure

The second step is performance of a mastoidectomy. Using large cutting drill (5~6 mm) with continuous irrigation and suction, cortex over the mastoid bone is removed. It is helpful to first outline the boundaries of the bone to be removed using the drill. The anterior border is a slightly curved line, extending from the top of the external auditory meatus to the mastoid tip. The superior margin is along a line roughly perpendicular to the first, extending from the root of zygoma posteriorly to the region of the asterion. These two lines form a skewed "T" that defines the anterior and superior margins of the mastoidectomy (Fig. 8.2a). The junction of these two lines generally marks the surface projection of the region of the mastoid antrum and lateral semicircular canal.

The bone cortex is removed within the boundaries of these lines, working anterior to posterior and superior to inferior. After drilling the cortical bone, air cells are encountered. Posteriorly, over sigmoid sinus, the bone will remain compact. In order to provide maximum exposure, wide cortical removal with cauterization should be performed prior to deeper penetration. Gentle, brushlike strokes with the drill will reveal the compact bone of the sigmoid sinus. Bone removal proceeds, 1 cm behind the sigmoid, maintaining a uniform depth as the sigmoid is exposed. When the sigmoid has been skeletonized, the mastoid air cells are drilled away to expose the temporal base dura (temporal tegmen) (Fig. 8.2b).

Moving anteriorly, the air cells will be removed to expose the compact bone of the bony labyrinth or the solid angle. The key landmark in this area is the mastoid antrum (Fig. 8.2c–e). This open space defines the anterior limit of bony removal and locates the lateral semicircular canal. Maintaining the same relative depth, air

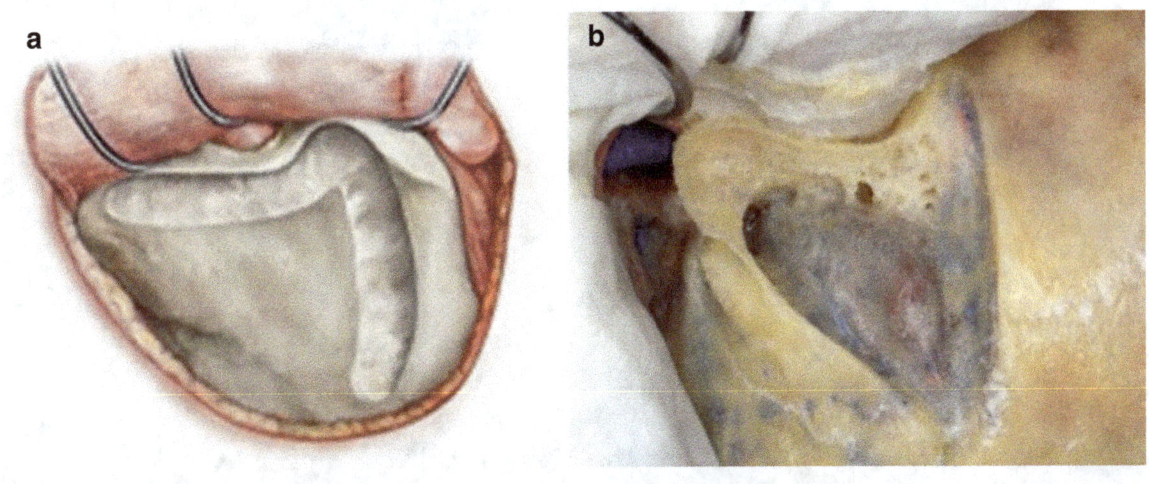

Fig. 8.2 (**a**) (*Left*) The anterior and superior margins of the mastoidectomy; (**b**) (*right*) the mastoid air cells are removed anteriorly and superiorly to expose the middle fossa dura (temporal tegmen). (**c–e**) Exposing the mastoid antrum. (**f**, **g**) Exposing the semicircular canal and the transverse sigmoid sinus. Cadaver (*left*) and drawing (*right*). (**h**) Skeletonizing of the sigmoid sinus, jugular bulb, the fallopian canal, and the entire course of the facial nerve through the mastoid bone

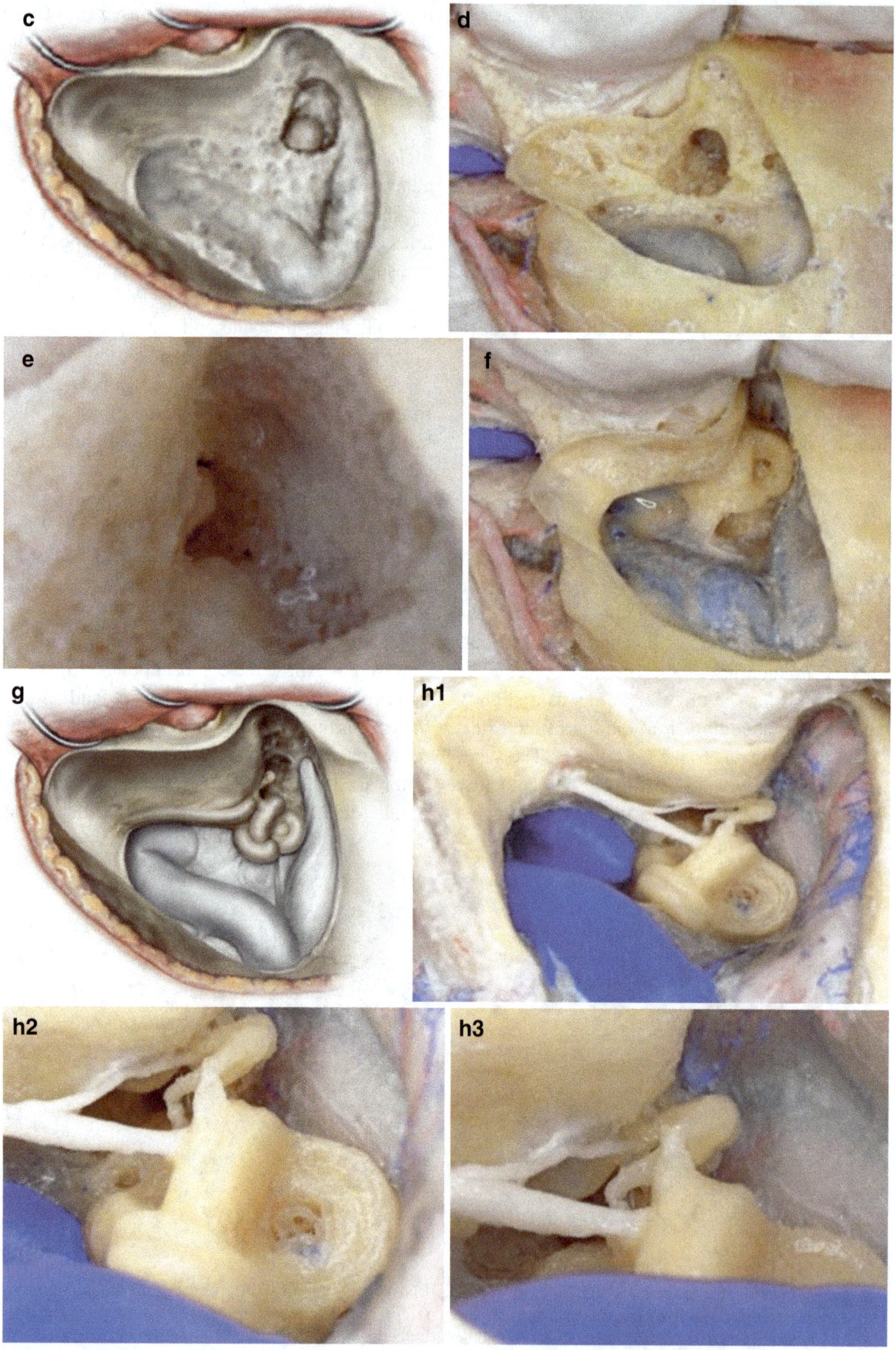

Fig. 8.2 (continued)

cell removal proceeds inferiorly toward the jugular bulb. After the air cells are drilled away, we will expose digastric ridge. Digastric groove defines the exit of facial nerve from the fallopian canal through the stylomastoid foramen. The stylomastoid foramen lies just medial to anterior edge of digastric ridge. At this point, middle fossa dura, presigmoid dura, and the sinodural angle should be skeletonized. Again, the technique of removing the bone to the point of leaving a thin shell which may be removed with a dissector is practiced to avoid damage to the dura and the venous structures. For maximal exposure in the retrolabyrinthine approach, the posterolateral portion of the bony part of labyrinth must be completely identified. Using medium diamond drill (2–3 mm), small air cells surrounding the labyrinth are removed. The ridge covering the lateral semicircular canal is first identified as the antrum is opened. The facial nerve will be located parallel and 1–2 mm in front of lateral semicircular canal at this point. Moving posteriorly, the posterior semicircular canal will be defined (Fig. 8.2f, g). Inferior to posterior semicircular canal, toward the jugular dome, lie the retrofacial air cells. They are drilled away to skeletonize jugular bulb. The dura is incised corresponding the presigmoid region and superior petrosal sinus. The dura is retracted anteriorly exposing CN VII and VIII in the CPA. Frequently the lower cranial nerves can also be visualized.

Anteriorly, approximately 12–15 mm medial to meatus acusticus external lies the fallopian canal. Therefore, bone removal in the anterior direction at this level must be done with extreme care to avoid violating the fallopian canal. Facial nerve, which lies anterior to labyrinthine structures, is carefully approached, again using the lateral semicircular canal as a landmark. The CN VII is skeletonized by using the diamond drill started at external genu inferiorly to stylomastoid foramen. Leave a thin layer of the bone around the facial nerve for protection. The drilling must be done with copious and constant irrigation to dissipate heat from the drill.

At this stage certain goals of bone removal should have been achieved, such as exposure of sigmoid sinus and jugular bulb. Exposure of presigmoid dura and middle fossa dura defines the lateral bony labyrinth, clearly visualizing the lateral semicircular canal (LSC) and posterior semicircular canals (PSC) and skeletonizing fallopian canal and exposing the entire facial nerve (Fig. 8.2h).

8.2.3 Translabyrinthine Drilling/IAC

The lateral and posterior semicircular canals (PSC) are first opened with the drill. The amputated, or anterior, end of LSC is carefully removed, bearing in mind close relationship of tympanic portion of facial nerve. Preservation of anterior wall of LSC will protect tympanic segment of VII nerve. Removal of superior segment of the posterior semicircular canal will expose the common crus which it shares with the SSC. The SSC is also opened by drilling superiorly and anteriorly. The amputated, or inferior, limb of the PSC is followed until the vestibule. Drilling in this area, lateral and inferior to the vestibule, will expose the vestibular aqueduct as it courses laterally toward the endolymphatic sac. The vestibule is now opened by continuing to remove the bone, following the common crus (Fig. 8.3a, b).

The wall of the vestibule which separates it from the internal auditory canal is only one very thin layer of the bone. The compact bone surrounding the internal auditory canal is identified by drilling along the canal at its superior and inferior edge. It is important in terms of maximizing the exposure, to remove the bone around the canal such that greater than one-half of the circumference of the canal is skeletonized. It is important to remove the bone superiorly and inferiorly so that the anterior-most extent of the canal is accessible. Bone removal inferior to the canal will in some cases expose the cochlear canaliculus which communicates with the CSF and perilymphatic spaces.

The bone around the internal auditory canal is then carefully removed. Beginning in the region of the porus acusticus, the compact bone surrounding the canal is thinned with a small diamond burr until only a thin, repressible shell remains. As the drilling proceeds laterally, bear in mind that dura only covers the canal contents for approximately two-thirds of the canal's length. As the bone is thinned at the lateral end of the canal, we will see transverse crest (thin bone) that lies between superior and inferior vestibular nerves. The paper-thin shell of the bone in the region of the porus acusticus is removed first with a fine dissector, with the bone over the lateralmost end canal saved for last. The superior lip of porus is generally the most difficult to manage because of the very close proximity of the facial nerve (Fig. 8.3c–e).

The dura is incised beginning just medial to the sigmoid sinus, 5–10 mm below superior petrosal sinus and continued in a line toward the midportion of the canal. At region of the porus, dural incision is extended superiorly and inferiorly. Using a #11 blade, the dura of the canal is cut to expose inferior and superior vestibular nerves. Sectioning of the nerves and then reflecting them laterally will reveal the cochlear and facial nerves. The latter two are separated from the superior and inferior vestibular nerves by Bill's bar at the lateral end (Fig. 8.3f, g).

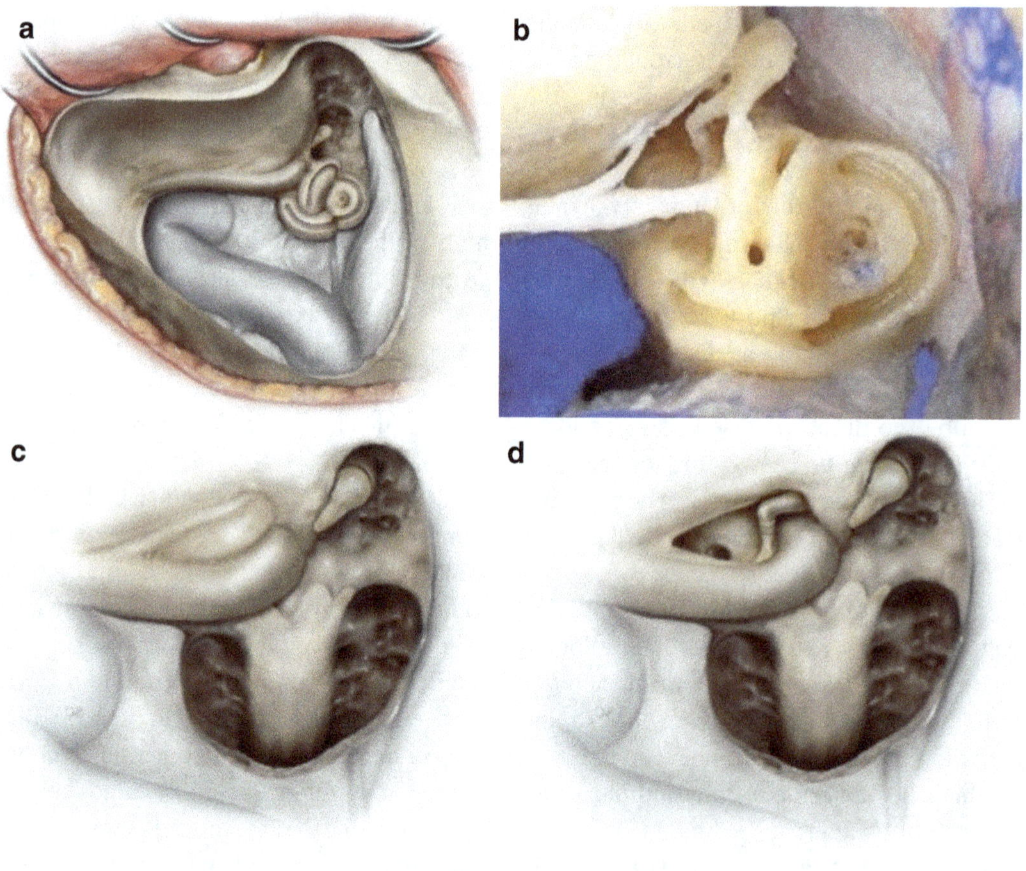

Fig. 8.3 (**a**, **b**). The vestibule is now opened by continuing to remove the bone, following the common crus. A (*left*) the drawing, B (*right*) the cadaver specimen. (**c**–**e**) The paper-thin shell of the bone in the region of the porus acusticus is removed first with a fine dissector, with the bone over the lateralmost end of the internal auditory canal saved for last. The superior lip of the porus is generally the most difficult to manage because of the very close proximity of the facial nerve. (**f**, **g**) Sectioning of the nerves and then reflecting them laterally will reveal the cochlear and facial nerves. The latter two are separated from the superior and inferior vestibular nerves by Bill's bar at the lateral end (*F* facial nerve, *C* cochlear nerve, *SV* superior vestibular nerve, *IV* inferior vestibular nerve)

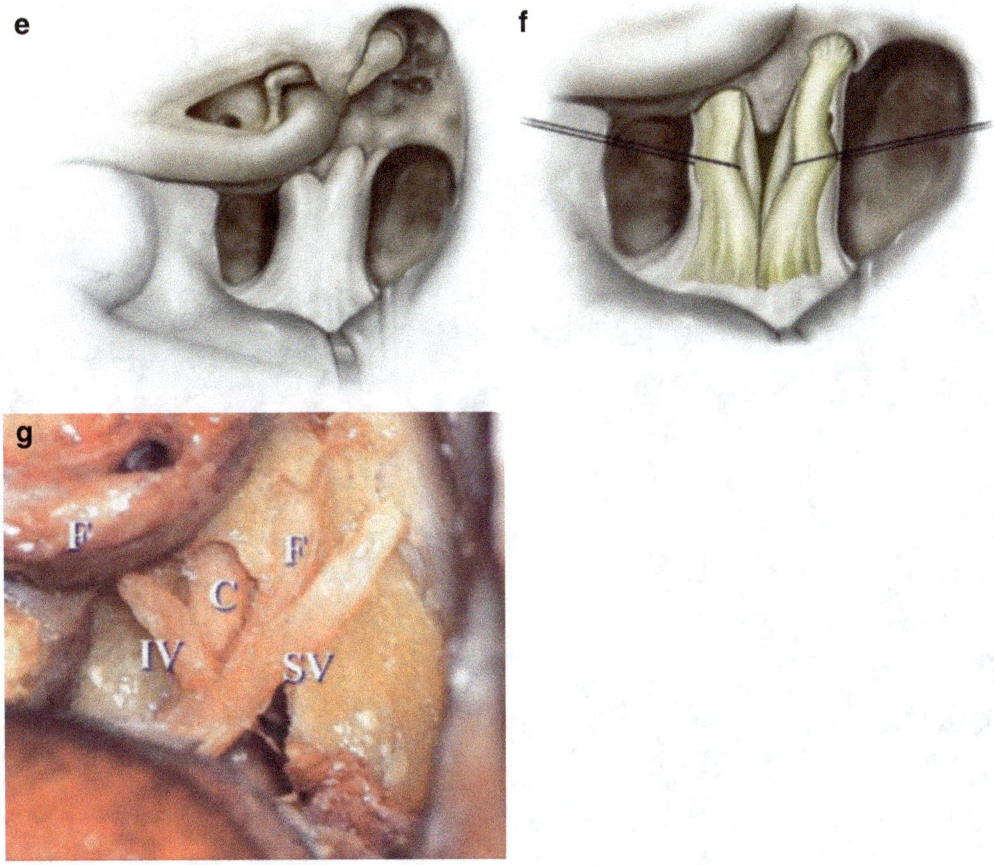

Fig. 8.3 (continued)

The wound is closed in the following manner. The incus is removed, and a piece of temporalis muscle is harvested and placed carefully through the epitympanum occluding the origin of the Eustachian tube. The removal of the incus and obliteration of the Eustachian tube entrance by the muscle reduces the possibility of CSF leakage. The dural incision is closed up to the canal, and carpets of autologous (abdominal) fat are positioned in the gaps of the dura so as to seal the CSF space. The previously fashioned musculofascial flap is closed tightly over the adipose graft, and the skin cut is closed in two layers.

8.2.4 Combined Transpetrosal Approach

The head is positioned (Fig. 8.4a) with the option for skin incision. Using the virtual computer image, it shows the transverse sigmoid junction until jugular vein, in the relationship with the labyrinth and its exposure that can be achieved with this approach (Fig. 8.4b). The next illustration (Fig. 8.4c) shows that dural opening, the neurovascular structure. Be aware that the dural opening is parallel to GSPN at the temporal skull base.

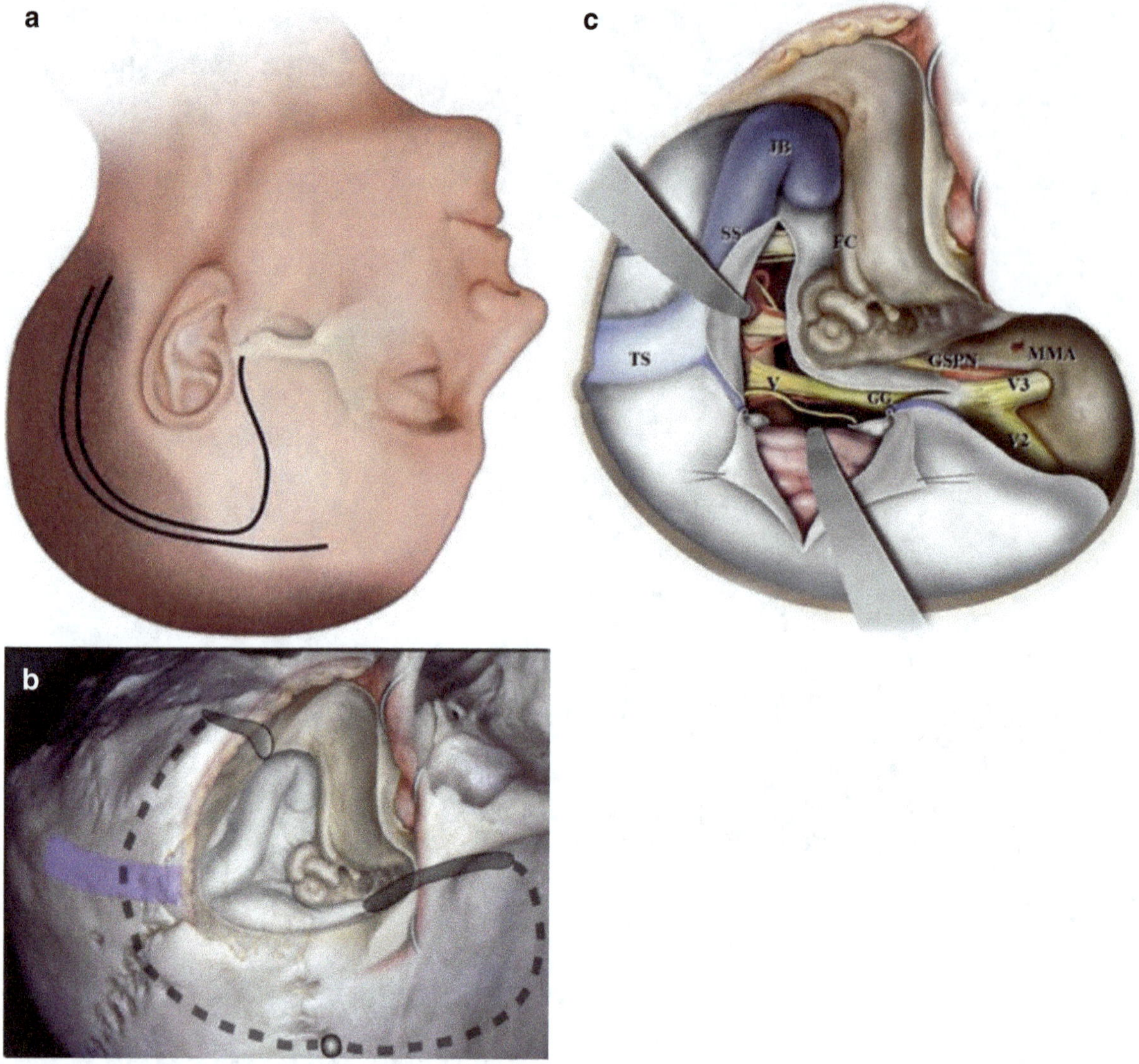

Fig. 8.4 (**a**) Head position and skin incision for combined transpetrosal approach. (**b**) The virtual computer image, showing the transverse sigmoid junction until jugular vein, in the relationship with the labyrinth. (**c**) The dural opening and neurovascular structure

References

1. Fukushima T, Sameshima T, Friedman A. Manual of skull base dissection. 2nd ed. Raleigh: AF Neurovideo; 2006.
2. Sameshima T, Mastronardi L, Friedman A, Fukushima T, editors. Fukushima's microanatomy and dissection of the temporal bone for surgery of acoustic neuroma, and petroclival meningioma. 2nd ed. Raleigh: AF Neurovideo; 2007. p. 84–114.
3. Tubbs RS, Griessenauer C, Loukas M, Ansari SF, Fritsch MH, Cohen-Gadol AA. Trautmann's triangle anatomy with application to posterior transpetrosal and other related skull base procedures. Clin Anat. 2014;27(7):994–8.
4. Aslan A, Mutlu C, Celik O, Govsa F, Ozgur T, Egrilmez M. Surgical implications of anatomical landmarks on the lateral surface of the mastoid bone. Surg Radiol Anat. 2004;26(4):263–7.

9 Dissection of Extended Middle Fossa and Anterior Petrosectomy Approach

Tetsuro Sameshima

9.1 Introduction

The extradural subtemporal approach through the middle fossa (MF) has become one of the most frequently used operative procedures in contemporary skull base of surgery. This approach is commonly used for exposing lateral wall of the cavernous sinus, to resect anterior petrous bone or to open the internal auditory canal. The MF surgery will be utilized for excision of intracanalicular acoustic neuromas, petrous and infracavernous chordomas, trigeminal neuromas, and small to medium size petroclival meningiomas. Full understanding of microanatomical structure of the cavernous sinus region, middle fossa, and the rhomboid construct is essential for this approach. Through this exercise the surgeon will acquire operative techniques to perform the anterior petrosectomy and also to expose the IAC through the middle fossa.

T. Sameshima
Department of Neurosurgery,
Hamamatsu University School of Medicine,
University Hospital, Hamamatsu city, Japan

9.2 Standard Middle Fossa Approach

9.2.1 Steps of the Surgery

9.2.1.1 Incision, Craniotomy, and Dural Elevation

The cadaver head is held with lateral position and surgeon at the vertex. The incision begins in the preauricular crease at the zygoma root and continues in a curvilinear fashion past the level of the squamosal suture. The incision extends and cuts the skin and subcutaneous layer to expose temporalis fascia (Fig. 9.1a).

Blunt dissection and a self-retaining retractor expose the temporal muscle. Temporal muscle is split along posterior margin of the skin incision and pulled using skin hooks to expose the temporal squama. A 5 cm by 5 cm temporal bone is cut which is placed two-third anterior and one-third posterior to the root of zygoma using a high-speed drill with suction irrigation (Fig. 9.1b). The inferior edge of the craniotomy, especially the inner table of temporal bone, is drilled away to make this opening even with the middle cranial fossa floor level along the zygoma root. Subtemporal inner plate at the middle fossa base must be shaved entirely flat (Fig. 9.1c, d).

The temporal lobe dura is dissected along the middle fossa floor starting from posterior to anterior. Foramen spinosum and foramen ovale are then skeletonized, and middle meningeal artery

J. July, E. J. Wahjoepramono (eds.), *Neurovascular Surgery*,
https://doi.org/10.1007/978-981-10-8950-3_9

(MMA) is coagulated and divided. The dura propria is elevated from trigeminal 3rd branch (V3) at the foramen ovale using No.15 blade scalpel and a sharp dissector. Identify the location of the geniculate ganglion and greater superficial petrosal nerve (GSPN). This dural elevation is important as 15% of geniculate ganglion lie under a dehiscence in the middle fossa floor. In surgery, the position of geniculate ganglion can be made sure by stimulation with a facial nerve stimulator. The surgeon needs to assume the approximate position of the cochlea and how far it is from the geniculate ganglion and the petrous carotid artery (C6). The petrous ridge is identified medially, and the Fukushima middle fossa rigid tapered retractor is positioned (Fig. 9.1e).

a

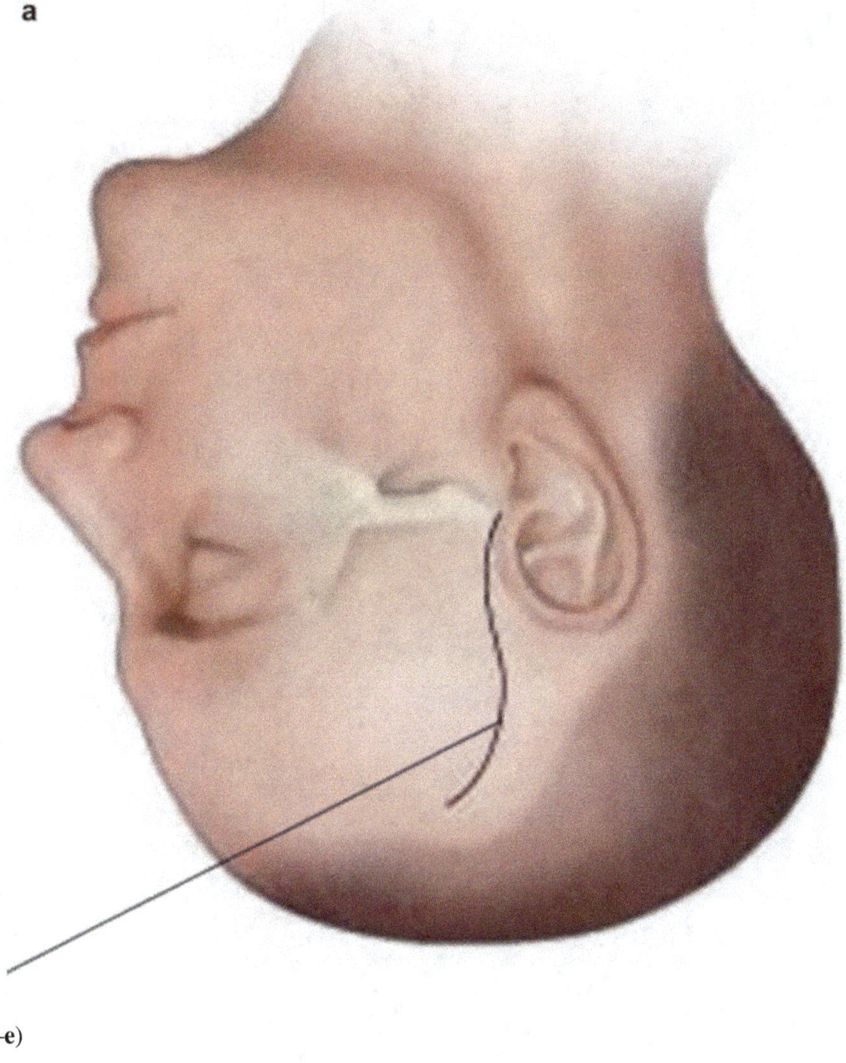

Fig. 9.1 (a–e)

Fig. 9.1 (continued)

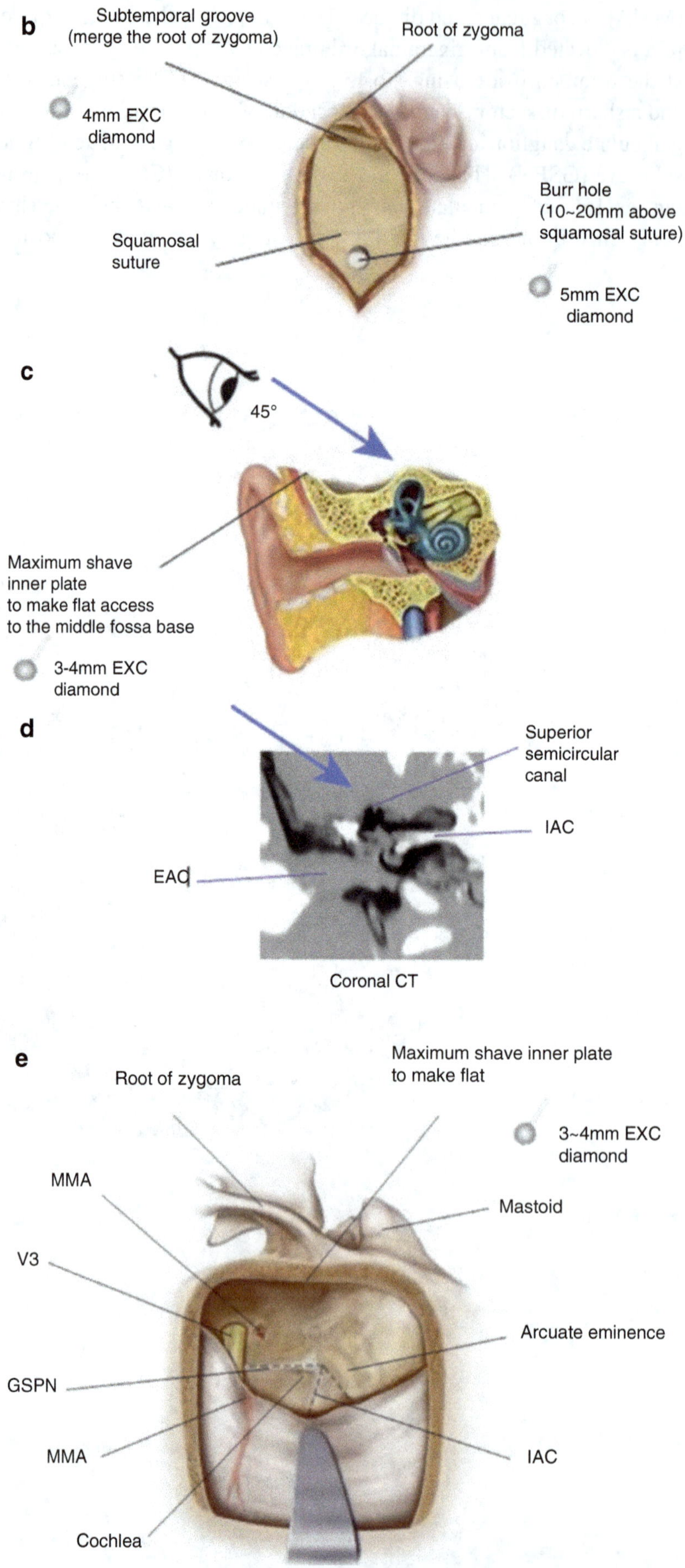

The arcuate eminence covering the superior semicircular canal is identified. The bone of the arcuate eminence is gently drilled off until the "blue line" of the superior semicircular canal is seen. Violating the canal will usually lead to deafness. In the fixed specimen, the line is not necessarily blue but green. Try to thin the denser cortical bone that surrounds the membranous labyrinth using a smooth diamond burr. Be careful that arcuate eminence is not always precisely overlying the canal. MF hemostasis must be complete and quick with diamond drill heat, touch spring coagulation, bone wax, bipolar, and surgicel.

9.2.1.2 IAC Drilling

Surface landmarks can be misleading. The surgeon must be oriented to the approximate location of IAC before drilling commences. The orientation of the IAC is a direct medial extension of the external ear canal (EAC). Identification of the GSPN provides a guide to the location of the geniculate ganglion and arcuate eminence, which can be used to approximate the location of the IAC.

Drilling starts anteriorly to and medially near the porus trigeminus along the petrous ridge. To facilitate a wider angle to the middle fossa with the microscope, we recommend using a pair of 2 mm and 4 mm tapered tip rigid steel retractor blades with the retractor tip wedged at the base between the petrous ridge and the dura. In that way we can retract effectively the temporal basal dura to obtain maximum surgical exposure toward the middle fossa. Gradual gentle drilling is recommended with constant cooling irrigation using a power diamond drill bit laterally toward the petrous carotid and posteriorly toward the arcuate eminence to expose the IAC (Fig. 9.2a–d).

There are four surgical techniques to identify the IAC during middle fossa approach. The classic technique described by William House follows the GSPN to geniculate ganglion and then approaches to labyrinthine segment of the facial nerve into the fundus of the internal auditory canal. Then continue to skeletonize the internal auditory canal (Fig. 9.2e). The technique popularized by Ugo Fisch is termed the meatal plane approach (Fig. 9.2f), in comparison to other approaches (Fig. 9.2e–h). In this technique, first identify superior semicircular canal which looked like a "blue line" (leaving a thin layer of bone on the top membranous labyrinth). At this step, a 60° viewpoint from the amputated part of the superior

a

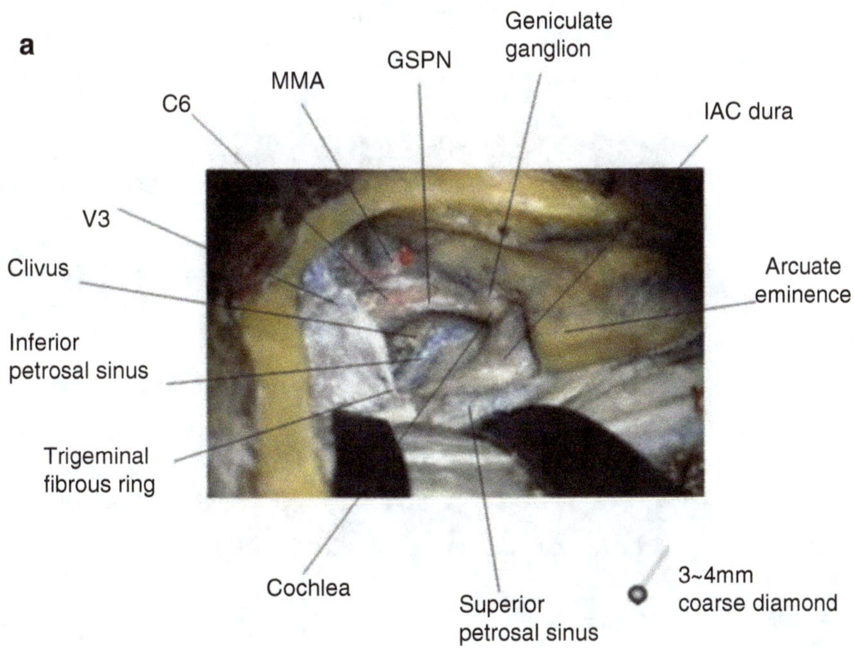

Fig. 9.2 (a–h)

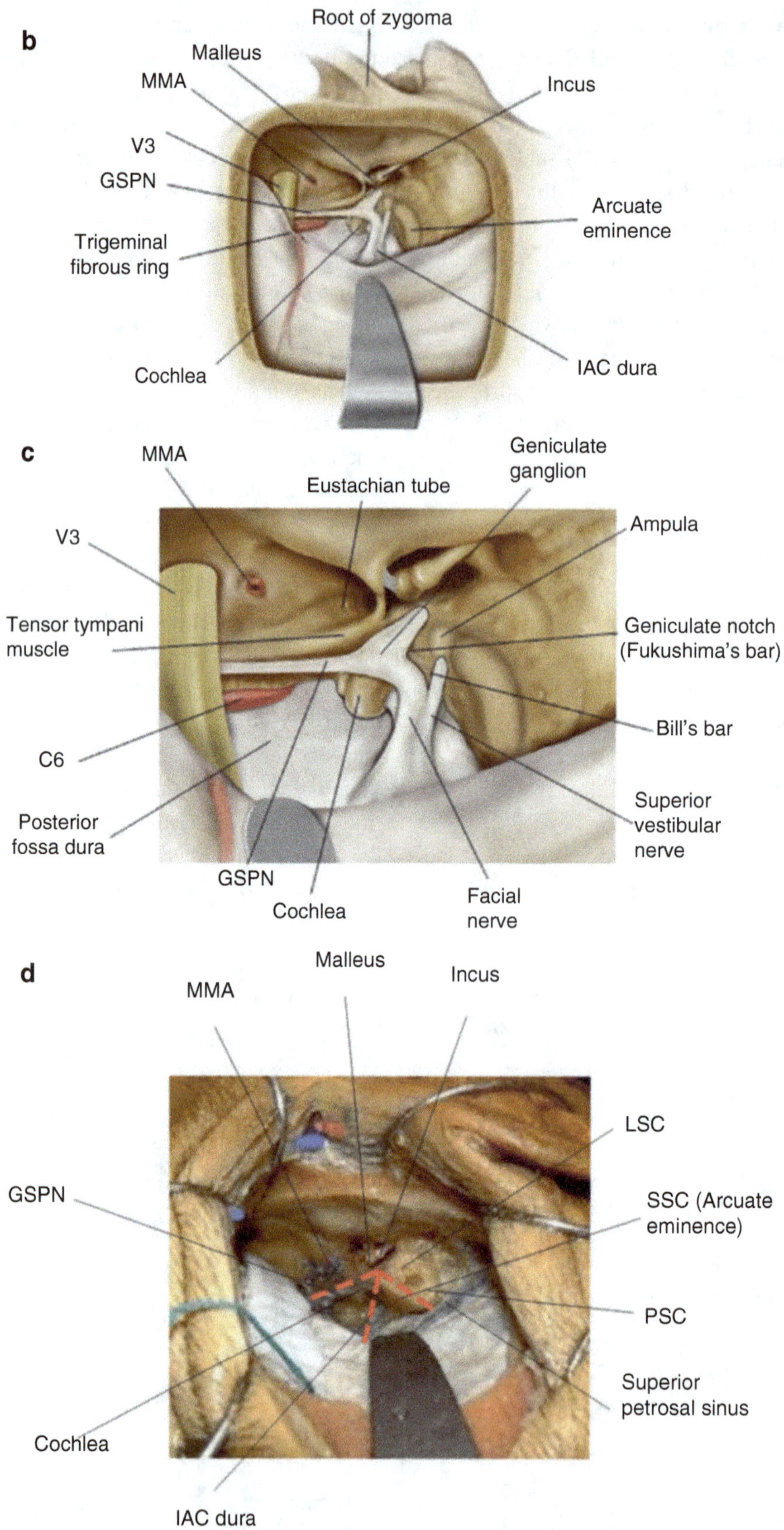

Fig. 9.2 (continued)

Fig. 9.2 (continued)

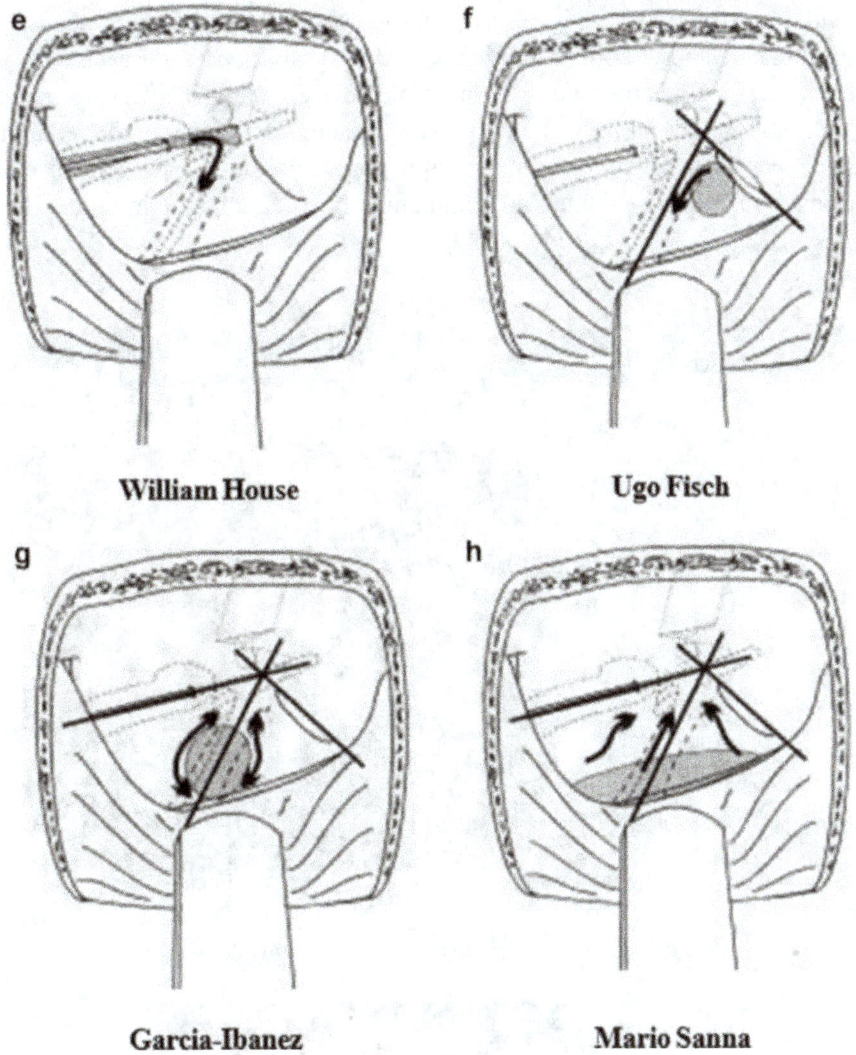

canal outlines a safe zone to drill the IAC. The third approach popularized by Garcia Ibanez is a medial drilling technique (Fig. 9.2g). After identifying the geniculate ganglion and arcuate eminence, the surgeon begins drilling medially on a line bisecting the angle between the arcuate eminence and the GSPN. It is safest to find the IAC by drilling close to the petrous ridge (Fig. 9.2h). Near the porus, the IAC dura is safe to be skeletonized around 270°. As the drill proceeds toward the fundus of the IAC, only the roof of the canal can be removed. Overly aggressive drilling of IAC fundus will disrupt cochlea anteriorly or the superior semicircular canal posteriorly. The latter technique is advantageous because the vulnerable inner ear part (cochlea and labyrinth) are away from the initial drilling prior to the IAC identification. While keeping in mind the location of the cochlea, the final drilling at the isthmus between the cochlea and arcuate eminence reaching toward Bill's bar is continued.

9.2.1.3 IAC Dura Incision and Tumor Removal

The dura should be maintained intact until the IAC exposure is complete. Drilling after opening the IAC dura risks damage to the IAC contents. After full skeletonization of the IAC (Fig. 9.3b), the dura is cut with reversed T shape along petrous ridge and then along the IAC. With the dural incision, be careful not to injure branches from the AICA vessel (Fig. 9.3a).

In acoustic tumor surgery, the dura is reflected anteriorly and posteriorly to expose the intracanalicular acoustic tumor (Fig. 9.3c). After locating the thin facial nerve both anatomically by the high magnification microscope and physiologically with 0.05 mA facial nerve monitor, we then start to dissect the facial nerve from the tumor capsule using a sharp knife, sickle knife, and angle-type hooks. The surgeon always identifies the meatal loop and eventually the labyrinthine artery. Almost always the most important key is the identification of the remaining vestibular nerve which forms a pseudocapsule tumor; and once the surgeon is able to identify this separation plane, the

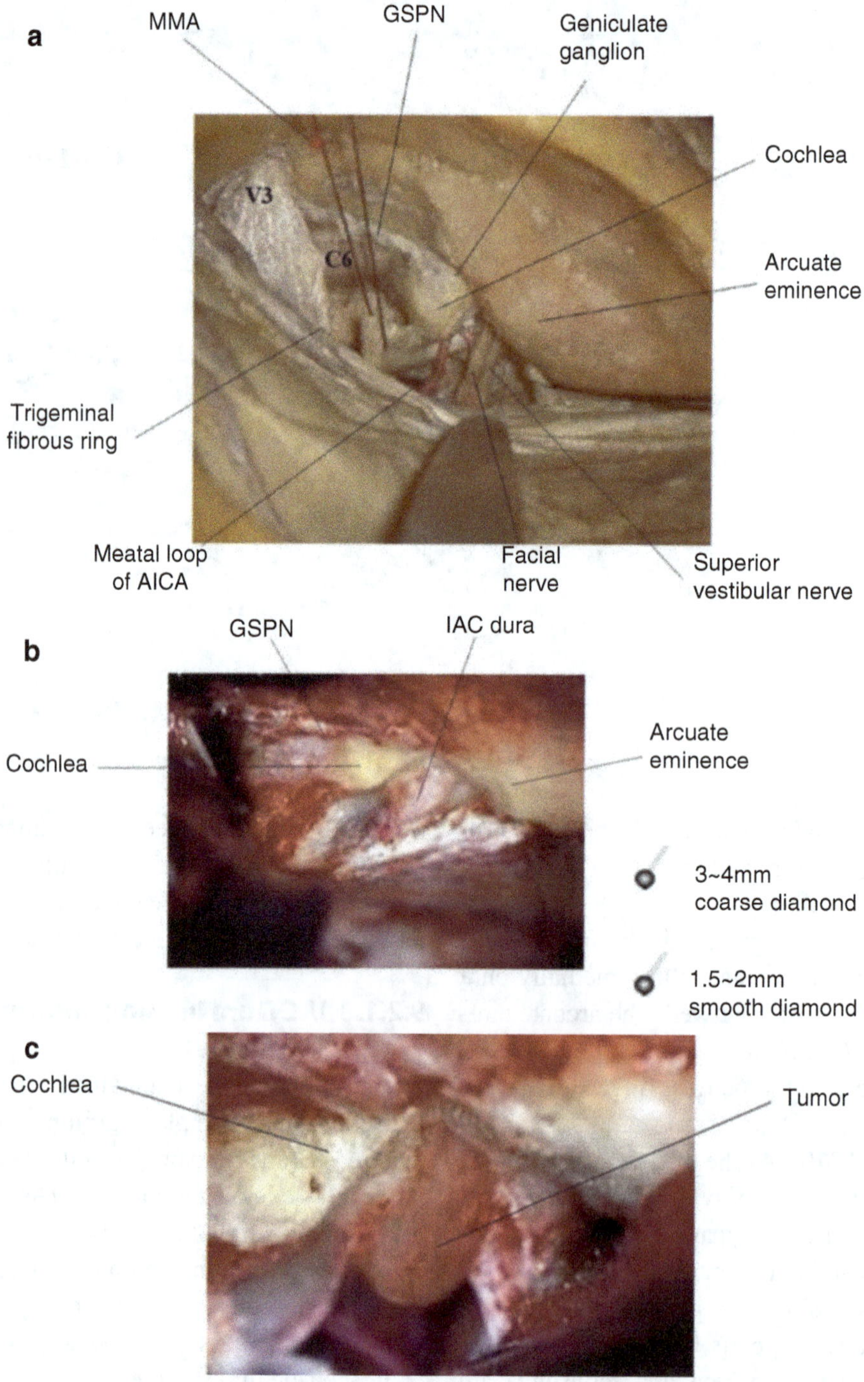

Fig. 9.3 (a–d)

Fig. 9.3 (continued)

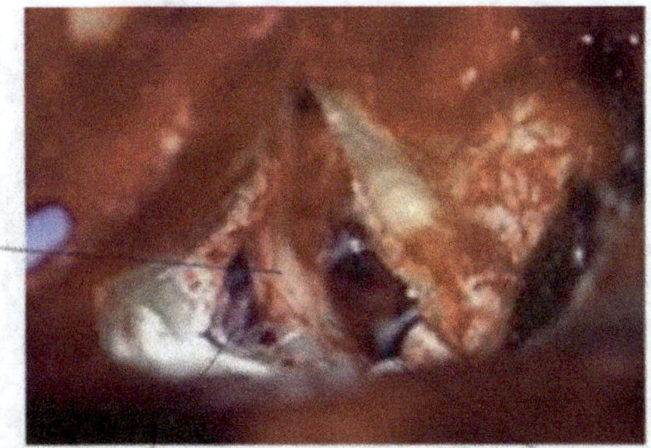

tumor capsule will be easily elevated using various supermicro CP angle instruments. The tumor's center has to be piecemeal removed, and then tumor portion at IAC can be elevated safely off from the thin facial nerve and then farther ventral and in the deeper part of surgical site from cochlear nerve. The most important technical tip is to maintain a bloodless, clean operative field with high magnification to keep the microanatomy (Fig. 9.3d).

9.3 Extended Middle Fossa and Anterior Petrosectomy Approach

Basically, start with middle fossa approach, and then extend the exposure to its anterior part. Petrous ridge is followed more anteriorly exposing porous trigeminus. Dura propria is detached from mandibular branch of trigeminal nerve. The drilling needs to be done at the rhomboid area (between IAC and ICA), exposing the ascending segment of the internal carotid and the whole path of abducens nerve including Dorello's canal. Here are some example cases that could be done with this approach (Fig. 9.4a–c).

9.3.1 Steps of the Surgery

9.3.1.1 Incision, Scalp Reflection, and Craniotomy

Place the cadaver head in the lateral position, and position yourself at the vertex. Make the skin incision in the shape of a question mark concave anteriorly, as illustrated (Fig. 9.4d). Incise the fascia overlying the root of the zygomatic process, and elevate it, using a periosteal dissector, from the lateral and medial surfaces of this structure. The goal is to free the temporal muscle from the zygomatic root, allowing the surgeon to mobilize the muscle anteriorly. This maneuver will help to provide a better view all the way at the floor of middle fossa, without needing to perform a zygomatic osteotomy.

Make a burr hole at superior to the squamosal suture, and drill a groove in the bone above the root of the zygoma using 4 mm extracoarse (EXC) diamond drill. Using a craniotome cut an approximately 5 cm × 5 cm four-sided bone flap; the position of the bone flap is about two-thirds in front of the external auditory canal (Fig. 9.4e). Using a small periosteal dissector, separate the dura from the bone along inferior edge of the craniotomy until the middle fossa floor is exposed. Using a cutting burr or a rongeur, remove any remaining bone to the level of the middle fossa floor. This will provide an unobstructed, flat view across the floor.

9.3.1.2 Dural Elevation and Identification of "Rhomboid" Structure

Retract the dura along the petrous ridge. The petrous ridge is composed of two ridges (medial and lateral). Identify the arcuate eminence as a primary landmark. After exposing the arcuate eminence, elevate the dura moving anteromedially to expose the greater superficial petrosal nerve (GSPN) and also tegmen tympani. The

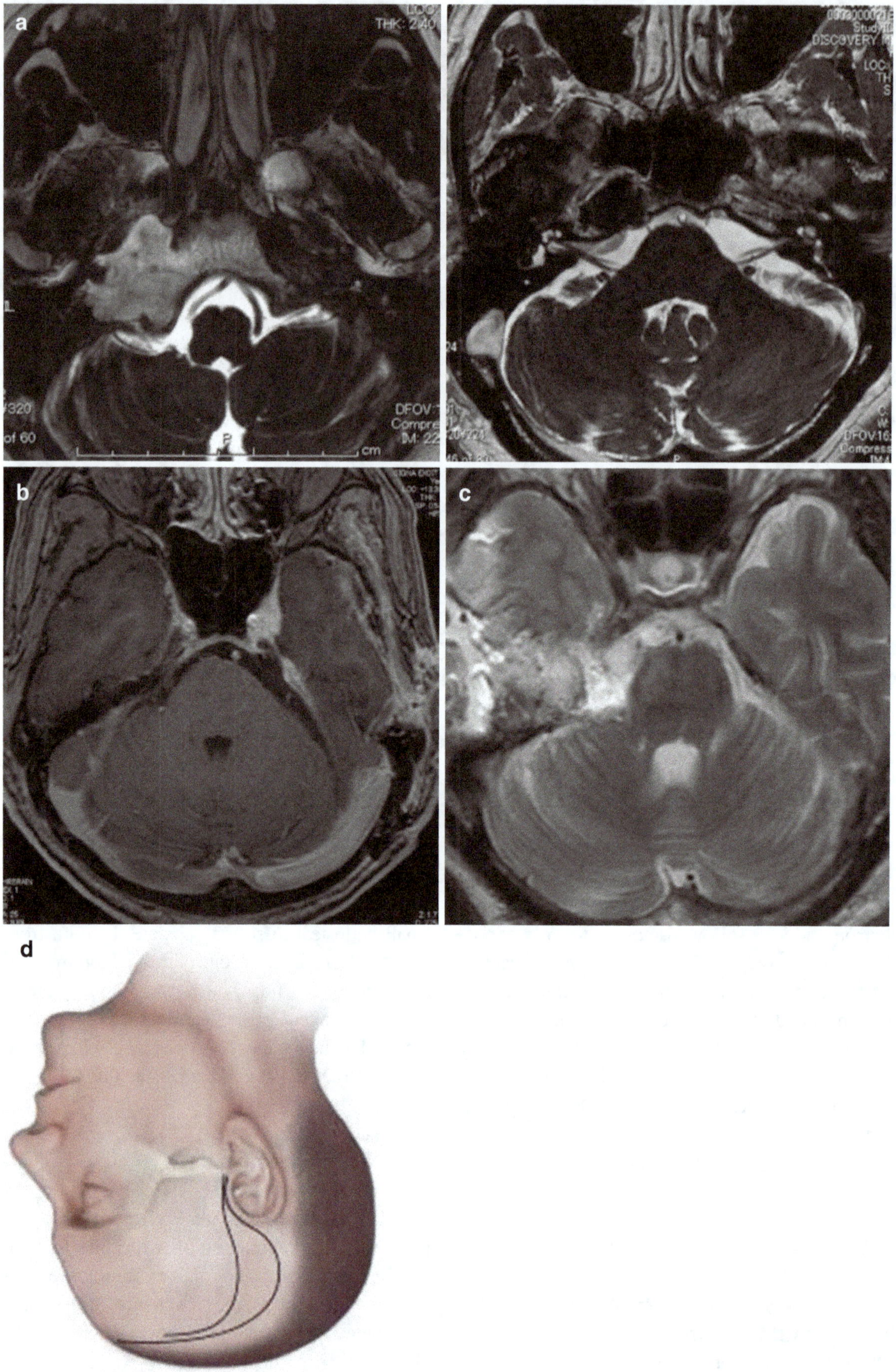

Fig. 9.4 (a–e)

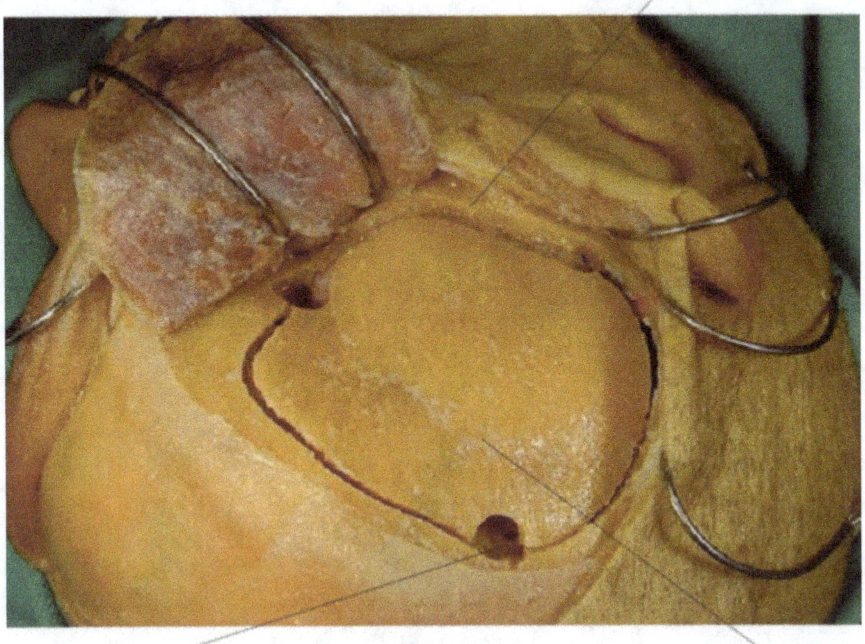

Fig. 9.4 (continued)

GSPN lies in the major petrosal groove and is shielded by thin layer of connective tissue, and it is continuous with the periosteum, which makes identification of the nerve dependent upon removal of this covering. Detach the dura to identify the middle meningeal artery that exits from foramen spinosum. Divide the artery at its entrance into the cranial vault. Now identify and expose third division of trigeminal nerve when it goes in to the foramen ovale.

Elevate the dura in posterior direction toward petrous ridge to expose bone between arcuate eminence and the trigeminal impression. Place two self-retaining tapered retractors to hold the temporal dura away from the middle fossa floor.

Sharply free the dura from the lateral trigeminal complex by developing the plane between the temporal dura and the connective tissue sheath of the nerve. This maneuver will increase the width of the extradural corridor through which the procedure is performed.

The middle fossa anatomical landmark that defines "rhomboid" complex now can be recognized (Fig. 9.5a, b). Few important parts are the intersections between GSPN and trigeminal nerve, between petrous ridge and arcuate eminence (AE), and between projected line along the axes of the GSPN and AE, and it is also very important to recognize the porus trigeminal.

This complex, projected obliquely toward the clivus through the petrous pyramid, delimits the volume of bone which will be removed.

9.3.1.3 Extradural Bone Removal

The goal of this stage of the operation is to create a maximal window in the anteromedial petrous pyramid while preserving the neural and vascular structures of the temporal bone. This objective is best accomplished by proceeding with the extradural bone removal in a precise, stepwise fashion.

Begin by drilling gently the medial two-thirds of IAC. Bisect the projected line along the axes of GSPN and AE. Start drilling by using 3 or 4 mm coarse diamond burr along midpoint of the bisection axis. We will find the dura that covers IAC

Fig. 9.5 (a, b)

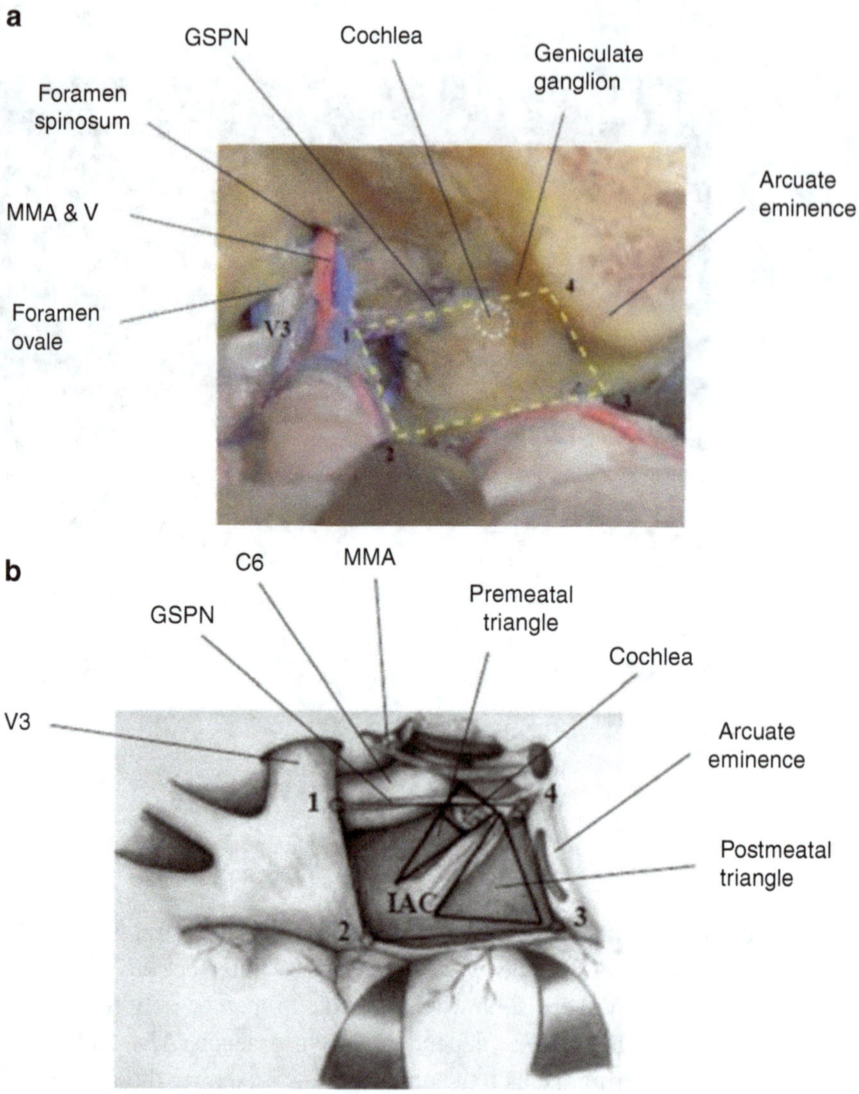

after we removed about 3–4 mm of the bone. Keep exposing and following dura that covers the medial IAC toward petrous ridge. The dura will flare at the porus acusticus, which will signal medial extent of the canal. Remove several millimeters of bone on the anterior side of the IAC, in the direction of the trigeminal complex.

Next, the GSPN and geniculate ganglion are addressed. The GSPN run through bony canal and come out at facial hiatus to continue its medial course in the major petrosal groove. With the medium diamond burr, the GSPN is gently exposed posteriorly to the facial hiatus, moving toward the geniculate ganglion. Expose the geniculate ganglion using light strokes with the smooth diamond burr, preserving a thin shell of bone over the ganglion. Uncover the entire IAC toward the geniculate ganglion. As you approach the fundus of the IAC, the opening should be no more than the width of the canal. Remember that the facial nerve sweeps upward to join the geniculate ganglion as it passes the cochlea. This moves the intracanalicular facial nerve more superficial as the fundus of the IAC is exposed.

Two of the three key landmarks, which locate the cochlea, are now identified: the geniculate ganglion and the porus acusticus. To identify the third important landmark used to avoid opening the cochlea (the intrapetrous carotid artery genu), uncover the internal carotid artery in the posterolateral triangle close to V3. Still using the medium diamond burr, expose the artery by removing the bone between the GSPN and the foramen spinosum. Divide the GSPN near its intersection with the trigeminal complex and reflect it posteriorly. Expose the carotid artery from where it crosses underneath the fifth nerve to lateral part where tensor tympani muscle crosses over the artery. At the point where the tensor tympani muscle and adjacent eustachian tube cross the artery lies the genu of the internal carotid artery. This completes the identify cation of the three defining landmarks of the premeatal triangle, where the cochlear resides (Fig. 9.6a–d).

Remove the soft, porous bone between the carotid artery and IAC, avoiding the posterior lateral volume of bone housing the cochlea. Surrounding bone of the cochlea is identified by its

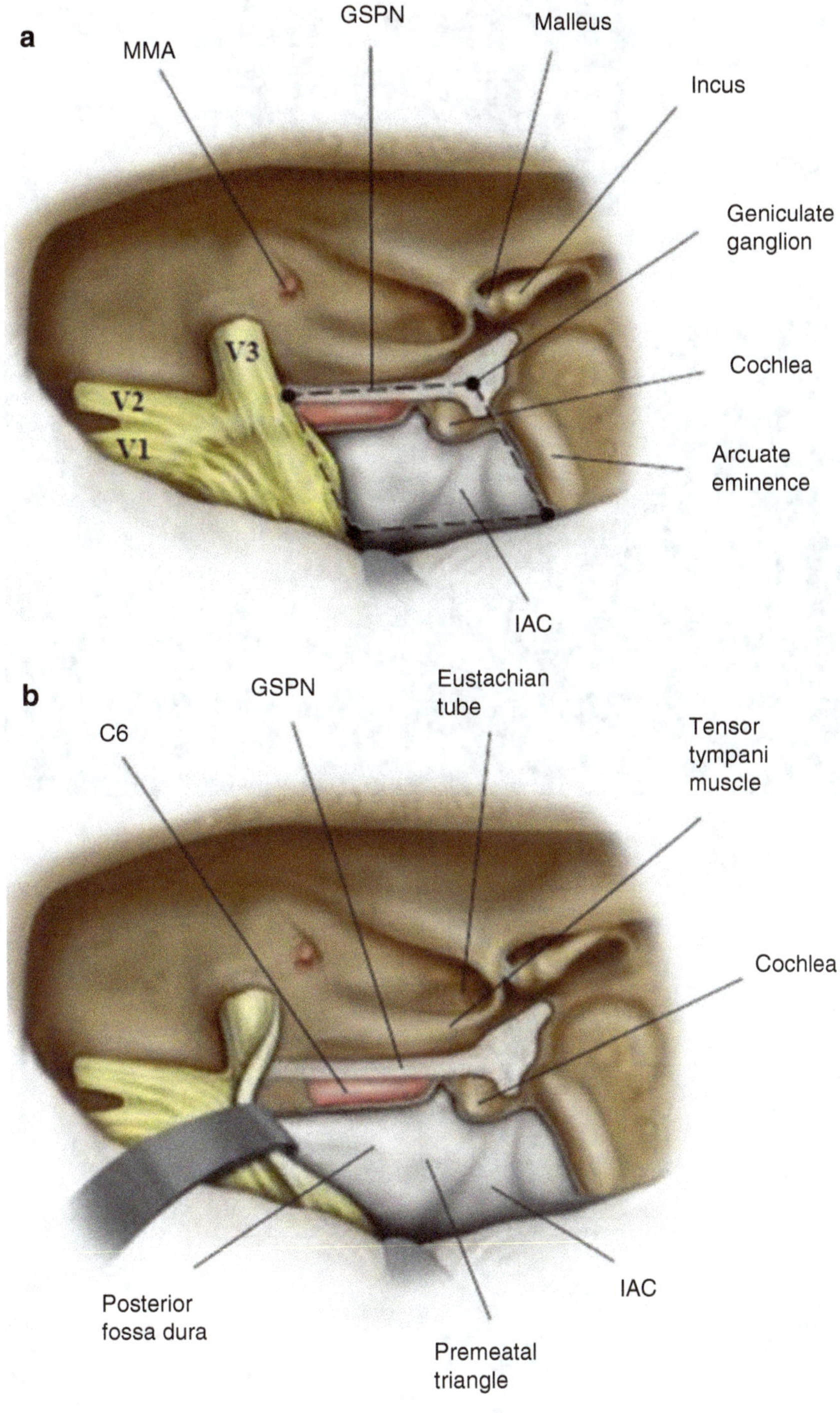

Fig. 9.6 (a–j)

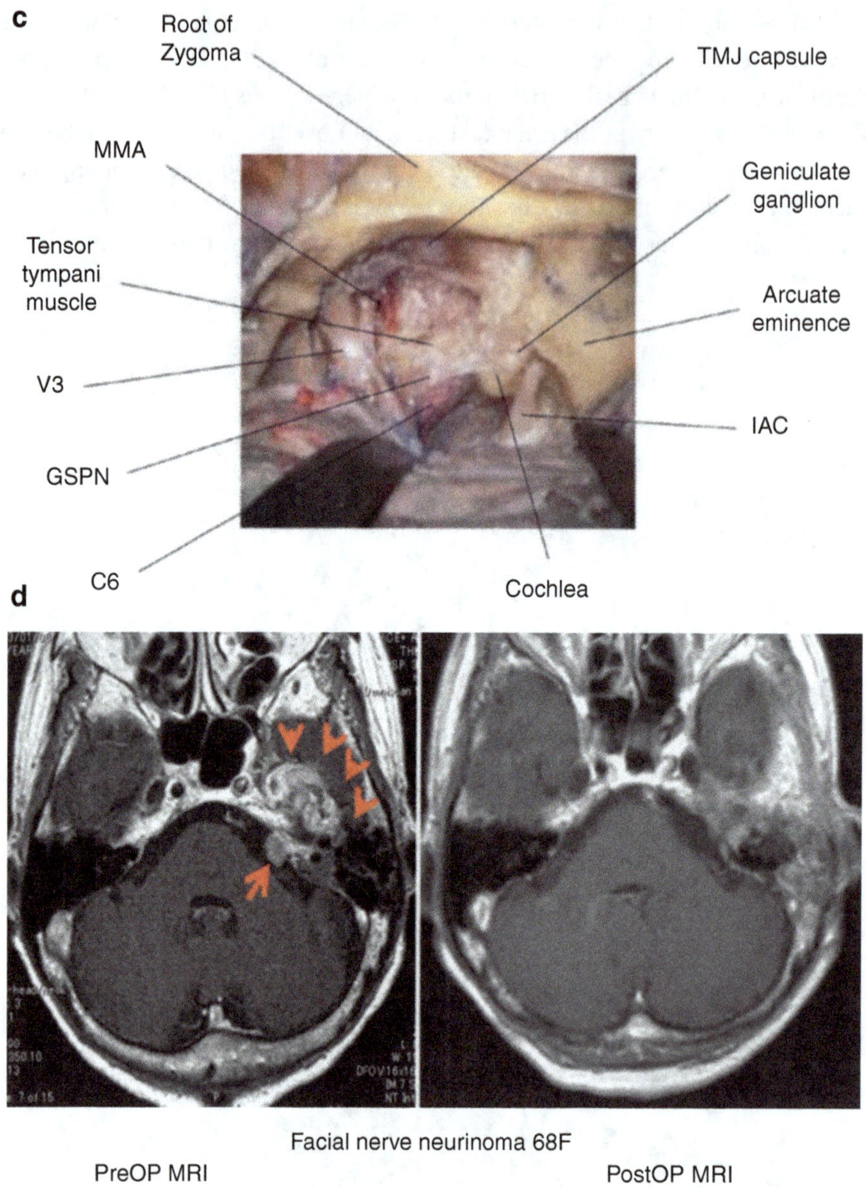

Fig. 9.6 (continued)

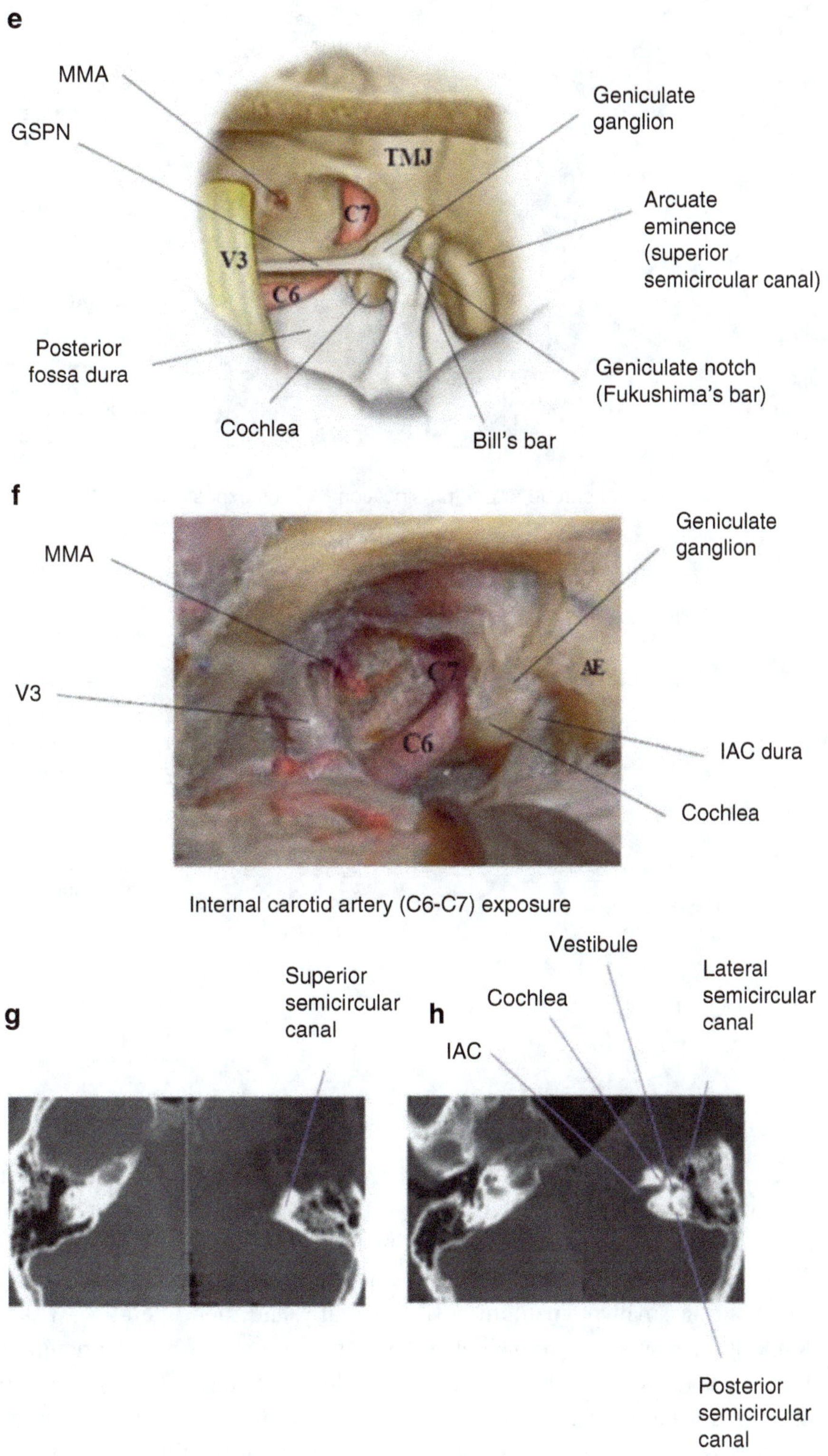

Fig. 9.6 (continued)

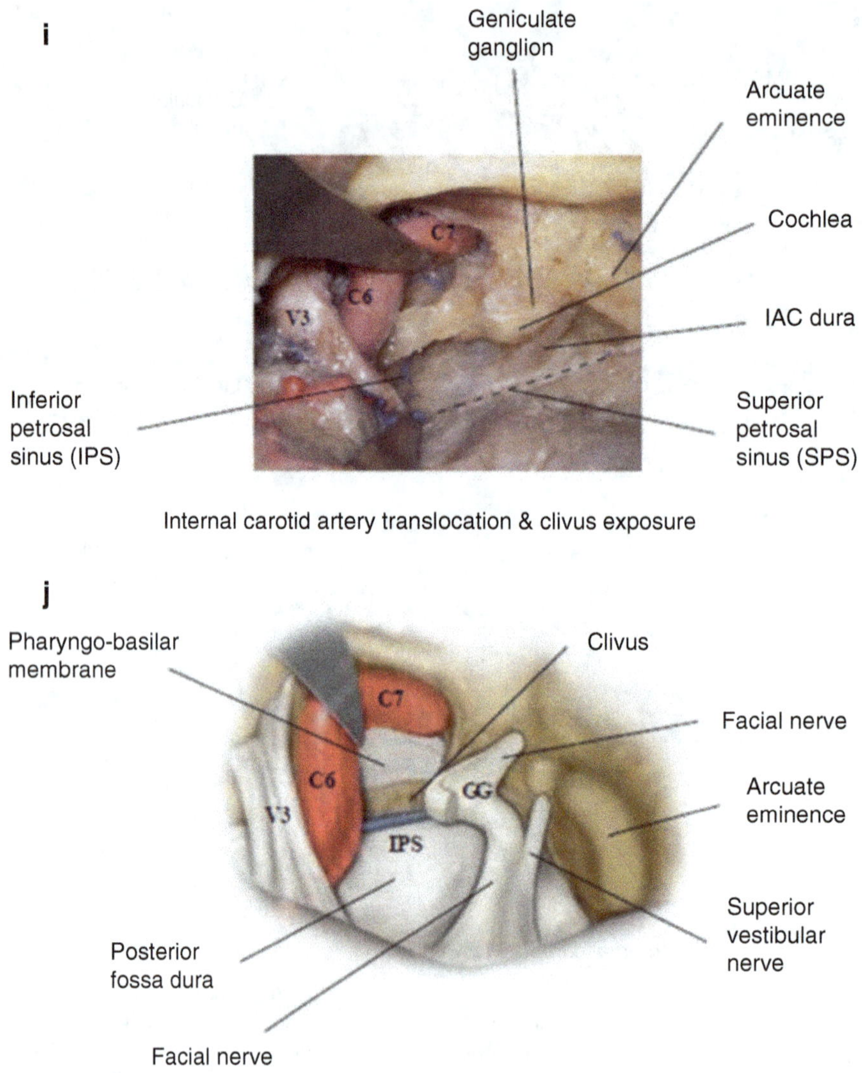

Fig. 9.6 (continued)

compact, nonporous nature. Dura of the posterior fossa is exposed medial and anterior to IAC by drilling away the wedge-shaped bone between superior semicircular canal and IAC (called "post-meatal triangle") using a small or medium diamond burr. Marking the superior semicircular canal with "blue line" color is very helpful, which usually lies under the arcuate eminence, in order to precisely define the lateral border of the triangle. Removal of this volume of bone will effectively unroof approximately 270° of the circumference of the IAC at the meatus (Fig. 9.6e, f).

Now the final stage of bone removal is performed: exposing posterior fossa dura inferior to IAC by removing the bone between the IAC and the intrapetrous carotid artery. First work medially and then laterally. At the lateral margin, the volume of bone containing the cochlea should be "undercut" in order to maximize exposure of the posterior fossa dura. The cochlea, lying within the basal half of the "pre-meatal triangle," is quite vulnerable to injury at this stage. Again, the change in the quality of the bone surrounding the cochlea must be recognized. Also note that the facial nerve lies in the anterior aspect of the IAC, so be especially careful in removing bone from the posterior pre-meatal triangle. Expose the dura moving inferiorly to expose the inferior petrosal sinus (IPS). Remove bone across this sinus until the cancellous bone of the clivus is reached.

At the anterior end, remove the bone of the petrous apex by coring out the apical bone next to the foramen lacerum. Staying within the cortical bone, thin the cortex until only a depressible shell remains. Dissect this shell away from the dura using a small sharp dissector. When the apex has been removed, the foramen lacerum will be opened posteriorly. Dissect the residual tip of bone free with a microdissector, and remove it with microrongeurs (Fig. 9.6g–j).

9.3.1.4 Dural Opening

Before opening the dura, we must interrupt superior petrosal sinus (SPS) at the porus trigeminus. Incise the dura superior to SPS starting from porus trigeminus to arcuate eminence. Make a second incision, parallel to the first, inferior to SPS in the posterior fossa dura. Ligate the sinus anteriorly at the porus trigeminus. Make a sagittal incision in the medial tentorium, 8–10 mm in length. Place a stitch in the lateral corner of the incised tentorium and retract this superiorly.

Open the dura surrounding the trigeminal root at the porus trigeminus. Now incise the posterior fossa dura, at lateral and medial margins of the exposure, toward inferior petrosal sinus (IPS). Incise the dura along the margin of the IPS to completely excise this section of posterior fossa dura. It is important to identify the basilar artery in the deepness of the exposure. The AICA origin should next be located and its course followed to the region of the porus acusticus. The sixth cranial nerve will be seen crossing over the AICA as it ascends toward Dorello's canal (tube). Dorello's canal is located inside the IPS far anteriorly. Note the differences in exposure by rotating the microscope through various angles from medial to lateral (Fig. 9.7a–e).

The extended middle fossa approach allows the surgeon to access the posterior fossa lesions that involve the CPA and extend anteriorly into the cavernous sinus and inferiorly along the pre-pontine region of the clivus. Simultaneous access is possible for transtentorial tumor extensions and hearing preservation. The major limitation of this technique is the amount of temporal lobe retraction necessary which can be much more extensive than that required for a standard middle fossa approach. Several examples of cases include trigeminal neurinoma, Meckel's cave meningioma, and basilar trunk aneurysm (Fig. 9.7f–h).

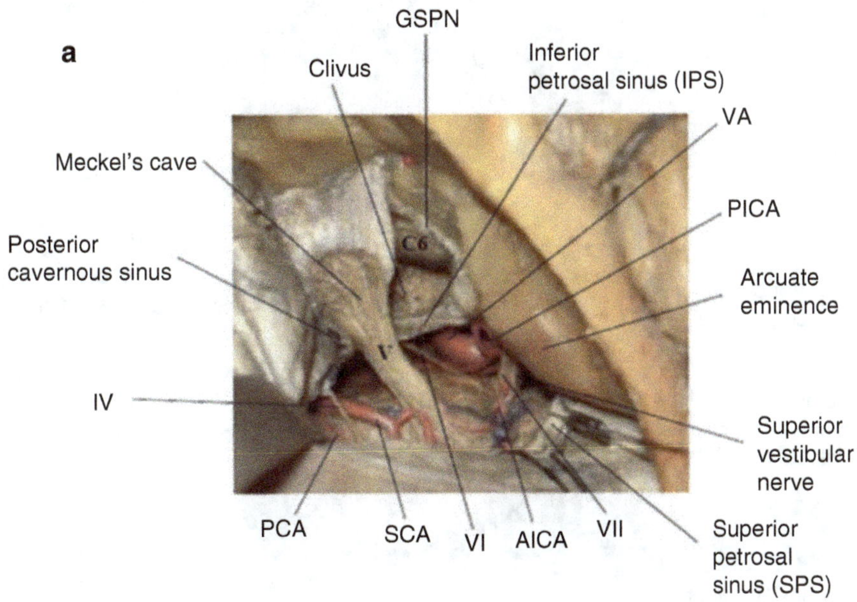

Fig. 9.7 (a–h)

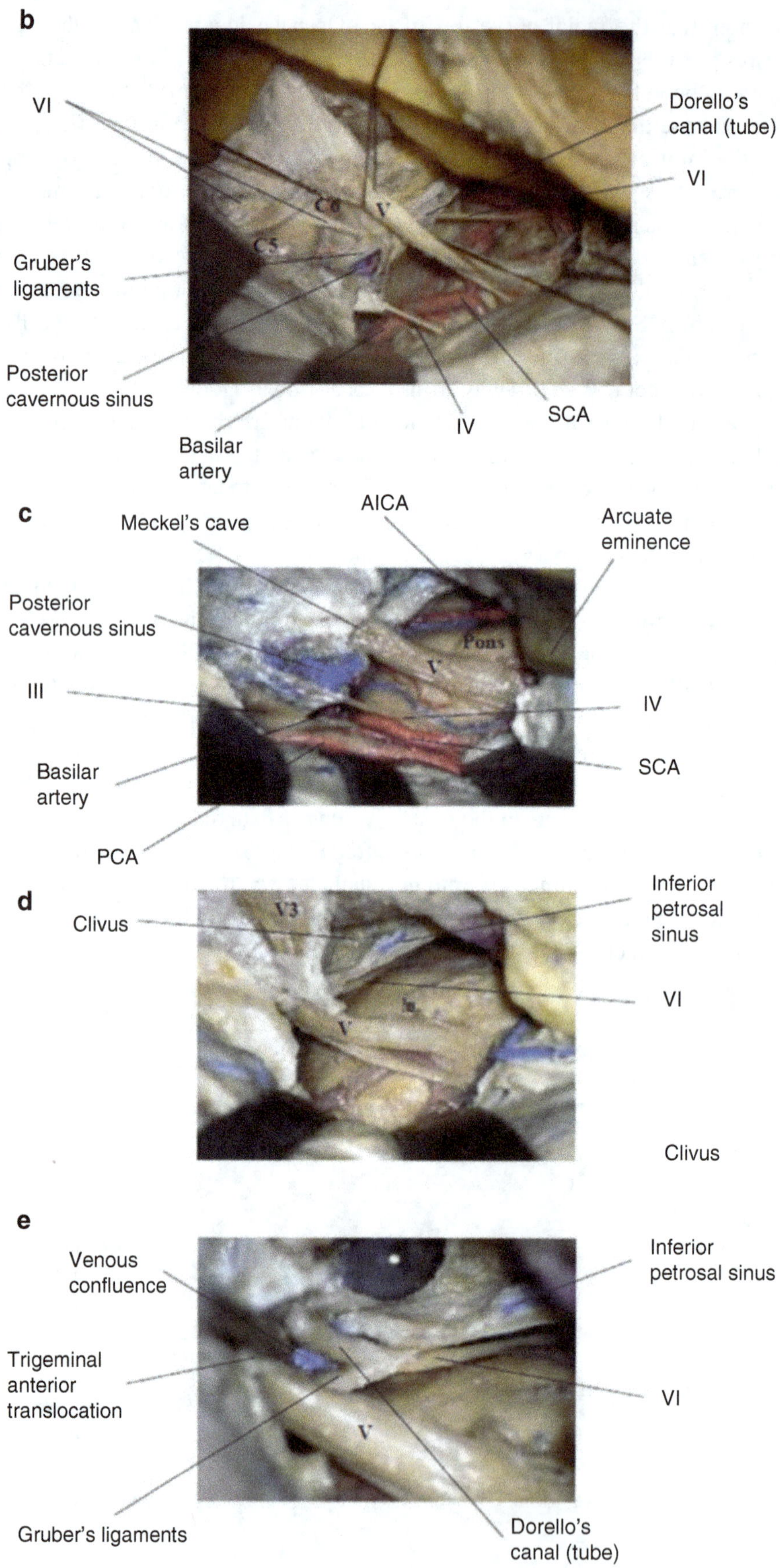

Fig. 9.7 (continued)

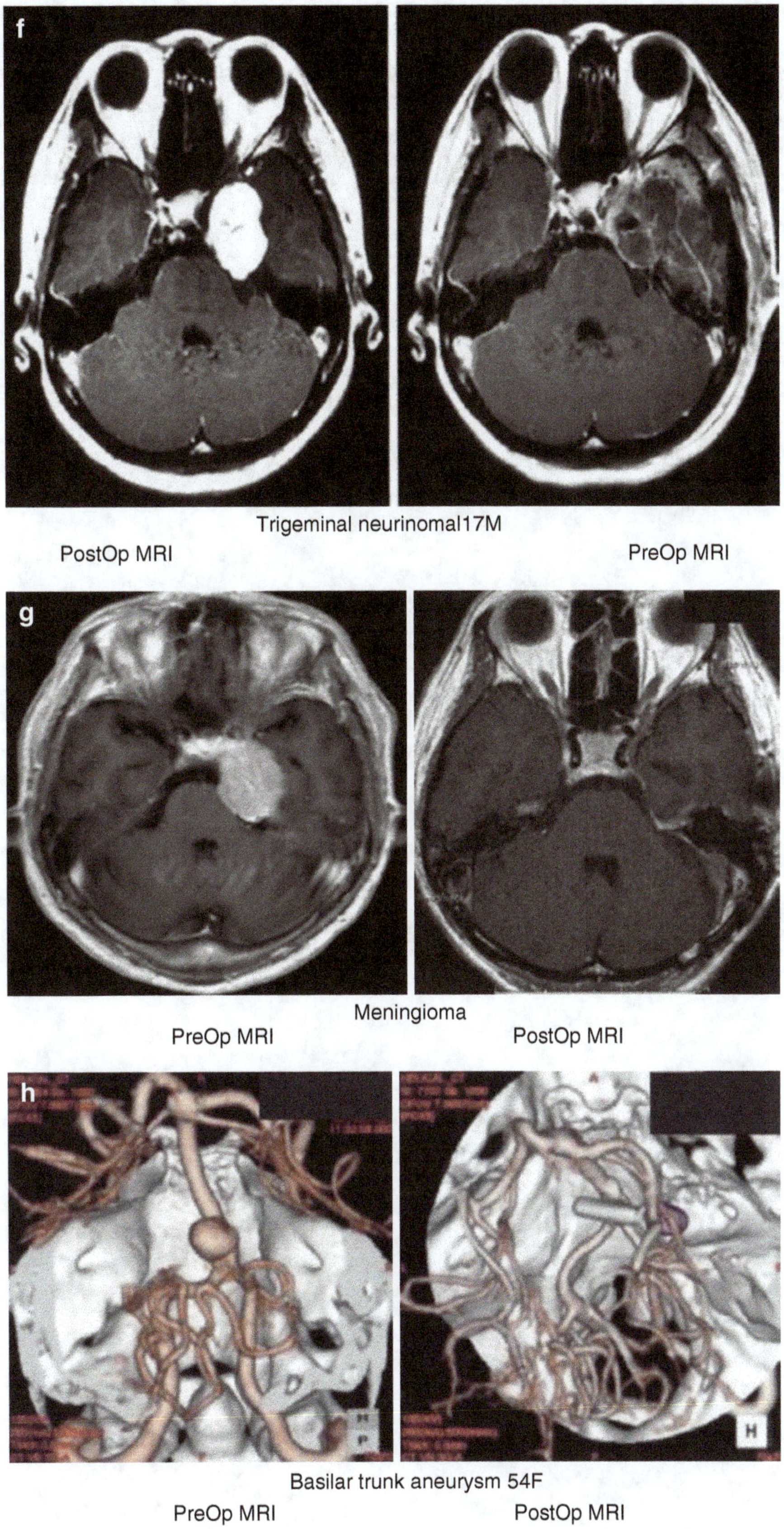

Fig. 9.7 (continued)

10 Basic Endovascular Technique for Aneurysm Coiling

Harsan

10.1 Introduction

Aneurysm coiling is a method to exclude the aneurysm from circulation. If the aneurysm can be excluded from the circulation, the thrombosis process will be initiated within the aneurysm, and lately it is hoped that there will be an endothelialization on the neck of the aneurysm.

This method is getting more popular and preferred by the patient as can be seen by the data from Lin N et al. [1] The number of patients with non-ruptured aneurysm that underwent coiling is increased from 20.6% in period before 2002 to 61.7% in period 2002–2007, while the number of patients with ruptured aneurysm is increased from 9.3% in period before 2002 to 42% in period 2002–2007.

10.2 Indication

According to the Guidelines for the Management of Aneurysmal Subarachnoid Hemorrhage [2] and Guidelines for the Management of Patients with Unruptured Intracranial Aneurysm [3], both clipping and coiling are effective treatment for aneurysm and considered for treatment. In ruptured case, coiling is indicated for elderly patient, patient in poor clinical condition and in those with aneurysm in the basilar apex.

10.3 Technical Aspect

There are some steps to follow to get a successful embolization of an aneurysm; these are preparation, vascular access phase, and intervention phase [4].

10.3.1 Preparation

This step is preparation of the patient and equipment that will be used in the procedures. Patient's preparation includes clinical/laboratory examination, neurologic examination, and radiologic/imaging examination.

In clinical examination, doctors have to check the general condition and vital sign of the patient; this condition determines the choice of anesthesia method during the coiling procedures. The main important laboratory tests are coagulation state and renal function study. Other clinical examination is neurologic state, especially if there is a focal neurologic sign.

After doing clinical study of the patient, available radiologic study had to be studied carefully, especially the exact location of the aneurysm and its correlation with the parent artery.

Harsan
Department of Neurosurgery, Faculty of Medicine Universitas Pelita Harapan (UPH), Neuroscience Centre Siloam Hospital Lippo Village, Tangerang, Indonesia

J. July, E. J. Wahjoepramono (eds.), *Neurovascular Surgery*,
https://doi.org/10.1007/978-981-10-8950-3_10

Before the treatment, the surgeon should start to prepare the tools and equipment for doing the embolization. A certain case requires special instrument such as balloon or stent, for balloon- or stent-assisted coiling.

There are several basic tools and equipment that need to be prepared prior to embolization, such as femoral puncture set; femoral (angiography) sheath; pressure bag (three to four sets); RHV (rotating hemostatic valve); three-way connector; guiding catheter; guidewire; microcatheter; microguidewire; coil (with its coil detacher), according to the size of the aneurysm; balloon; and stent. When all of the equipment is ready, the procedures can be started.

10.3.2 Vascular Access Phase

For coiling an aneurysm, the patient is usually in general anesthesia. After patient is anesthetized and positioned, the procedure is started by setting the pressurized flushing to give continuous irrigation to the catheter system.

Preferred vascular access is right common femoral artery. The Seldinger technique was used to cannulate femoral artery and followed by placing 6 Fr femoral sheath. Then, angiography is performed to get newest image of the aneurysm, including 3D rotation angiography. This 3D image will guide interventionist to select the best projection to see the correlation of the aneurysm with parent artery.

Once the working projection is selected, the vascular access is continued by inserting 6 Fr guiding catheter with RHV (rotating hemostatic valve) on its proximal that allow continuous pressure irrigation (Fig. 10.1).

The rotating hemostatic valve is a specific "three-way" with controlled valve on its proximal side which prevents leakage of blood or fluid irrigation but can be opened when needed to insert device (like guidewire or microcatheter). The RHV should be set up with the three-way connector, the fluid irrigation, and the contrast flushing during the treatment (Figs. 10.2 and 10.3).

The guiding catheter advances to the location of aneurysm as close as possible to the aneurysm

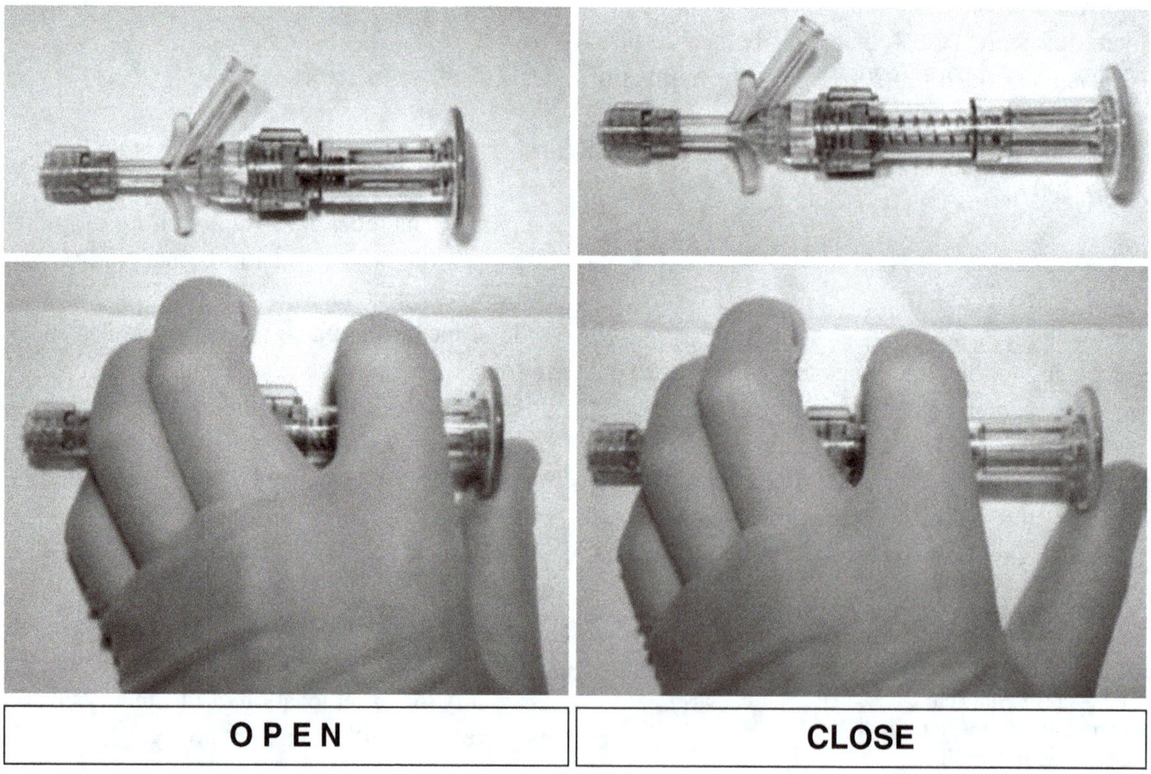

Fig. 10.1 The rotating hemostatic valve should be checked prior to the treatment

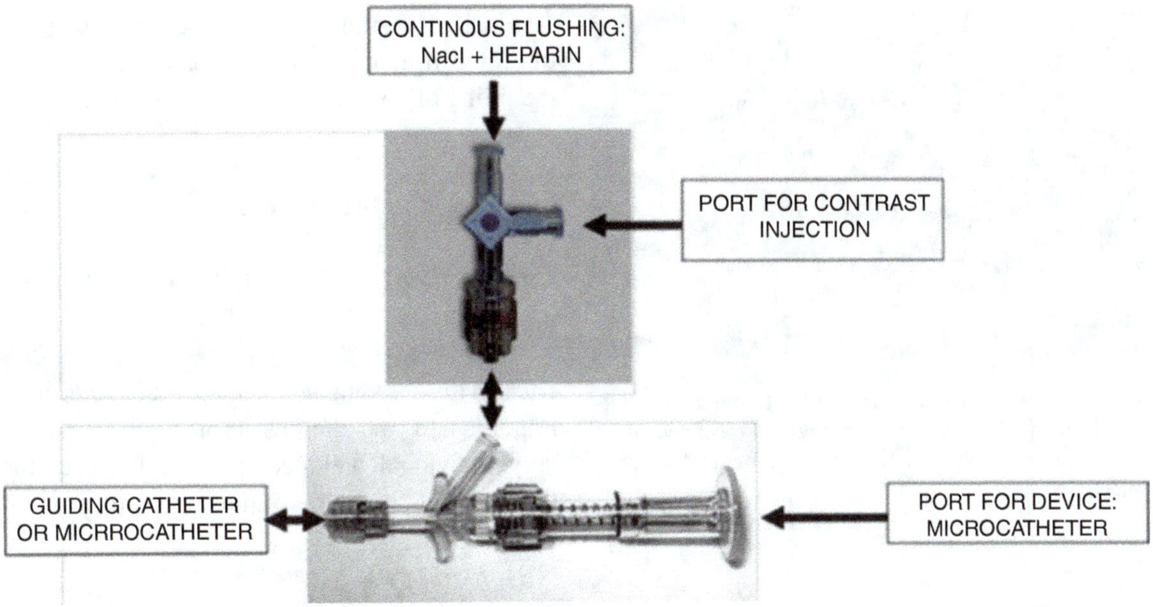

Fig. 10.2 The three-way connector is placed at the RHV side to allow the heparin flushing and contrast injection during the treatment. The microcatheter is inserted through the "port for device"

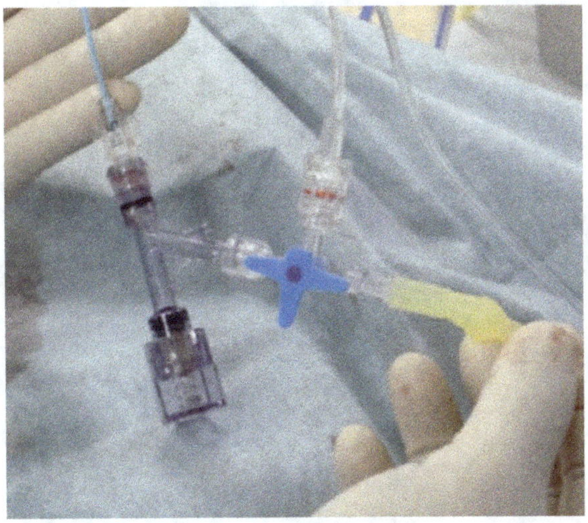

Fig. 10.3 Any device for endovascular is inserted to the catheter/guiding catheter through Y-connector. Three-way is connected to Y-connector to give continuous flushing and contrast injection

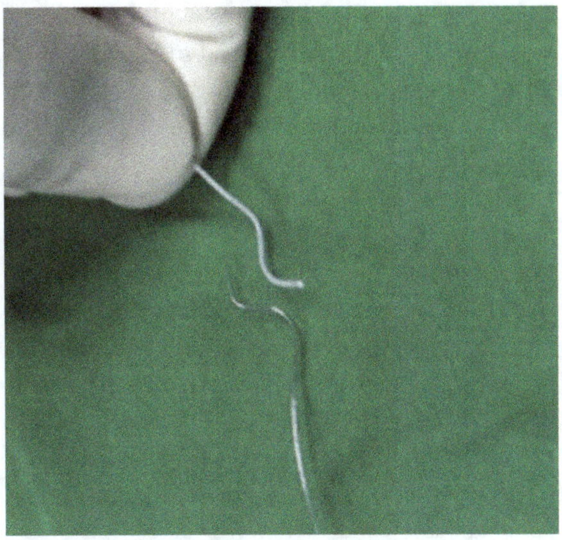

Fig. 10.4 The microcatheter is shaped

but stays extracranial. In the meanwhile, the microcatheter and microguidewire are prepared. The microcatheter can be shaped with the shaping mandrel and heated with steam, while microguidewire is shaped with blunt needle (Fig. 10.4).

The rotating hemostatic valve was put on the proximal part of the microcatheter to give continuous irrigation with heparinized saline. Microguidewire was inserted to the microcatheter through RHV. Microcatheter and microguidewire are then inserted to the guiding catheter through the RHV attached on the proximal end of the guiding catheter (Fig. 10.5).

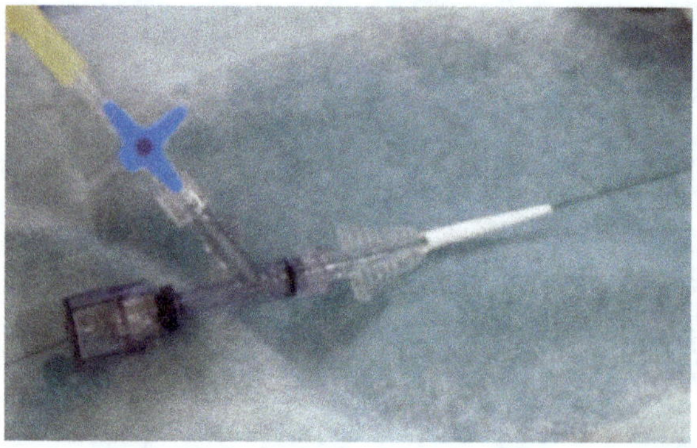

Fig. 10.5 Microguidewire is inserted to the microcatheter through Y-connector. Three-way is connected to Y-connector to give continuous flushing and contrast injection

10.3.3 Intervention Phase

After the guiding catheter was placed in desired position, intervention/coiling phase is started. The X-ray tube was adjusted to working position, and angiography to make "road map" imaging is done. Microcatheter and microguidewire is navigated to aneurysm location, guided by road map image. The ideal position of the tip of microcatheter is between one-third and two-thirds on the aneurysm sac.

Heparin 3000–5000 units IV is given once the microcatheter reaches the aneurysm sac in desired position, before starting coiling (50–70 units/Kg). Some authors prefer to give this heparin after the first coil is inserted in the aneurysm.

The first coil to deploy is usually a coil with 3D shape and called "framing" coil to cover the entire wall of the aneurysm. Then coiling is continued by "filling" the aneurysm sac with 2D coil until adequate packing is achieved.

Final angiogram is made to see the final position of coil and condition of parent artery, also the filling of contrast to the aneurysm sac.

10.4 Case Illustration

Case 1 (Figs. 10.6, 10.7, and 10.8)Case 2 (Figs. 10.9, 10.10, and 10.11)

During the attempt to do the coiling, it's very important to find the best projection view. It is very individual and necessary to tailor to the location and projection of the aneurysm.

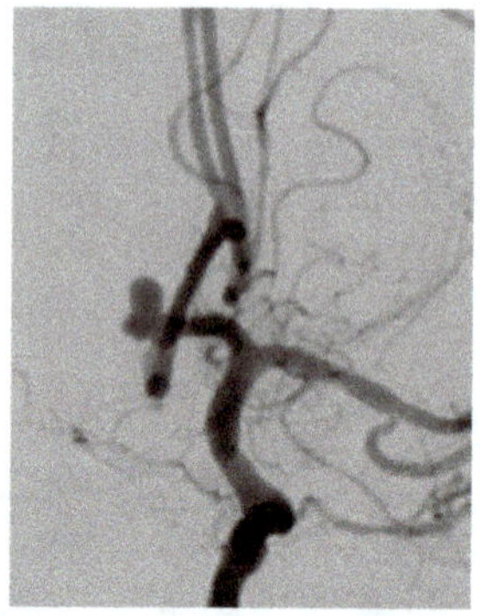

Fig. 10.6 It's a com aneurysm. It's done through the left side. The best projection is RAO 21 CRAN 10

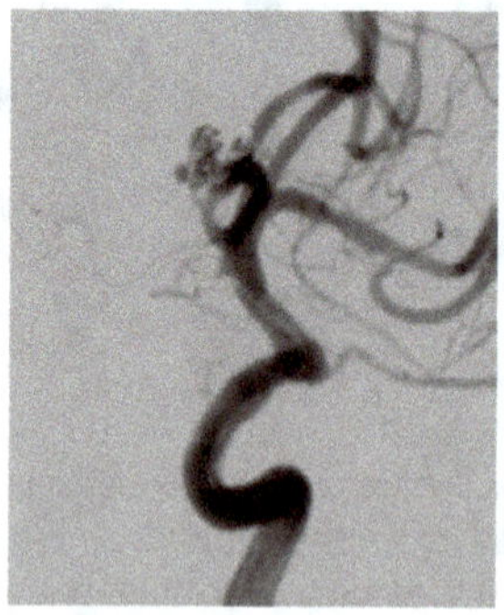

Fig. 10.7 During framing

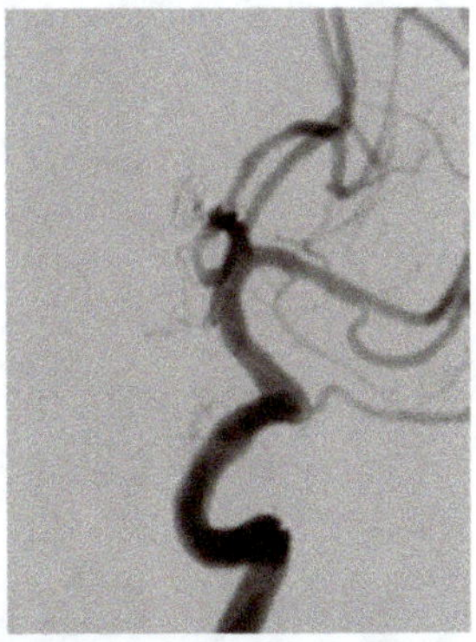

Fig. 10.8 The final angiography after coiling

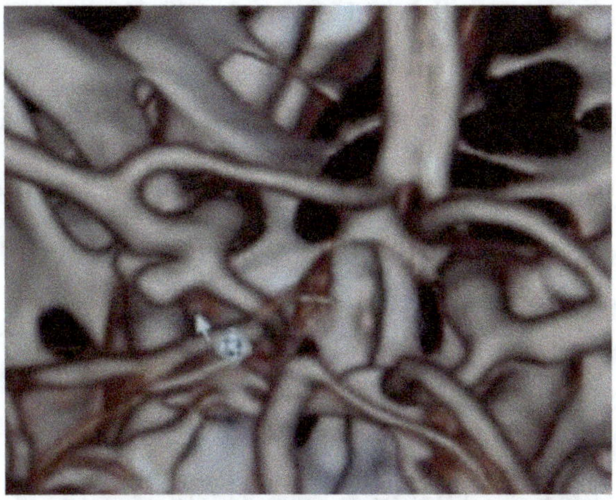

Fig. 10.9 Three-dimensional (3D) CT angiography is showing left IC-P-com aneurysm

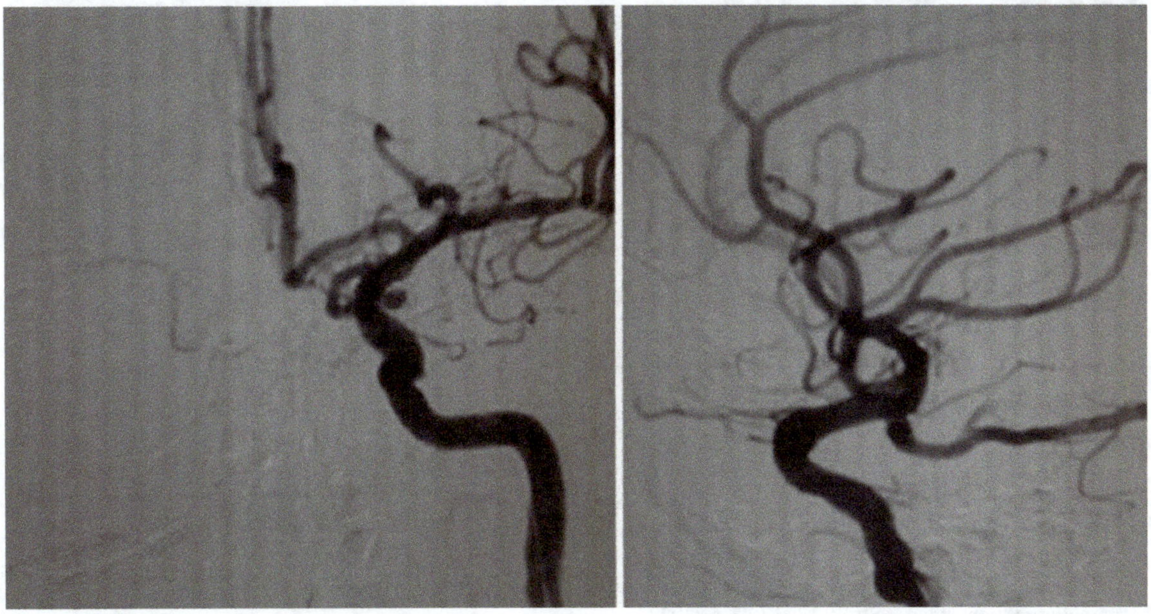

Fig. 10.10 The angiography of left IC, *left*, AP view, and *right*, lateral view. Both are not the best projection

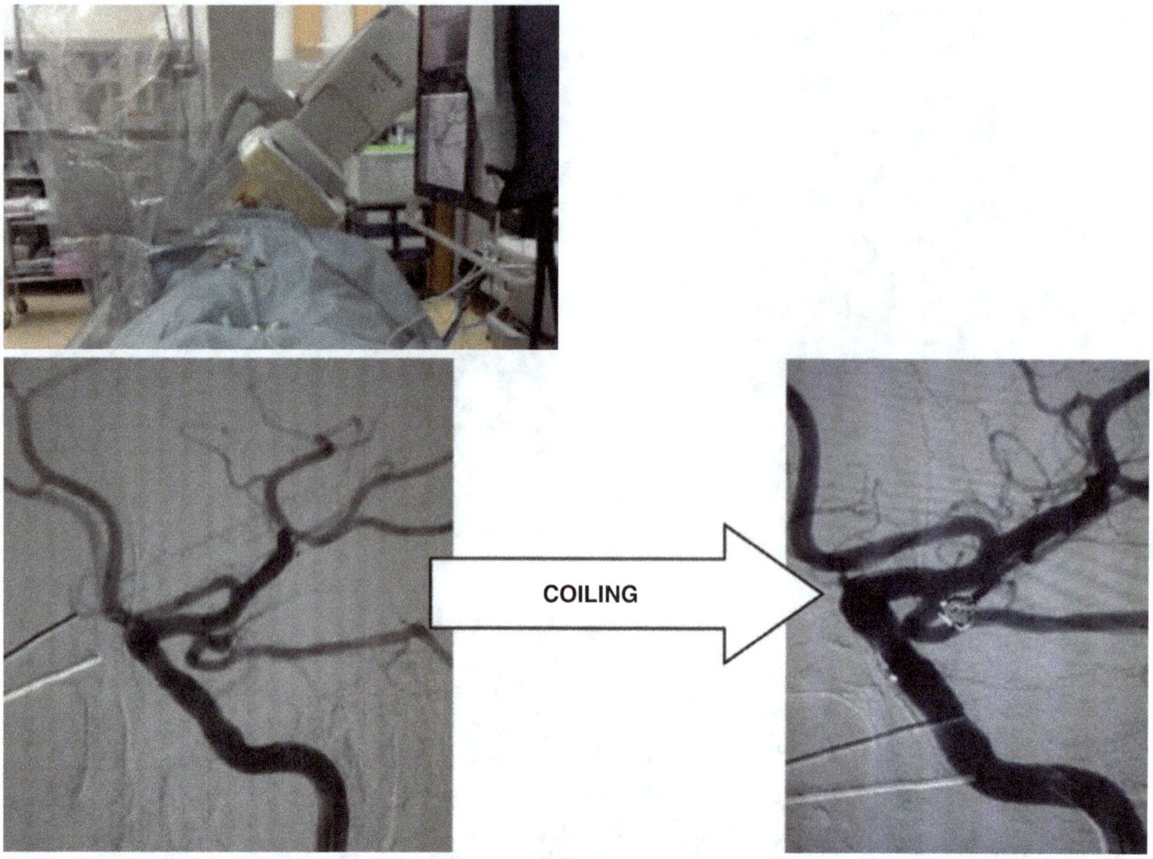

Fig. 10.11 The best projection view is LAO 45° caudal 5°. *Lower*: it is showing before and after coiling

References

1. Lin N, Cahill KS, Frerichs KU, et al. Treatment of ruptured and unruptured cerebral aneurysm in the USA: a paradigm shift. J NeuroIntervent Surg. 2012;4:182–9.
2. Connolly ES, Rabinstein AA, Carhuapoma JR, et al. Guidelines for the management of aneurysmal subarachnoid hemorrhage. Stroke. 2012;43(6):1711–37.
3. Thompson BG, Brown RD, Amin-Hanjani S, et al. Guidelines for the management of patients with unruptured intracranial aneurysms. Stroke. 2015;46:2368–400.
4. Harrigan MR, Deveikis JP. Handbook of cerebrovascular disease and neurointerventional technique. Dordrecht: Humana Press; 2009.

Part II

Surgery for Specific Location of Vascular Lesion or Specific Pathology

11 Surgery of Posterior Communicating Artery Aneurysm

Julius July

11.1 Sign and Symptoms

Posterior communicating artery (PCoA) aneurysm is the aneurysm that arises at junction of internal carotid (IC) and PCoA. This aneurysm accounts for 15–25% of all intracranial aneurysm [1, 2]. If the aneurysm neck arises along the PCoA itself, it's called "true" PCoA aneurysm, and this accounts more or less 1.3% of all intracranial aneurysm and 6.8% of all PCoA aneurysm [3].

This aneurysm usually presents with subarachnoid hemorrhage that commonly distributed at the Sylvian fissure and basal cistern but also can be higher up at the Sylvian fissure mimicking the middle cerebral artery rupture. They also can present with oculomotor nerve palsy (34%) [4], spontaneous subdural hemorrhage (1.72%) [5], intracerebral hemorrhage at the temporal lobe, and even intraventricular hemorrhage [6].

Although this aneurysm is located at the anterior end of the PCoA, they probably behave more like the posterior circulation aneurysm. ISUIA study finds the rupture risk from PCoA aneurysm is following the posterior circulation (<7 mm (2.5%), 7–12 mm (14.5%), 13–24 mm (18.4%), >25 mm (50%)), which is higher compared to anterior circulation [7]. From the ISUIA study, it seems that the smaller the aneurysm the less likely to rupture. But some study also shows that 87.5% of ruptured PCoA aneurysm have the size less than 10 mm and even 40% of them have the size less than 5 mm [8].

J. July
Department of Neurosurgery, Faculty of Medicine Universitas Pelita Harapan (UPH), Neuroscience Centre Siloam Hospital Lippo Village, Tangerang, Indonesia

11.2 Investigation and Imaging

Since the era of CT angiography (CTA), it is unnecessary to routinely use the intervention angiography for diagnostic purpose of intracranial aneurysm. Current CTA could provide a three-dimension reconstruction of the vessel, and the imaging is sufficient and very useful for surgical planning.

Several things that the surgeon needs to consider as part of the surgical planning for IC-PCoA aneurysm are the following.

11.2.1 The Size of the PCoA Itself

The size of the PCoA needs to be evaluated preoperatively and also its relationship to the aneurysm neck. Sometimes during the clipping, surgeon has to incorporate the PCoA into the clip, although it could be done without the risk of morbidity, but this have to be anticipated prior to surgery. Preoperative evaluation becomes very essential to have a safe surgery. The size of the

J. July, E. J. Wahjoepramono (eds.), *Neurovascular Surgery*,
https://doi.org/10.1007/978-981-10-8950-3_11

PCoA can range from very small (not visualized on the CTA) to a large artery as big as P2 segment of posterior cerebellar artery (PCA), and usually the P1 segment of the same side is hypoplastic. Such condition is known as fetal PCoA (Fig. 11.1). The surgeon should not compromise such PCoA during the clipping because the major supply to the P2 is mainly coming from the IC. The surgeon has to take this information for the surgical planning, including the decision to choose open surgery over the endovascular technique.

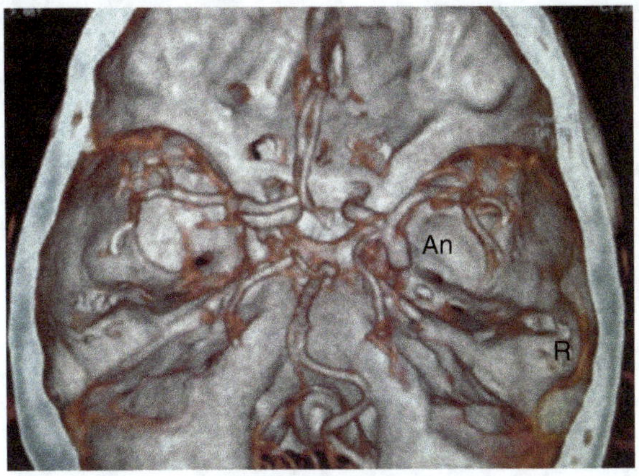

Fig. 11.1 3D reconstruction CTA female 66 years old shows right (R) IC-PCoA aneurysm (An) with ipsilateral fetal PCoA variant. Notice that the P1 segment ipsilateral is hypoplastic; PCoA diameter is as big as P2 segment. The main feeder of right P2 segment is coming from right IC

11.2.2 The Direction of Aneurysm Dome

Simplified classification of the PCoA aneurysm based on dome direction, modified from previous published study [9, 10], is divided into two groups, lateral and medial. The classification is based on the line that is drawn parallel with the sagittal plane and the other perpendicular line horizontally. The cross of both lines is located at the IC-PCoA junction (Fig. 11.2). It is not an absolute line and only used as an additional consideration while planning for surgery.

Lateral direction of the dome has higher rupture rate, and try to avoid temporal lobe retraction in the beginning of dissection. The surgeon may apply the temporal retraction gently, after he/she exposes the IC. Anterolateral direction of the dome is often blocking our view to the PCoA origin. Special precaution is needed for such

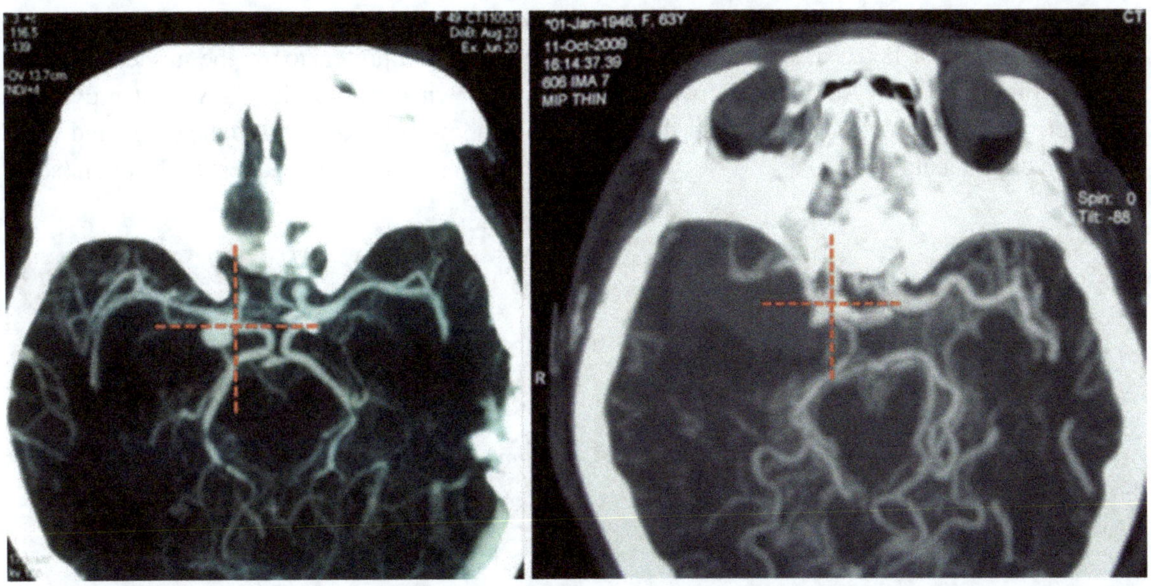

Fig. 11.2 CT angiography of two patients. *Left*: female 49 years old, with right IC-PCoA aneurysm, dome projecting to lateral and have fetal PCoA bilaterally, and presented with subarachnoid hemorrhage. *Right*: Female 49 years old, with right IC-PCoA aneurysm, dome projecting to lateral, and presented with temporal ICH (intracerebral hemorrhage) and required urgent surgery

case because some variation of branches from PCoA are supplying important structure such as optic chiasm, oculomotor nerve, mammillary body, tuber cinereum, cerebral crura, ventral thalamus, and rostral portion of the caudate nucleus [3, 10].

11.2.3 Anterior Clinoidectomy

Anterior clinoidectomy is not necessarily done routinely. A study by a Korean group, looking at the anterior clinoidectomy for IC-PCoA aneurysm, found that only 6 of 94 cases require anterior clinoidectomy [11]. They found three factors based on imaging study (CTA and four vessels angiography) that may help surgeon to estimate whether anterior clinoidectomy is necessary. The distance between aneurysm neck and anterior clinoid process may serve as a simple measure for clinical setting. In the study, the group that requires anterior clinoidectomy (6 patients) was shorter (mean 4.4 ± 0.7 mm, median 4.7 mm), and the group without anterior cinoidectomy (88 patients) was longer (mean 7.2 ± 1.4). Statistically, surgeon should consider anterior clinoidectomy if the distance between the aneurysm neck and anterior clinoid process is less than 4.7 mm. It is rarely required if the distance is more than 5.8 mm (Fig. 11.3). If the distance is less than 4.7 mm, often the aneurysm neck is covered by the anterior clinoid process, or it blocks the clip while the clipping attempt.

11.3 Steps of the Surgery

11.3.1 Position, Skin Incision, and Craniotomy

Patient head should be positioned in order the surgical view and trajectory of the dissection are almost perpendicular to the direction of the dome. This position should allow the surgeon to approach the neck of the aneurysm from the opposite direction of the aneurysm dome/fundus (Fig. 11.4). The head should be elevated 30–45° above the heart to enhance the brain relaxation because of optimal venous return from intracranial.

The head is fixed with either Sugita or Mayfield or other system of head holder. The skin incision and the craniotomy are planned according to surgeon preference, either pterional approach, lateral supraorbital approach (LSO), or keyhole supraorbital approach.

11.3.2 Dural Opening and Dissection

The dura is opened with curve incision with the base toward the skull base and hold with tenting suture silk 3/0 round needle (Fig. 11.5a). The brain is covered by a layer of wet surgicel or cottonoid. Author prefers to use the surgicel for some reasons; when the surgicel is wet, it provides a smooth layer of protection to the brain, and when we remove it, it does not adhere to the brain (some

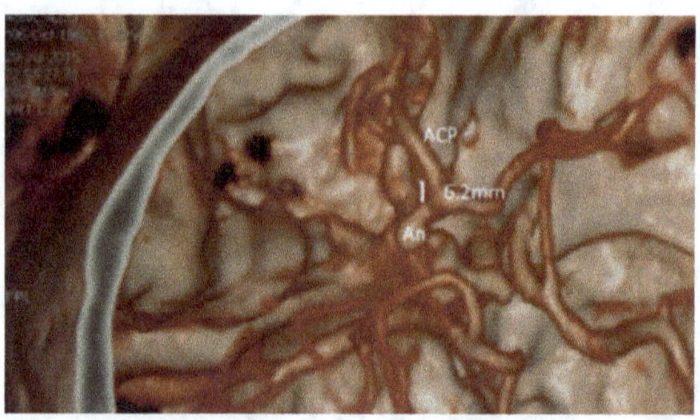

Fig. 11.3 CTA of 52 years old female with left PCoA, the distance of anterior clinoid process (ACP), and the proximal neck of the IC-PCoA aneurysm (An) is 6.2 mm (*white line*). In this case, we don't need the anterior clinoidectomy

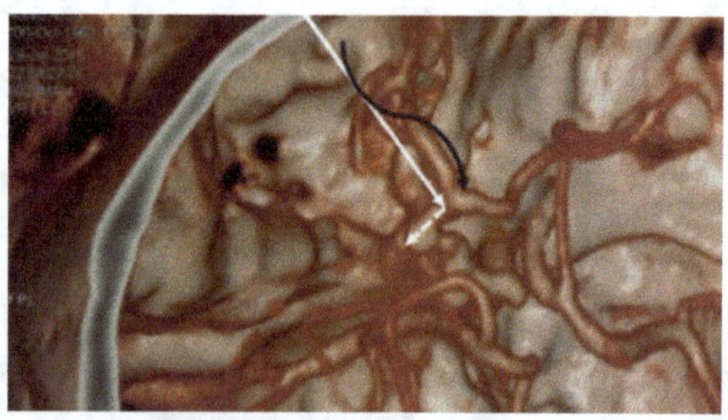

Fig. 11.4 Same patient on Fig. 11.3; the white arrow shows the surgical trajectory that is perpendicular to the direction of the dome (*dash arrow*). The dissection should avoid the dome of aneurysm and approaching the neck from the opposite direction of the dome

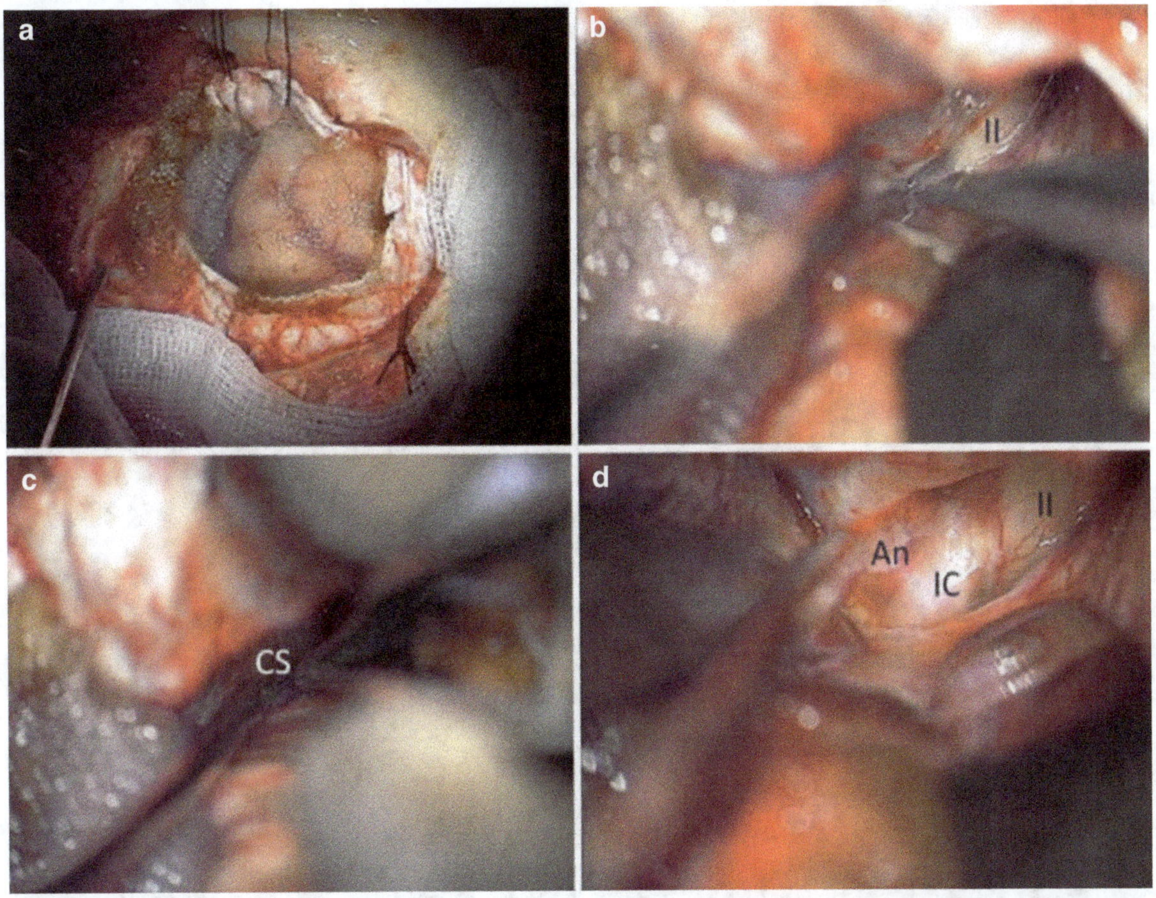

Fig. 11.5 (a) After the craniotomy, the dura is opened with curve shape toward the skull base, and it is tented with silk suture to the muscle. The brain is covered with a wet surgicel. (b) Gently retract the brain and try to reach the chiasmatic cistern, open the arachnoid with micro-scissor, and release the CSF. (c) The CSF is released and the surgeon will get more working space. (d) Sharply dissect the arachnoid, and identify the optic nerve (chiasm) and internal carotid artery (IC), and we usually will see part of the aneurysm (An)

cottonoid may adhere to the brain tissue and may cause bleed when we try to remove it). Firstly, try to reach the chiasmatic cistern and open the arachnoid with micro-scissor (Fig. 11.5b). Once it opened, release the CSF, and the brain will slowly relax, and surgeon will get more space for more dissection (Fig. 11.5c). Always try not to pull anything, and it is better to do sharp dissection all the time. Pulling will increase the chance of premature rupture of the aneurysm.

It is a basic principle to avoid the dome until the surgeon is able to secure the parent artery and the neck of the aneurysm (Fig. 11.5d). A study looking at the risk of intraoperative rupture found that IC-PCoA aneurysm had the second highest rate of rupture (9.3%) after the anterior communicating artery (AComA) aneurysm, among the anterior circulation aneurysms [12].

After the surgeon exposes the parent artery and the neck, he/she may continue dissection to identify the PCoA itself, release the neck from the surrounding arachnoid, and identify the anterior choroidal artery. The surgeon has to minimize the manipulation to the dome of the aneurysm while doing the dissection (Fig. 11.6). Sometimes we could find more than one anterior choroidal artery. After we identify all nearby structure, then the clip may be applied with both legs of the clip adequately squeezing the aneurysm neck. It is important to check all nearby branches are patent. Sometimes, the surgeon may open the lamina terminalis if there is a hydrocephalus on the CT scan.

Nowadays we could check the patency of the branches, the complete clipped of aneurysm, by using the indocyanine green (ICG), but we need to have a special microscope.

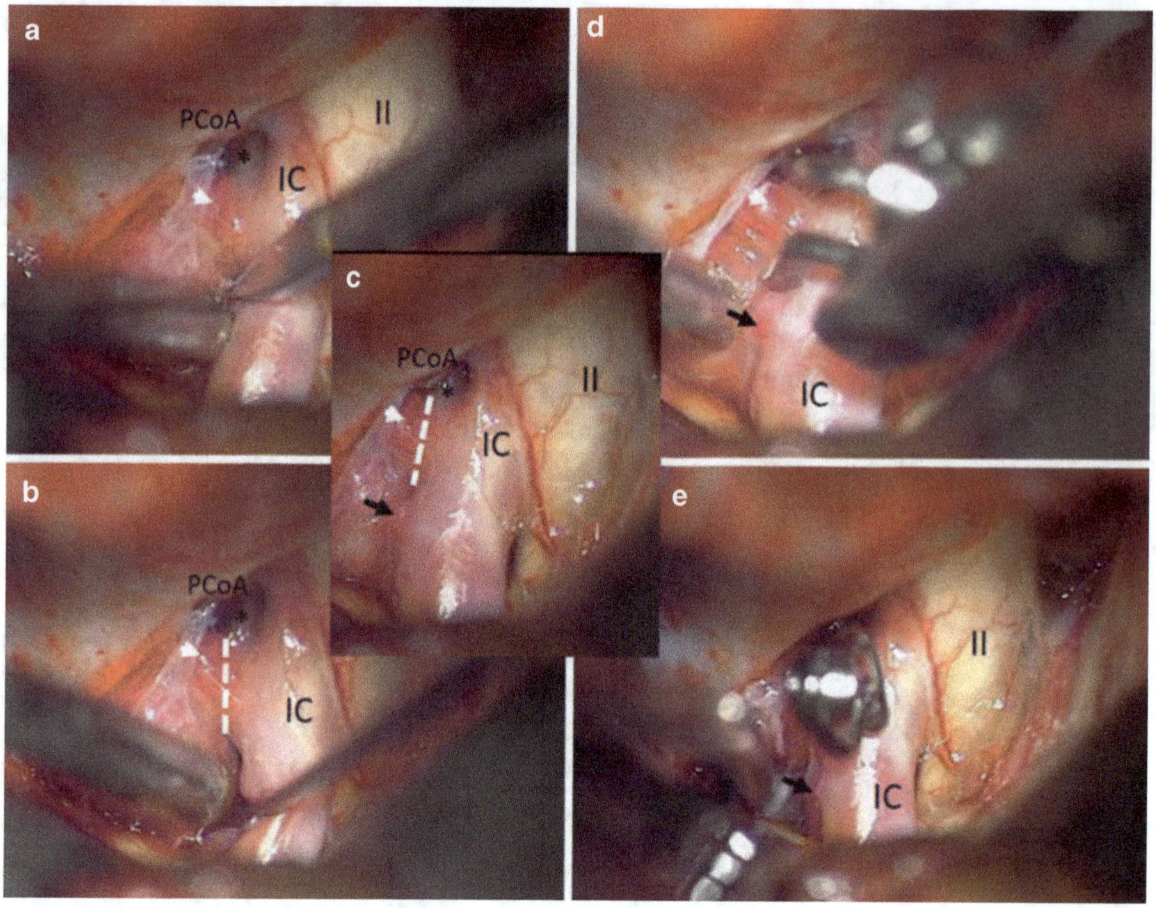

Fig. 11.6 (**a–c**) The sharp dissection exposes the internal carotid artery (IC), optic nerve (II), PCoA (*asterisk*), and the neck of the aneurysm (*dash line*); sometimes we found the bleb on the aneurysm (*white arrow*) and the anterior choroidal artery (*black arrow*). (**d**) The clip is slowly applied to the aneurysm; in such case we choose bayonet clip. (**e**) After the clip application, we should make sure the anterior choroidal artery and PCoA are patent

11.3.3 Closing

It is better to close the dura mater with watertight closure, tenting the dura mater against the craniotomy edge and using subcutaneous vacuum drain for 24 h. All this effort will minimize the complication and enhance the wound healing.

11.4 Expert Opinion/Suggestion to Avoid Complication

All aspect of surgery is important, starting from the planning based on the investigation and imaging study until the postoperative care. During the preparation of surgery, we need a good anesthetic team that will anesthetize the patient without blood pressure (BP) fluctuation. Injection of local anesthetic at the head holder pin site will avoid pain, thus no BP changes.

Head positioning is very important, not only for surgical trajectory and view, but it is also contributing to the brain relaxation. The use of mannitol, CSF drainage either at lumbal or ventricular, and PCO_2 monitoring are tools that surgeon may use to enhance the brain relaxation. Opening the bone, the duramater and applying the retractor have to be done gently. If we need to remove the anterior clinoid process, try to avoid manipulation of the nearby dura mater, because the dome of the aneurysm might be adhered to the dura mater and manipulation of the dura may cause premature rupture of the aneurysm.

Sharp dissection is a must, and never pull anything during dissection because it may cause remote bleeding that obscures the view and causes brain swelling or it may trigger premature rupture of the aneurysm. All the efforts have to be done to prevent premature rupture.

During clip application, simulation is an important part of successful clipping. The surgeon have to always remember that clip revision is very dangerous and often causes catastrophic bleeding and the surgery ends up with higher morbidity and mortality. Always try to avoid clip revision.

Closing is as important as opening. Meticulous closing may reduce the postoperative complication such as epidural hematoma and subdural hematoma.

11.5 Things to Be Observed and Postoperative Care/Follow-Up

After the surgery, hydration is important and also the electrolyte level should be checked. Subarachnoid hemorrhage (SAH) is often followed by cerebral salt wasting syndrome (CSWS) due to the brain natriuretic peptide (BNP) that is released during the SAH. Sodium loss will be followed by water depletion, and the sodium level in the blood will be decreasing. The loss should be replaced and maintained, and sometimes it requires weeks to get it over.

References

1. Morita A, Kirino T, Hashi K, Aoki N, Fukuhara S, Hashimoto N, et al. The natural course of unruptured cerebral aneurysms in a Japanese cohort. N Engl J Med. 2012;366:2474–82.
2. Ojemann RG, Crowell RM. Surgical management of cerebrovascular disease. 2nd ed. Baltimore: Williams and Wilkins; 1988. Internal carotid artery aneurysms; p. 179–98.
3. He W, Gandhi CD, Quinn J, Karimi R, Prestigiacomo CJ. True aneurysms of the posterior communicating artery: a systematic review and meta-analysis of individual patient data. World Neurosurg. 2011;75:64–72.
4. Soni SR. Aneurysms of the posterior communicating artery and oculomotor paresis. J Neurol Neurosurg Psychiatry. 1974;2013:475–84.
5. Gelabert-Gonzalez M, Iglesias-Pais M, Fernandez-Villa J. Acute subdural haematoma due to ruptured intracranial aneurysms. Neurosurg Rev. 2004;27:259–62.
6. Golshani K, Ferrell A, Zomorodi A, Smith TP, Britz GW. A review of the management of posterior communicating artery aneurysms in the modern era. Surg Neurol Int. 2010;1:88.
7. Wiebers DO, Whisnant JP, Huston J III, Meissner I, Brown RD Jr, Piepgras DG, et al. Unruptured intracranial aneurysms: natural history, clinical outcome, and risks of surgical and endovascular treatment. Lancet. 2003;362:103–10.
8. Forget TR Jr, Benitez R, Veznedaroglu E, Sharan A, Mitchell W, Silva M, et al. A review of size and location of ruptured intracranial aneurysms. Neurosurgery. 2001;49:1322–5.
9. Fukuda H, Hayashi K, Yoshino K, Koyama T, Lo B, Kurosaki Y, Yamagata S. Impact of aneurysm projection on intraoperative complications during surgical clipping of ruptured posterior communicating artery aneurysms. Neurosurgery. 2016;78(3):381–90.
10. Matsukawa H, Fujii M, Akaike G, Uemura A, Takahashi O, Niimi Y, Shinoda M. Morphological and clinical risk factors for posterior communicating artery aneurysm rupture. J Neurosurg. 2014;120(1):104–10.
11. Park SK, Shin YS, Lim YC, Chung J. Preoperative predictive value of the necessity for anterior clinoidectomy in posterior communicating artery aneurysm clipping. Neurosurgery. 2009;65:281–5.
12. Leipzig TJ, Morgan J, Horner TG, Payner T, Redelman K, Johnson CS. Analysis of intraoperative rupture in the surgical treatment of 1694 saccular aneurysms. Neurosurgery. 2005;56:455–68.

12 Surgery of IC-Anterior Choroidal Aneurysms

Thomas Kretschmer, Christian Heinen, Julius July, and Thomas Schmidt

12.1 Signs and Symptoms

Anterior choroidal artery aneurysms (AChAA) are comparatively rare and appear with a frequency from around 2–4% to 10% in larger series, e.g., M Lawton personal series of 2500 clipped aneurysms: $n = 98$ AChA = 4% [1]. Number of AChAA in treated aneurysms group of BRAT study 2.2%, median aneurysm size 7 mm, total 9 cases of 408 treated; 209 were clipped and 199 were coiled [2]. Kuopio aneurysm data base from 1977–2005, consist of 3005 patients with 4253 aneurysms, there were 99 (10%) AChAA in 70 (8%) patients [3].

There are no characteristic clinical findings for unruptured AChAA. Not infrequently they are detected during work-up of other ruptured or non-ruptured aneurysms. AChAA already can rupture at small size due to their characteristics of thin wall and orientation aligned along the main blood jet from the ICA. Rupture of AChAA can lead to blood distribution favoring the ipsilateral side and basal cisterns, comparable to PCoA aneurysm rupture.

T. Kretschmer (✉) · C. Heinen · T. Schmidt
Department of Neurosurgery, Evangelisches Krankenhaus Oldenburg, Oldenburg, Germany

J. July
Department of Neurosurgery, Faculty of Medicine Universitas Pelita Harapan (UPH), Neuroscience Centre Siloam Hospital Lippo Village, Tangerang, Indonesia

Ruptured AChAA usually will show blood at lateral suprasellar and ambient cisterns [3]. Very rare it presents with subdural or intracerebral blood collections despite proximity of the aneurysm to the temporal lobe. Intraventricular breakthrough of hemorrhage will be more prominent in temporal horn. Cranial nerve deficits seem to be infrequent; however oculomotor insufficiency has been described in ruptured or unruptured cases [4].

There are specific aspects about the AChA aneurysms especially the anatomy and its variant.

12.1.1 Anatomy

The AChA is a phylogenetically "old," respectively, early vessel, which is prominently developed until the 5th week during human embryology (choroidal stadium). The anterior circulation supplies almost the whole brain during this phase. Over hemispheric growth additional supply by the vertebrobasilar system is necessary. As a consequence the brain volume supplied by the AChA is progressively reduced. The AChA may show various anatomical variations.

The AChA originates 2–4 mm distal of PCoA on the posterolateral part of ICA, almost always, lateral to optic tract. Its diameter is only about 1 mm (0.5–1.5 mm). The artery then runs below the optic tract from lateral to medial. It courses

J. July, E. J. Wahjoepramono (eds.), *Neurovascular Surgery*,
https://doi.org/10.1007/978-981-10-8950-3_12

along the perimesencephalic cistern (**cisternal segment**), entering temporal horn of lateral ventricle at choroidal fissure ("plexal point"). Within ventricle (**choroidal segment**), it runs along the choroid plexus to anastomose with branches of the lateral and medial posterior choroidal artery (PChA).

Despite its relative small size and short length, it supplies some major *territories*: AChA perforators supply the optic tract, optic radiation, crus cerebri, hippocampus, corpus amygdaloideum, substantia nigra, globus pallidus, lateral thalamus, and the posterior crus of the internal capsule. Along its course AChA may send off as many as 16–20 separate branches.

In proximity to the AChA origin, there may be one or several perforator branches to the temporal lobe. The optic tract gets blood supply from perforator of anterior choroidal artery that passes medially and turns around the optic tract and then penetrates the tract superiorly. There are also variants where perforators go through the optic tract and supply internal capsule and globus pallidus. Other perforators pierce peduncle and supply red nucleus and substantia nigra. Following the peduncle, the lateral geniculate and the pulvinar are crossed before entering the lateral ventricle choroid plexus.

12.1.2 Variants

AChA may be duplicated in 4% of cases. Ectopic ramification with AChA originating from posterior cerebral artery (PCA) or middle cerebral artery (MCA) has been described. Origins of AChA and PCoA usually are 3–4 mm apart and, however, on occasion may be simultaneous or only 1–2 mm apart. Very rarely the AChA comes off the ICA proximal of the PCoA origin. Rare variants, whereby AChA supplies the occipital lobe, including the calcarine cortex, were described.

12.2 Preoperative Investigation

AChAA may be hard to differentiate from PCoA aneurysms on angiograms. In comparison to PCoA aneurysms, they project in a more lateral direction and may point into the uncus of the temporal lobe. It is crucial to identify the AChA as such and to determine whether it arises as a single trunk or as multiple branches.

CT and thin slice CT angiography with 3D reconstruction will raise suspicion for an AChAA; however it does not suffice to clearly depict details of vessel-to-aneurysm topography and exact site and course of emanating branches. As such, contrary to some of the other aneurysm locations, we feel catheter angiography is precondition to further treatment decision. Depending on the result of imaging studies, branching pattern, age, and condition of the patient, we decide whether to clip or coil. Angioarchitecture at the aneurysm neck plays an important role in that decision, with branching directly at the neck favoring aneurysm clipping and clip reconstruction of the AChA.

3D rotational angiography is a very valuable tool to dismantle the true topography. Frequently the aneurysm will project laterally and straight to caudal with respect to the ICA. So AP and lateral views are very important to resolve the aneurysm sac projection. The AChA itself will best be seen in a lateral and sometimes basal view and needs to be discerned from the PCoA (Fig. 12.1). From its origin on the lateral ICA aspect, the artery courses posteriorly for 4–5 mm and short medially to optic tract to follow its course laterally around the peduncle. This curvature can easily be detected on a lateral view. The differentiation is more difficult on an AP view: here the AChA describes a medial curve, to then turn laterally and upward, to make a sudden kink at the plexal point.

12.3 Presurgical Preparation

We do prepare as for any other aneurysm clipping. One exemption being an additional reciprocating saw (with very slender blade) and chisels in the rare occasion, we plan to place an orbital extension of the standard lateral supraorbital approach (LSO). Patients will have a CV line (central venous line); we do not routinely order blood products in unruptured cases. After patient

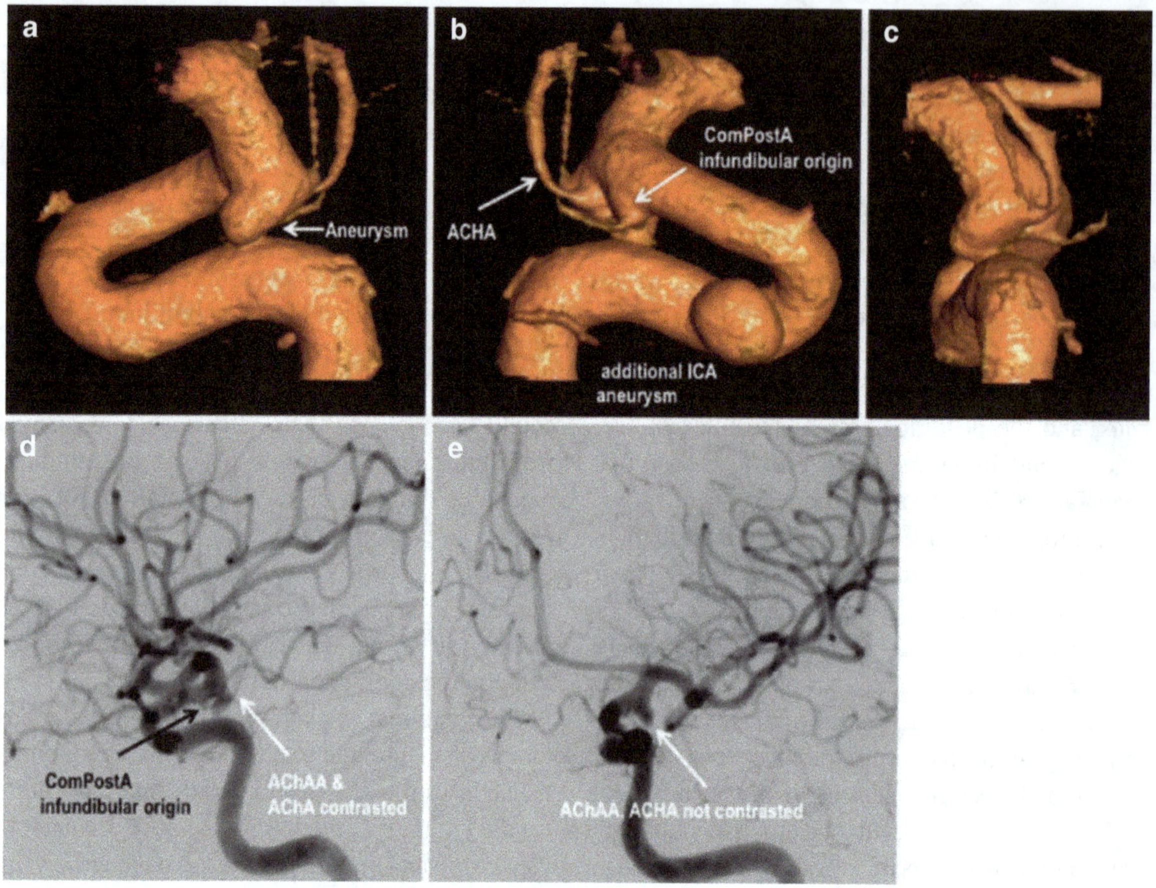

Fig. 12.1 (**a–e**) Preoperative imaging. Angiographic depiction of an AChAA from different views including 3D reconstruction (upper row). (**a**) Lateral view on aneurysm with AChA emanating from dorsal neck. (**b**) Medial view of AChAA neck, with infundibular PCoA close to aneurysm. Extradural aneurysm of ICA, as secondary finding. (**c**) Dorsal view on aneurysm and emanating AChA. PCoA and ACA (A1) can also be depicted. (**d**) Lateral view of angiographic image, infundibular PCoA branches off close to AChA, as well as the more distal (flow direction) broad-based AChAA neck and AChA emanating from there. (**e**) Slightly oblique AP view. With this alignment only the aneurysm is perceptible, however, not the branching AChA. To depict the AChA in this case, images turned further are necessary

and head clamp positioning, the patient is prepped and draped. During this procedure, he will receive 1 g/KG of mannitol if not the kidney is not compromised. Standard trays for craniotomy and vascular microsurgery are prepared. We have a standard clip sieve on the table, which is assembled to our needs. It contains the clip forms and sizes we use most of the time; only "exotic" clips will be directly unpacked as needed. A straight aneurysm clip and two types of temporary clips (7 mm bent and straight) are taken out of the sieve and placed ready on the instrumentation table for cases of premature rupture. Adenosine (for induction of temporary cardiac standstill) as well as indocyanine green (ICG) will be available on the anesthesiology side before we start. Anesthesiology will be prepared to enable temporary clipping by bolus administration of thiopental with 100% inspiratory oxygen concentration at any time during the procedure. Imaging studies are depicted; monitors for anesthesiology and OR care are available to follow the procedure.

12.3.1 Approach

The initial microsurgical strategy is similar to those of PCoA aneurysms, as these arteries emanate in close vicinity. However, as the AChA and

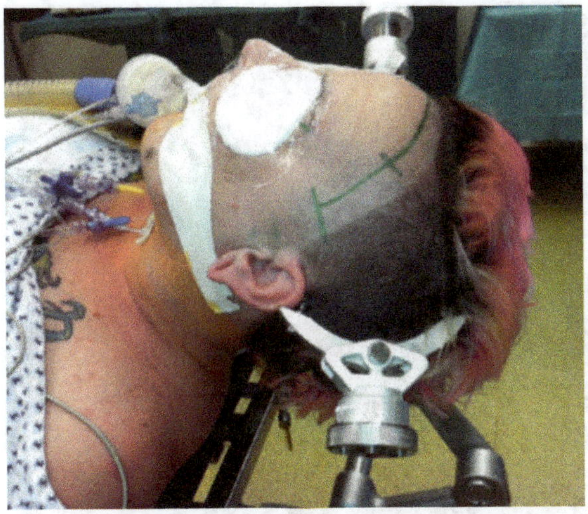

Fig. 12.2 Positioning. Head elevated well above heart level, slightly reclined toward the floor, and only minimally turned toward the right shoulder (about 20°). Planned incision for lateral supraorbital approach (LSO) with orbital deroofing. For LSO incision is at hairline margin, starting 2–3 cm above zygoma (if such a frontally placed incision is chosen, it needs to end well above the zygoma; otherwise the facial nerve is jeopardized); length of incision depends on the approach chosen and hairline distance from eyebrow. For simple LSO 6–8 cm suffice

its perforator takeoff are hidden by aneurysm sack and ICA, the specific anatomy with high likelihood of perforators directly emanating at the aneurysm neck makes its treatment more challenging. Standard approaches such as pterional, lateral supraorbital (LSO), and supraorbital keyhole are used most frequently. Our personal choice is standard LSO [5]. In cases of expected obtunded view on AChA origin, we might choose an orbital extension of the LSO in the form of a combined one-piece orbital rim deroofing to gain some extra degrees of surgical dissection corridor (cranio-orbital approach).

Patient is placed supine, and the head is higher than heart level, moderately reclined, and minimally turned to the contralateral side by about 20° (Fig. 12.2). If the head is turned too much, the temporal lobe is rotated over the aneurysm in the visual trajectory of the surgeon. Correct head position avoids the need for a fixed retraction device in particular for temporal lobe retraction.

The incision is placed at the hairline and begins 2.5–3 cm above the zygoma. Six to seven centimeters of length usually suffice if galeal flap is well retracted by spring or rubber-connected fishhooks (Fig. 12.3). It is important to expose zygomatic process of frontal bone in order to enable a craniotomy cut down to the fronto-sphenoidal base.

For the standard LSO, we place one burr hole below superior temporal line, 2–2.5 cm posterior to the zygomatic process, as we do not see the need for the so-called keyhole burr hole. A mini-craniotomy is fashioned without additional burr hole cut very precisely to the cranial base. The inner bony rim (internal tabule) and cranial base are flattened out to enable unimpeded vision with a drill or the unguarded craniotomy burr.

12.4 Surgical Steps

Following craniotomy, dura is incised to create a frontally based flap that is pulled over the frontal base and fixed with dural stitches. Low-profile craniotomy and low dural opening enable for a comfortable subfrontal dissection corridor. After introducing the operating microscope, a first subfrontal dissection trajectory starting from the frontal "zygomatic process pillar" in a perpendicular direction will directly lead to the ipsilateral optic nerve and optic cistern (Fig. 12.4a).

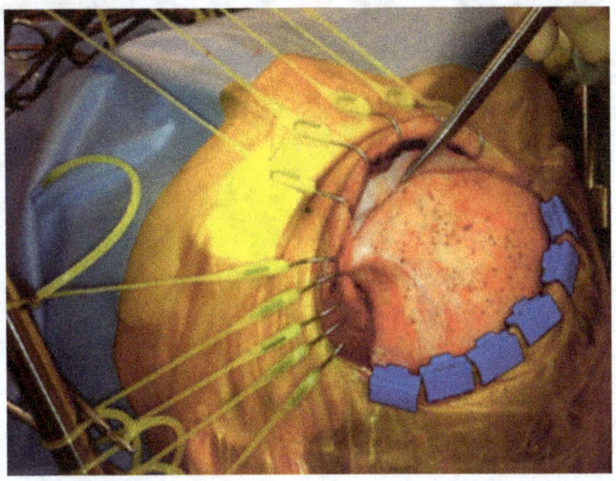

Fig. 12.3 Incision and exposure. Exposure after a 7 cm skin incision and having raised a combined galeal-muscle flap by incising through fascia and muscle. Muscle is carefully stripped from bone to prevent later atrophy. In this case orbital rim was fully exposed for cranio-orbital approach. In routine LSO it is not necessary to detach that far down; to expose beginning of zygomatic process of os frontale is enough to cut craniotomy flush with the frontal base

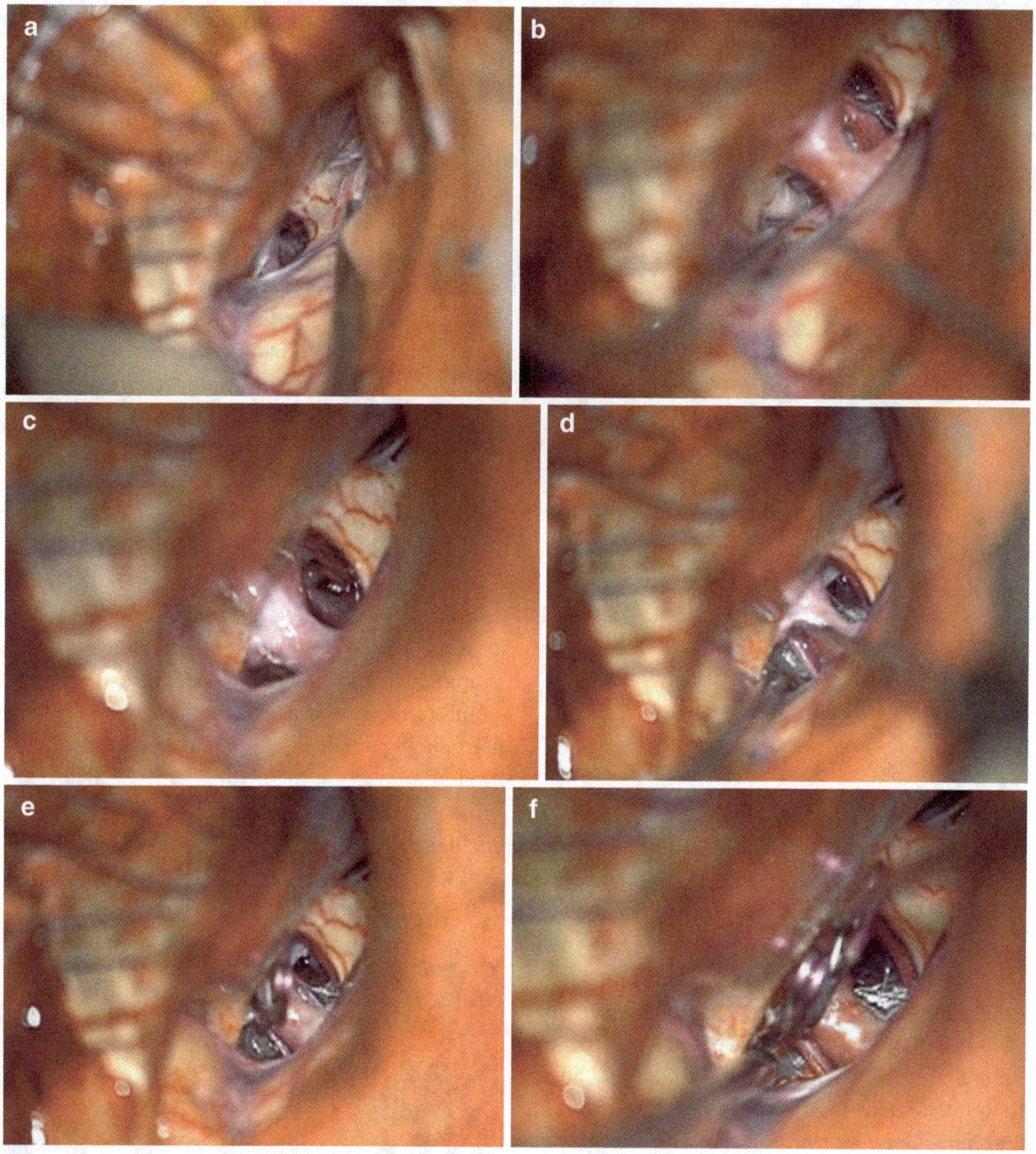

Fig. 12.4 (**a–f**) Aneurysm clipping. (**a**) Beginning of intradural part. Subfrontal exposure and opening of optic cistern. (**b**) Distal ICA after head has been lowered depicts bifurcation and A1. (**c**) Distal part of aneurysm neck. ICA hides AChA. (**d**) After deflecting the ICA with dissector, AChA can be seen. (**e**) As neck area and AChA have been identified, safe clipping is now possible. (**f**) Second smaller clip is needed for neck area to reconstruct beginning of AChA wall

The optic cistern, medial to optic nerve, is safer to be opened first, as compared to the optico-carotid cistern on the lateral side in ruptured cases. CSF drainage via the cistern will further relax the brain and progressively open a subfrontal corridor by using gravity without any fixed retraction. After opening the optico-carotid cistern, subfrontal adhesions are progressively loosened. Although the ICA is the target and will readily be in the operative view, additional freeing of the temporal and frontal lobe, allowing them to fall back, opens the available dissection space. However, microsurgical dissection should begin without any temporal lobe retraction to avoid premature aneurysm rupture by opening first the optic and then the optico-carotid cistern to gain a surgical corridor sufficient for ACI dissection. The superomedial surface of the ICA is safe for dissection. Once the proximal ICA is freed and centered in the obtained view, additional room can then be gained by splitting carefully just the beginning of the proximal Sylvian fissure overlying the carotid T.

After the more distal ICA is freed from arachnoid adhesions, the PCoA and the oculomotor nerve can be identified (Fig. 12.4b). The aneurysm should be located distally to the PCoA origin (Fig. 12.4c). Once the AChA is identified, it needs to be determined if the AChA arises as a single trunk or multiple vessels (Fig. 12.4d). AChAA may arise from a proximal or distal segment. Large or giant AChAA (quite rare) might be adherent to the uncus of the temporal lobe or rarely to the oculomotor nerve. Frequently the aneurysm sac or the ICA itself (Fig. 12.4d) will hide the AChA that is emanating behind the sac. Safe clip application necessitates maneuvers that ascertain direct view on the ICA at the aneurysm neck and AChA takeoff. Sometimes this might only be possible by use of a transient dynamic maneuver displacing the main trunk with a microdissector. This might encompass active compression or displacement of the aneurysm dome with a microdissector to gain sight to potentially hidden perforators (only in unruptured aneurysms). All these maneuvers are potentially dangerous as they do bear a high risk of premature rupture but might be the only means to directly assess the "takeoff area." Besides experiencing their use necessitates heightened awareness for premature rupture and knowledge of "bailout" strategies, e.g., temporary clipping, cardiac standstill, handling of ICA lacerations, use of fenestrated clips, and vessel wall reconstruction techniques with clips. Measures to gain view and change trajectory also include turning of the OR table in the longitudinal axis of the patient and lowering of the OR table head/backpiece. Escalated measures are short cardiac standstill by adenosine (one dose will give 20–40 s), sometimes even temporary ICA clipping (only very short tolerance time, if possible needs to be avoided by full use of other alternatives).

After optimal aneurysm exposure, preparation for clip application is undertaken. Temporary and permanent clips should be readily available. A potential site for temporary clip application and choice of the temporary clip is chosen. For clipping the shortest clip amenable should be chosen. In uncomplicated aneurysms a straight or slightly laterally bent clip might be appropriate. Complex aneurysm architecture at the neck might necessitate clip combinations to reconstruct the AChA and/or perforator takeoff (Fig. 12.4e, f). At times it is warranted to place a pilot clip to secure the dome first, before the neck is reconstructed. Small branches adherent to the aneurysm wall not amenable to dissection might be excludable from clipping them off by use of a tandem technique with a fenestrated and a straight clip.

If a complex branching pattern or obtunded view can be foreseen, we are inclined to use a one-piece mini-cranio-orbital extension of the standard LSO from the start of the craniotomy (Fig. 12.5). This will add several degrees of dissection corridor (from a caudal to cranial direction in the sagittal plane) and allows to lower the headpiece of the OR table further, as the orbital rim is not in the field of view. However, an optimal view on the branching site cannot always be achieved.

Adjuncts to delineate the neck and perforator situation after clipping might be an angled endoscope (however we mostly find it too bulky in that location), ultrasound mini-Doppler, and ICG. To avoid misinterpretation of results, it is advisable to test already before clipping.

After clipping and ICG/ultrasound control of perfusion, we fill the operative site with Ringer's and close dura. The wound is closed meticulously in layers. We separate adaption of the muscle and fascia as we do prevent drains. Also in a mini-cranio-orbital approach in small incisions (ca. 7 cm), prevention of swelling, hematoma, and pristine, unchanged cosmetic are obtainable with careful handling of soft tissue and bone (Fig. 12.6a, b).

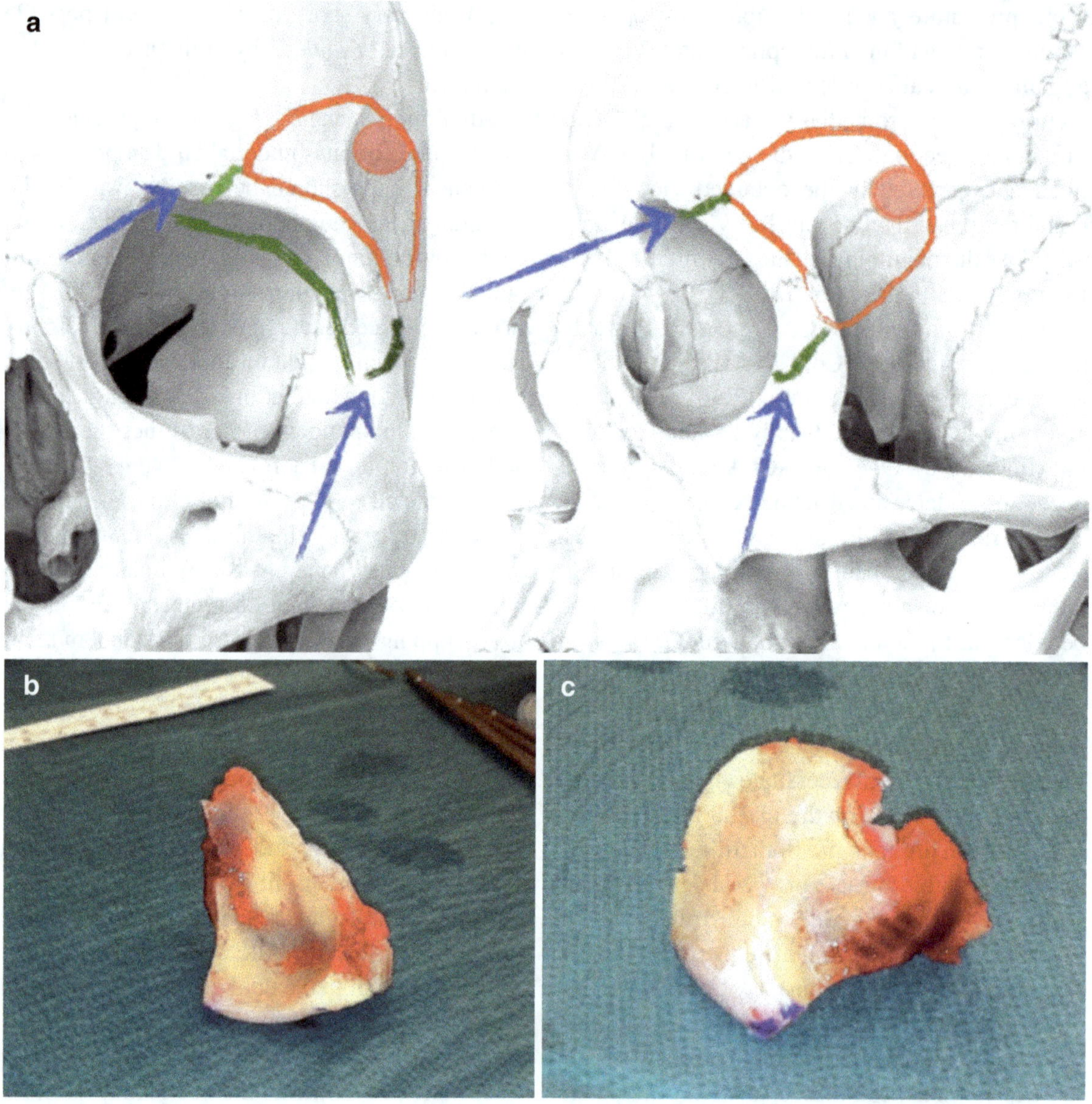

Fig. 12.5 (**a–c**) Craniotomy. Usually a standard LSO (red line) will suffice. In this we prefer to place one burr hole below superior temporal line and then cut a craniotomy down to the frontal base and across the sphenoid bone. In the depicted case, however, a one-piece mini-cranio-orbital approach was chosen with orbital deroofing (green line, instead of red frontal base line). (**b**) Shows inner side of the orbital roof. We prefer to incise medial and lateral orbital roof with very thin reciprocating saw (blue arrows in **a**) to have a sharp cut with minimal bone loss and split the rest with small chisels that will create a triangular shape (green line in **a**). (**c**) Shows the outer side with burr hole, corresponding to (**a**) right side

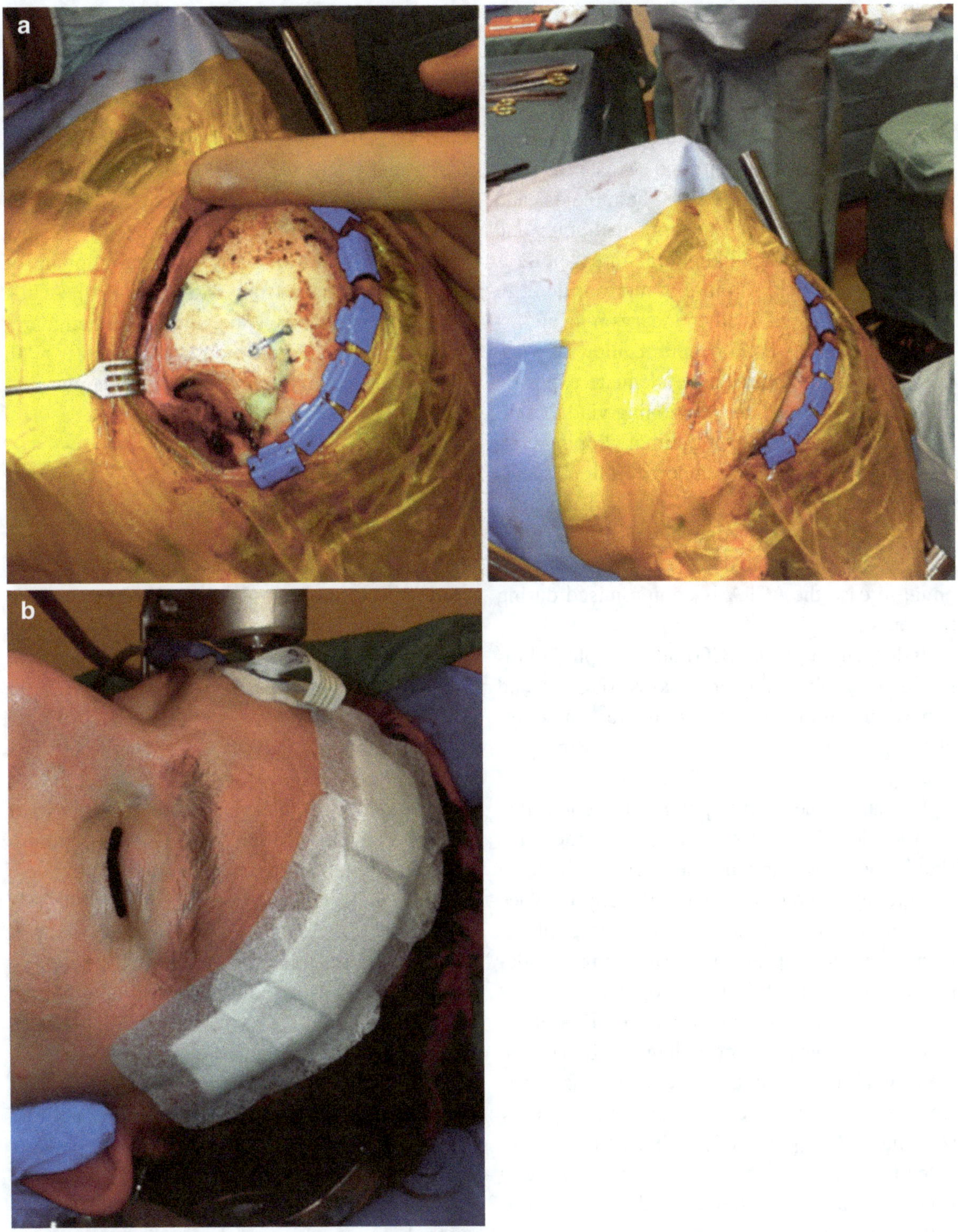

Fig. 12.6 (**a**, **b**) Closure. (**a**) Bone flap is repositioned and secured in place with mini-plates. Craniotomy groove and burr hole have been sealed with bone cement, followed by meticulous suture in layers (muscle and fascia separately, galea, skin). We do not routinely use drains. (**b**) Demonstrates cosmetic result with absence of orbital hematoma or swelling

12.5 Complication Management and Avoidance

Treatment of AChAA bears a far higher risk for complications. The main risk is inadvertent occlusion of the AChA with the devastating consequences of hemiparesis to hemiplegia and hemianopia. This applies to surgical clipping and interventional coiling alike. Premature rupture is another severe risk. Rupture is more difficult to handle as compared to other aneurysm locations.

Meticulous dissection, optimization of view trajectory by combination of adequate exposure around ICA, and patient positioning via table tilt are necessary to preset for optimal clipping conditions. Provisions for temporary clipping/cardiac arrest should have been made in advance, before skin incision. Median nerve SEP monitoring is a valuable tool to detect early signs of ischemia, in case the AChA is compromised during the course.

Indocyanine green (ICG) angiography, ultrasound (US) mini-Doppler to assess outflow, and papaverine/nimodipine irrigation after temporary clipping are adjuncts to assess vessel patency or treat spasm.

Premature aneurysm rupture can be controlled with a pilot clip across the aneurysm sac. This should then give enough time to assess the local topography in order to reapply the clip or place an additional one. If this is not feasible, placement of a pilot clip under pharmacological adenosine cardiac arrest is another option.

In case of devastating rupture of ICA/aneurysm neck, which cannot be handled by suction alone within the above-stated time constraints, we recommend to assess the tear by temporary clipping of ICA (preferably within 30 s to 2 min). If the ICA lumen cannot be clip reconstructed, a small circular cotton wrap around ICA is placed and secured in place with an angulated aneurysm clip. If bleeding does not cease after the circular cotton sheath in place, additional absorbable fibrin sealant patch (TachoSil®) is added. Small rents can be sealed with tiny TachoSil® pledgets and cottonoid in a first attempt. All in all it will be very difficult to save the AChA in such a circumstance.

In cases of inadvertent closure of AChA by embolus, emergent bypass or open embolectomy is not really feasible at this location and thus do not represent realistic bailout options.

The incidence of procedure related to permanent AChA syndrome after surgical clipping of an AChAA ranges from 5 to 16% [4, 6]. AChA syndrome manifests with contralateral hemiparesis to hemiplegia and more inconsistently with contralateral hemianesthesia or hemianopia.

12.6 Postoperative Care and Follow-Up

We do not use drains on a routine basis. The wound is closed meticulously in layers to prevent blood accumulation (temporalis muscle and fascia are closed separately). Skin is closed with staples or suture that will be removed after 7 days.

ICG angiography is used on a routine basis intraoperatively; however it has no power to reliably rule out residual perfusion. Regardless of intraoperative evaluation, we do perform postoperative catheter angiography to confirm complete clipping in every aneurysm case regardless of location (Fig. 12.7). In our own practice, this will be done in the direct postoperative period. In non-ruptured cases catheter angiography will be performed within the next 2 days to enable early discharge of the patient.

The patient is discharged within 3–7 days after surgery in non-ruptured cases. Length of stay in subarachnoid hemorrhage (SAH) patients is dictated by the course of the disease, length of intensive care treatment, overcoming of the spasmic phase, sequelae of hemorrhage, and also availability of a rehabilitation placement.

The first follow-up on our clipped patients will be 3 months after discharge at our outpatient clinic.

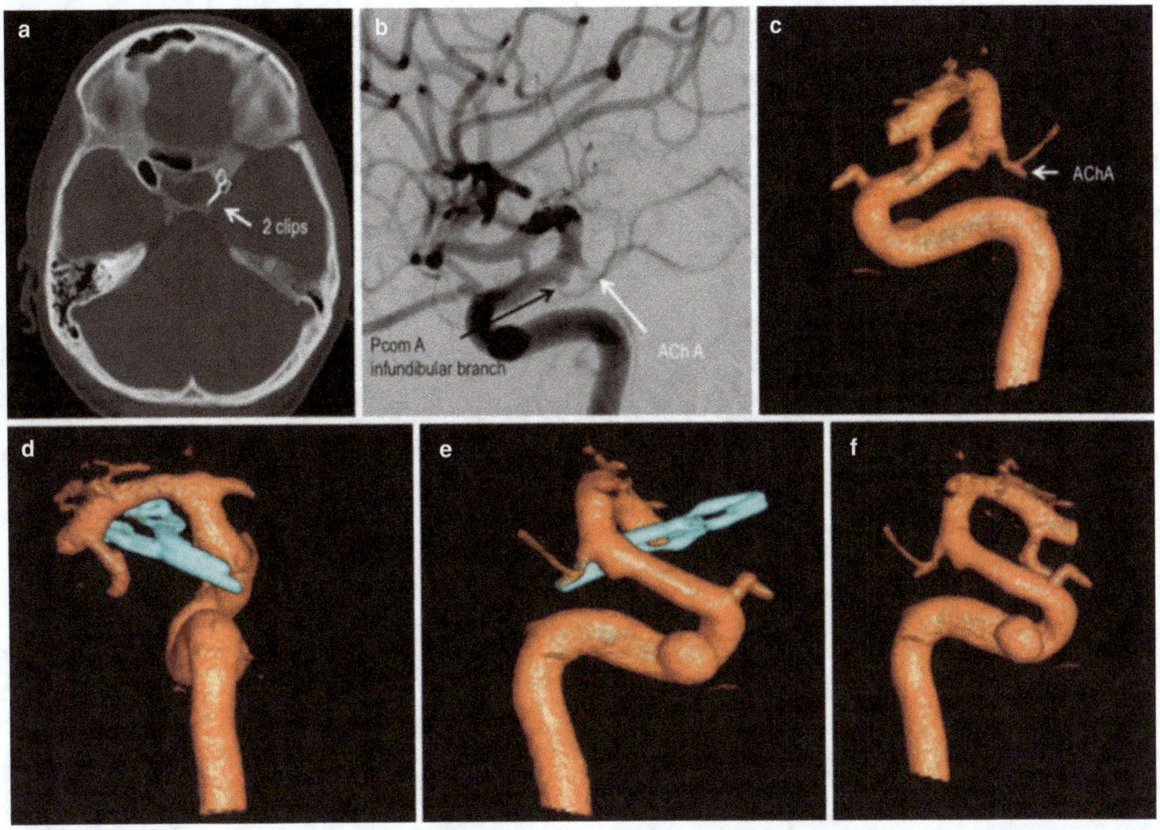

Fig. 12.7 (**a–f**) Postop imaging. Clip position in relation to bony skull base on CT, postop angio, and 3D rotational angio reconstructions with and without clips. (**a**) Basal view on placed clips in CT. (**b**) Lateral view of ICA with infundibular PCoA, clipped aneurysm, and reconstructed AChA. (**c**) 3D reconstruction of (**b**). (**d**) Posterior view on clip tips. (**e**) Medial view with depiction of reconstructed AChA. (**f**) Same view as (**e**) without clips

12.6.1 Pearls

AChAA are rare but bear a higher risk of rupture and are more difficult to treat. They are frequently thin walled and have the main AChA branch in direct vicinity to or emanating from the aneurysm neck. As such the risk of ischemic complications due to surgery is comparatively high.

References

1. Lawton MT. Seven AVMs. Thieme;2014.
2. Spetzler RF, McDougall CG, Albuquerque FC, Zabramski JM, Hills NK, Partovi S, et al. The barrow ruptured aneurysm trial: 3-year results. J Neurosurg. 2013;119(1):146–57.
3. Lehecka M, Dashti R, Laakso A, van Popta JS, Romani R, Navratil O, et al. Microneurosurgical management of anterior choroid artery aneurysms. World Neurosurg. 2010;73(5):486–99.
4. Lee Y-S, Park J. Anterior choroidal artery aneurysm surgery: ischemic complications and clinical outcomes revisited. J Korean Neurosurg Soc. 2013;54(2):86–92.
5. Hernesniemi J, Ishii K, Niemela M, Smrcka M, Kivipelto L, Fujiki M, Shen H. Lateral supraorbital approach as an alternative to the classical pterional approach. Acta Neurochir Suppl. 2005;94:17–21.
6. Friedman JA, Pichelmann MA, Piepgras DG, Atkinson JL, Maher CO, Meyer FB, Hansen KK. Ischemic complications of surgery for anterior choroidal artery aneurysms. J Neurosurg. 2001;94(4):565–72.

13 Surgery of Paraclinoid Aneurysm

Naoki Otani, Terushige Toyooka, and Kentaro Mori

13.1 Signs and Symptoms

Paraclinoid aneurysm is defined as an aneurysm that originates at the internal carotid artery (ICA) distal to the proximal dural ring (PDR) and proximal to the posterior communicating artery (PCoA), which means both ophthalmic and clinoidal segments of the ICA. Patients with these aneurysms present with retro-orbital or supraorbital pain and varying degrees of visual field constriction and/or visual acuity decline which is associated with compression of optic nerve. This nerve is typically pushed superiorly and medially, which manifests as a unilateral inferomedial (lower nasal) quadrantanopsia [1]. In addition, paraclinoid aneurysms may manifest as progressive diplopia due to compression of the cranial nerves involved in ocular movement caused by aneurysm growth. Unruptured paraclinoid aneurysm has a low risk of rupture compared to other types of cerebral aneurysm. The surgical indications for unruptured paraclinoid aneurysm should consider this low rupture risk as well as several other factors such as the aneurysm shape, the aneurysm size, and how old the patient.

13.1.1 Case Illustration One

A 56-year-old female was admitted to our service due to the progressive visual field deficit consisting of inferomedial quadrantanopsia (Fig. 13.1) with retro-orbital pain. We ordered a 3D-CT angiography, and it demonstrated a right ICA aneurysm with the dome projecting superiorly (Fig. 13.2).

13.1.2 Case Illustration Two

A 64-year-old female was brought to the hospital due to a severe retro-orbital pain. 3D-CT angiography demonstrated a large left ICA-ophthalmic artery aneurysm (Fig. 13.3a). The aneurysm dome projected medio-superiorly. Postoperative 3D-CT angiography showed complete clipping was achieved (Fig. 13.3b).

N. Otani (✉) · T. Toyooka · K. Mori
Department of Neurosurgery, National Defense Medical College, Tokorozawa, Saitama, Japan
e-mail: naotani@ndmc.ac.jp; toyo@ndmc.ac.jp; kmori@ndmc.ac.jp

J. July, E. J. Wahjoepramono (eds.), *Neurovascular Surgery*,
https://doi.org/10.1007/978-981-10-8950-3_13

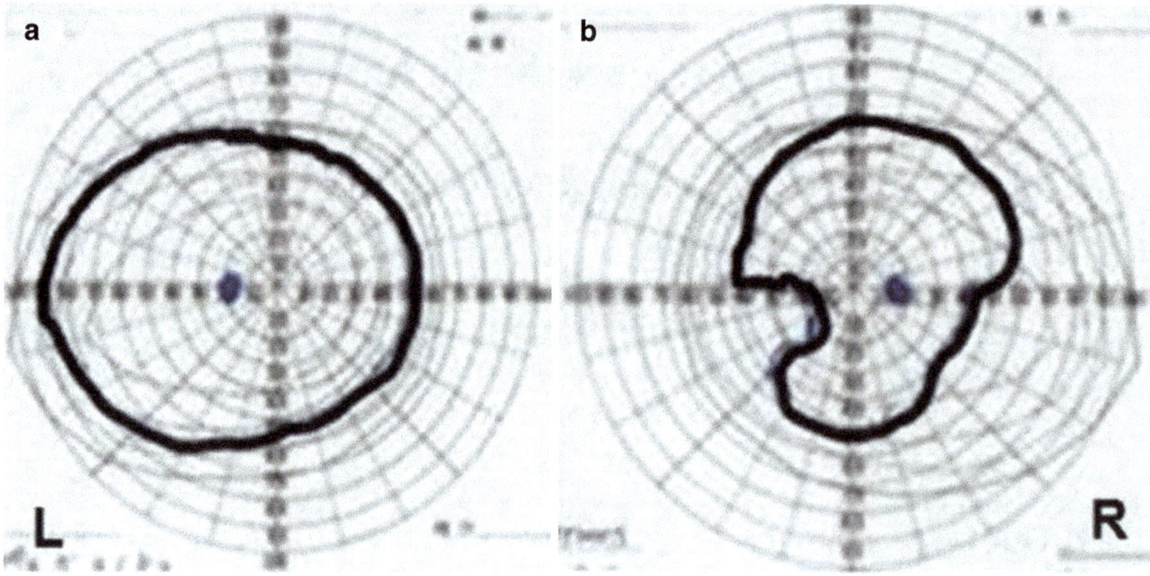

Fig. 13.1 Case 1. Visual field examination showing unilateral inferomedial quadrantanopsia on the right (**b**). Normal visual field on the left (**a**)

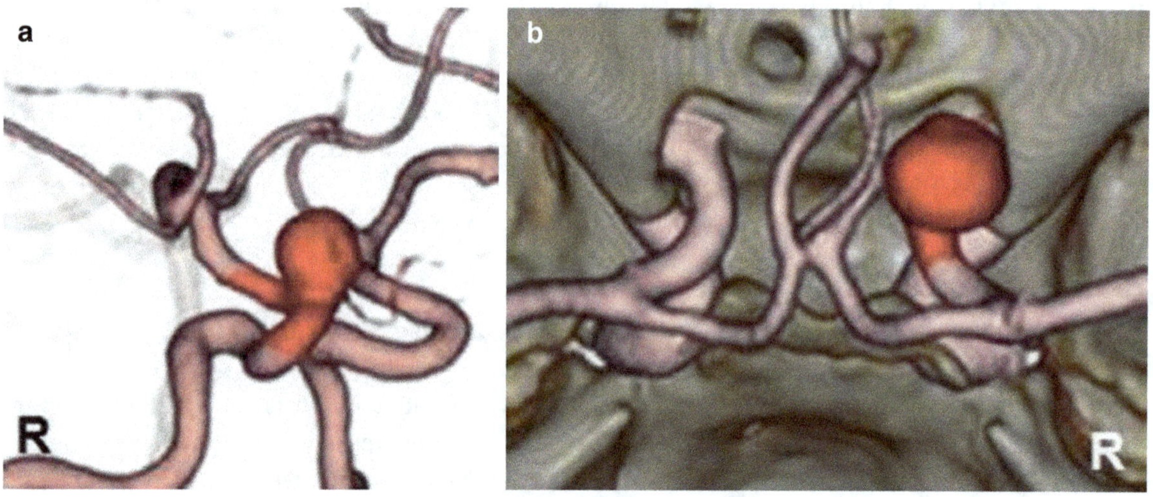

Fig. 13.2 Case 2. Three-dimensional computed tomography angiograms showing a paraclinoid aneurysm. (**a**) Oblique view. (**b**) superior view

13.2 Investigation

The ICA that is located along the anterior clinoid process (ACP), between proximal and distal dural ring (DDR), is called clinoid segment (usually referred as C3). After passing the distal dural ring (DDR), the ICA actually runs in the subarachnoid space. From DDR to the origin of the PCoA is called ophthalmic segment. In order to make it clear, the term paraclinoid aneurysm is the aneurysm that originates from the ICA between the PDR and the PCoA (or in the other

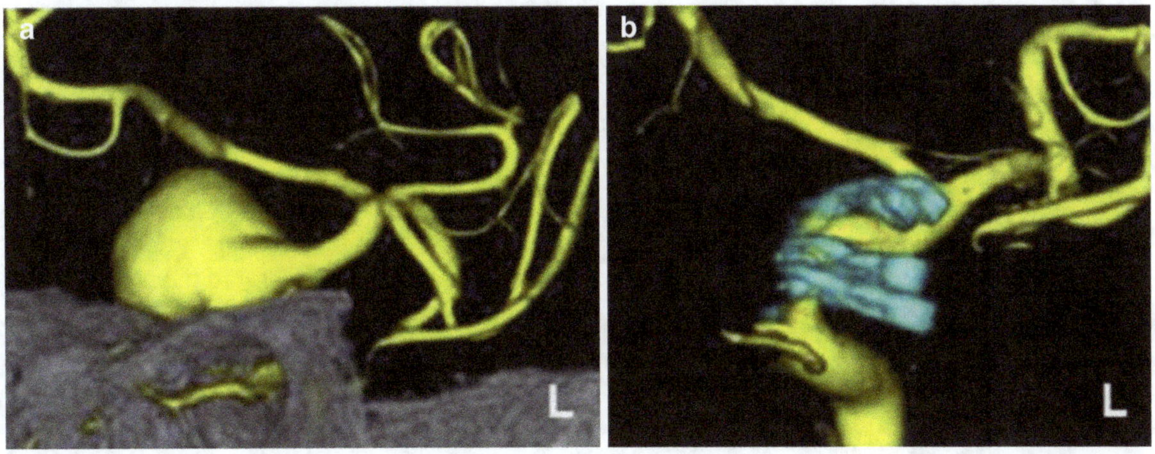

Fig. 13.3 Case 2. (**a**) Preoperative three-dimensional computed tomography angiogram showing a paraclinoid aneurysm. (**b**) Postoperative three-dimensional computed tomography angiogram showing complete clipping of the aneurysm

words, between the clinoid and ophthalmic segments). Paraclinoid aneurysms can be classified as ophthalmic aneurysm (which arise from superior part of ICA), superior hypophyseal aneurysm (which arise from the inferomedial part of ICA), supra-clinoid aneurysm which arise from anterior wall of ICA, and the infra-clinoid aneurysm which arise from posterior wall of ICA. These aneurysms are usually surrounded by bony and neurovascular anatomy, namely, ophthalmic artery, optic nerve, oculomotor nerve, and ACP (Figs. 13.4 and 13.5). The most important step in the dissection for this aneurysm is to release the aneurysm dome from optic nerve and ACP.

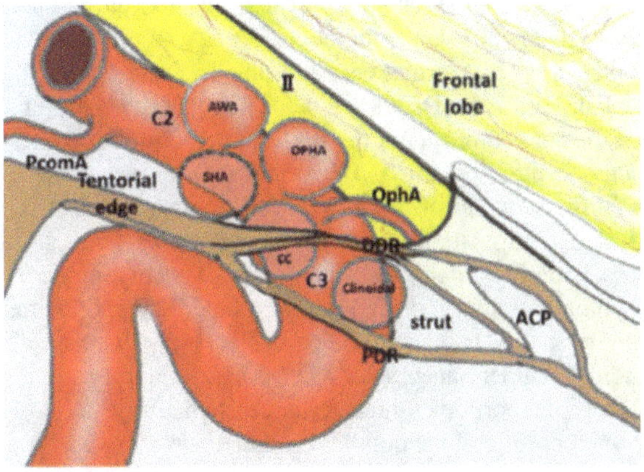

Fig. 13.4 Illustration of paraclinoid aneurysm. The clinoid segment (C3) of the internal carotid artery (ICA) runs along the anterior clinoid process (ACP), passing between the proximal (PDR) and distal dural rings (DDR), and the ophthalmic segment (C2) courses from the DDR to the posterior communicating artery (PCoA). Paraclinoid aneurysm originates from the ICA between the PDR and the PCoA (clinoid and ophthalmic segments). Paraclinoid aneurysms are classified as ophthalmic, anterior wall type located on the anterior wall of the ICA, superior hypophyseal, carotid cave type, and clinoidal segment aneurysms located on the infero-medial wall of the ICA, and variant aneurysms. Paraclinoid aneurysms are surrounded by many important osseous and neurovascular structures such as the ACP, optic nerve (II), oculomotor nerve, ICA, and ophthalmic artery (OphA). *AWA* anterior wall aneurysm, *OphA* ophthalmic artery aneurysm, *SHA* superior hypophyseal artery aneurysm, *CC* carotid cave aneurysm, *clinoidal* clinoidal segment aneurysm, *strut* optic strut

13.3 Preoperative Preparation

13.3.1 Neuroimaging Examinations

Bone CT is useful to investigate paraclinoid aneurysm. The size, shape, and pneumatization of the ACP and surrounding sinus, such as sphenoid and ethmoid, all should be assessed for safe clinoidectomy. Calcification of the proximal ICA should be examined for safe proximal control just before clip application.

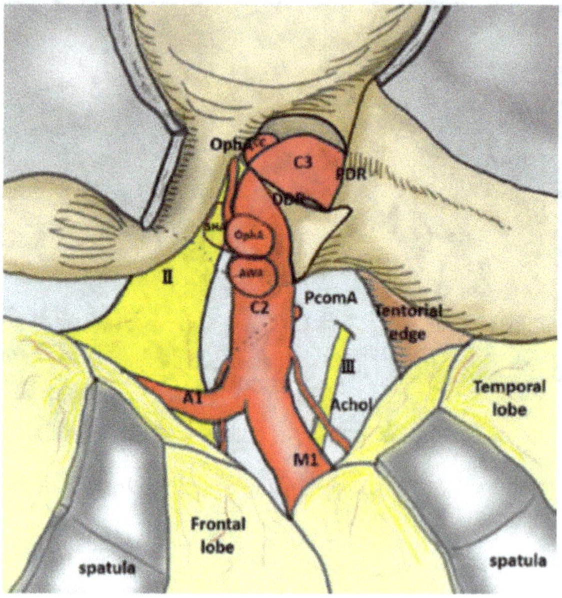

Fig. 13.5 Illustration of treatment of paraclinoid aneurysm via the anterolateral approach. Incision of the falciform ligament to the optic nerve is made to mobilize the optic nerve (II). Additional incision is made across the distal dural ring (DDR) to expose and identify the origin of the ophthalmic artery (OphA) and to mobilize the internal carotid artery (ICA). *III* oculomotor nerve, *C2* ophthalmic segment of the ICA, *C3* clinoid segment of the ICA, *PCoA* posterior communicating artery, *Achol* anterior choroidal artery, *AWA* anterior wall aneurysm, *OphA* ophthalmic artery aneurysm, *SHA* superior hypophyseal artery aneurysm, *CC* carotid cave aneurysm, *clinoidal* clinoidal segment aneurysm, *PDR* proximal dural ring, *A1* horizontal portion of the anterior cerebral artery, *M1* horizontal portion of the middle cerebral artery

Few contraindications to do anterior clinoidectomy extradurally are caroticoclinoid foramen (Fig. 13.6a) and the interclinoid ligament (Fig. 13.6b); both should be assessed preoperatively [2]. 3D-CT angiography with or without DSA are mandatory to investigate paraclinoid aneurysm. Meningo-orbital artery (MOA) forming the main collateral to the retinal artery cannot be resected. The development of the superficial Sylvian vein and the circulation pattern of the sphenoparietal sinus should be evaluated in the venous phase, which may show contraindication for dural peeling of the lateral cavernous sinus in extradural anterior clinoidectomy. The role of (MR) imaging is helpful to show the relationship of the dome and the optic nerve, using constructive interference in steady-state sequence.

13.3.2 Suction Decompression

Suction decompression via the cervical carotid artery and detachment of aneurysm from the nearby anatomical structures (e.g., optic nerve) are necessary for big and giant aneurysm. We also may prepare the carotid at cervical level to use it as a proximal control or angiography during surgery (Fig. 13.7).

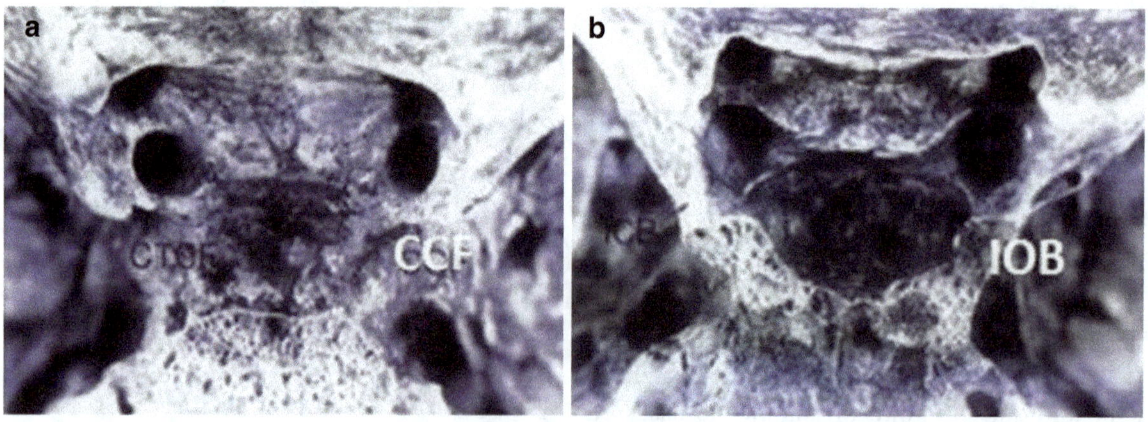

Fig. 13.6 Contraindications for anterior clinoidectomy such as caroticoclinoid foramen (**a**, CCF) and interclinoid osseous bridge (**b**, IOB) should be assessed preoperatively

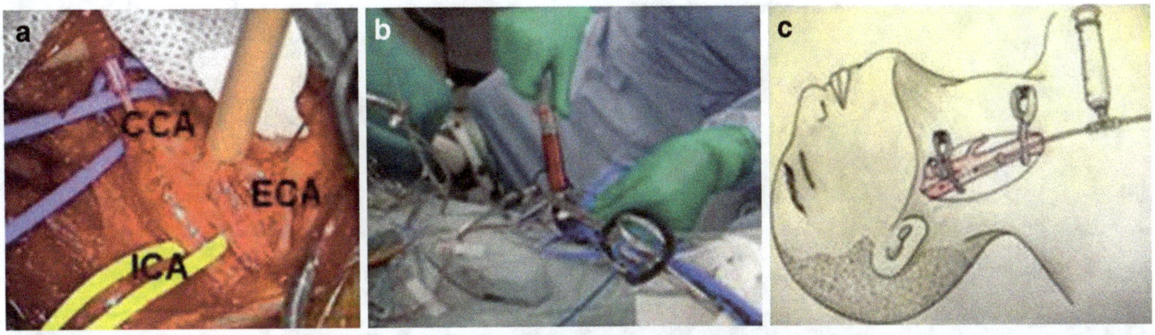

Fig. 13.7 Suction decompression (**b** and **c**) to expose and secure the cervical carotid artery (**a**) also helps proximal control of the internal carotid artery (ICA). *CCA* common carotid artery, *ECA* external carotid artery

13.3.3 Bypass Procedure (Revascularization)

High-flow bypass should be prepared, if necessary. If the aneurysm cannot be clipped for any technical reasons, either it calcified at the neck area or sclerotic, then bypass surgery is necessary from extracranial carotid artery to M2 segment of MCA; we may use the radial artery or saphenous vein.

13.3.4 Intraoperative Angiography

During surgery, it is necessary to confirm complete secure of the aneurysm and also needs to confirm the preservation of branches and parent artery flow, by using the intraoperative angiography. Therefore, the radiolucent Mayfield head clamp is helpful.

13.3.5 Spinal Drainage

There is some advantages of spinal drainage to enhance the brain relaxation during surgery, which enable to get more wide epidural space during extradural surgical procedure. In addition, these procedures may reduce the occurence of CSF leakage postoperatively.

13.3.6 Intraoperative Monitoring

Intraoperative monitoring of the motor-evoked potential (Fig. 13.8b) and visual-evoked potential (Fig. 13.8a) is mandatory for safe clipping.

13.3.7 Instruments for Anterior Clinoidectomy

A 6-mm coarse burr drill is useful for removing the lateral part of sphenoid bone. Sharp dissectors are needed for gently detaching lateral wall of cavernous sinus. A 2-mm or 3-mm coarse burr drill is useful for drilling of the ACP. In addition, an irrigation suction system, micro-rongeur, and micro-punch are necessary to minimize mechanical or avoid heating the optic nerve.

13.3.8 Approach

As mentioned before, removing of ACP is one of the very important steps to have a safe clipping of paraclinoid aneurysm. The pterional trans-Sylvian approach with intradural anterior clinoidectomy and the Dolenc approach of combined extradural and intradural clinoidectomy are usually used to treat paraclinoid aneurysms, but both approaches have advantages and

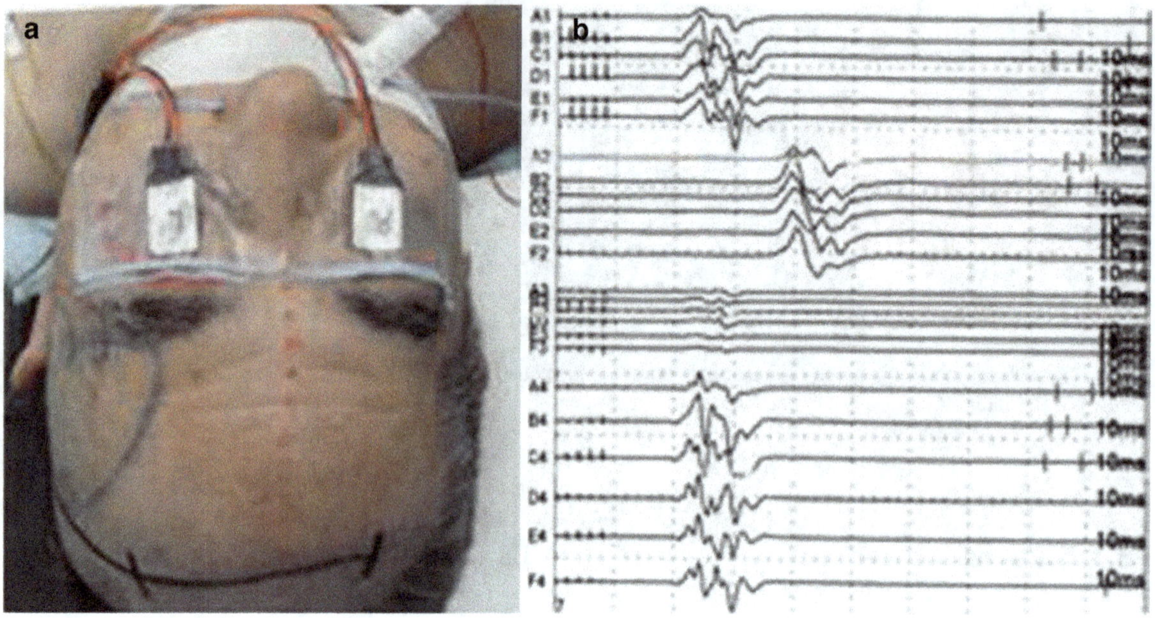

Fig. 13.8 Preparation for intraoperative visual-evoked potential (**a**) and motor-evoked potential monitoring (**b**)

disadvantages [3]. The pterional trans-Sylvian approach with intradural anterior clinoidectomy has the advantage of adequate exposure to dissect the aneurysm but carries a critical risk of destructive injury of the ICA, optic nerve, and aneurysm, even if protected by the dural flap. The extradural temporopolar approach is an epidural approach involving the moving of temporal lobe posteriorly with the dura mater [4, 5] and includes extradural anterior clinoidectomy, optic canal opening, detaching lateral wall of cavernous sinus, and then retraction of temporal lobe over the dura mater. Such epidural temporal lobe retraction is less likely to cause temporal lobe contusion and critical injury during anterior clinoidectomy.

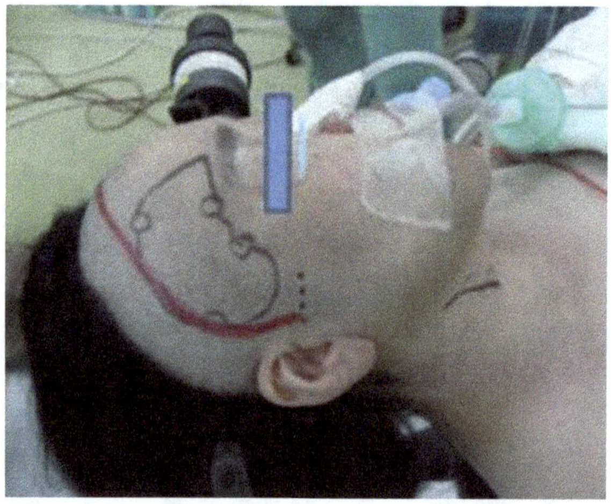

Fig. 13.9 Scheduled skin incision and frontotemporal craniotomy

13.4 Steps of the Surgery

13.4.1 Patient Position

After the patient was put to sleep and placement of the lumbal drain for CSF aspiration, the patient is placed in supine position and head rotated to contralateral side of operative field about 30°, slightly extended to have the anterior cranial fossa perpendicular to the floor. Neck should be slightly extended and elevated to avoid venous congestion. Additional slight lateral extension of the head helps to expose the carotid ICA (Fig. 13.9).

13.4.2 Skin Incision

The skin is cut half coronal and then inter-fascial separation is performed. Retract the temporal muscle to inferior without incision. The cervical common carotid artery, ICA and ECA will be prepared for many purposes later on such as proximal control, angiography during surgery, suction decompression if necessary, or even high-flow bypass if the patient needs it.

13.4.3 Craniotomy

Frontotemporal (pterional) bone flap is opened until supraorbital notch, the squama part of the temporal bone is removed until we expose the middle cranial floor, and on top of that we could add osteotomy of orbitozygomatic, if orbitozygomatic approach is needed for a large or giant aneurysm. It is easier to cut the orbitozygomatic bar in the two-piece method. Subperiosteal dissection is done for frontal and temporal. Then drill the lesser wing of the sphenoid until it becomes flat, and combine with the use of a rongeur; it is necessary to expose the meningo-orbital band. Keep dissecting the dura, and expose the superior orbital fissure (SOF) and foramen rotundum (Fig. 13.10). After the roof of the SOF is exposed, we need to identify intersection of periosteal dura and dura propria of temporal lobe. The bone around the meningo-orbital band needs to be drilled, and then incise the band about 4-mm length (Fig. 13.11). Gently detach the dura propria from the lateral wall of the SOF in order to expose ACP from extradural (Fig. 13.12). It is important to preserve sphenoparietal sinus while detaching dura propria and stop detaching at location where the cavernous sinus receives the blood from the sphenoparietal sinus. It is done to avoid venous congestion postoperatively.

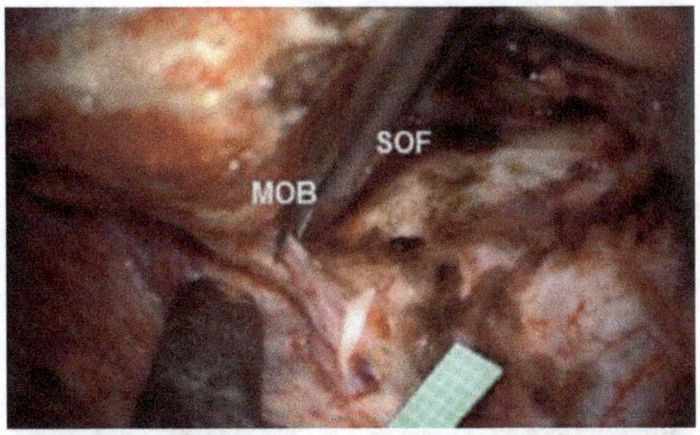

Fig. 13.11 Cutting the meningo-orbital band (MOB). *SOF* superior orbital fissure

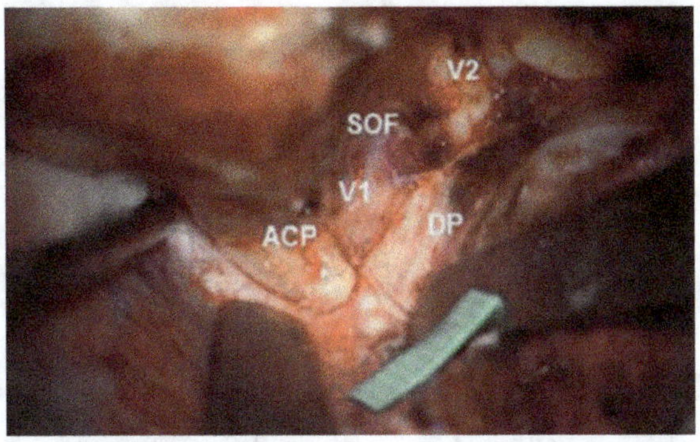

Fig. 13.12 After peeling of the dura propria (DP) of the temporal dura mater and epidural exposure of the anterior clinoid process (ACP). *V1* ophthalmic branch of the trigeminal nerve, *V2* maxillary branch of the trigeminal nerve, *SOF* superior orbital fissure

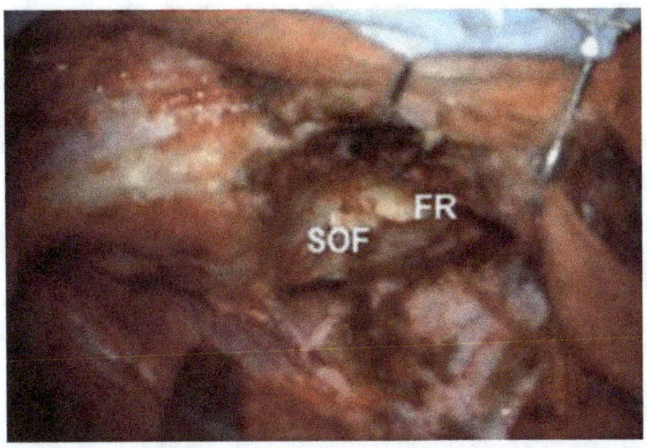

Fig. 13.10 After frontotemporal craniotomy. The foramen rotundum (FR) and superior orbital fissure (SOF) are exposed

13.4.4 Opening the Optic Canal and then Complete Removal of ACP

Orbital roof is drilled gently until it is as thin as the eggshell layer. Following the SOF laterally, identify the base of ACP, and then open the orbit at its posterior part. Expose the periorbital, and detach it from inside of orbit with preservation of the periorbital fat. The optic nerve is identified as it exits the optic canal. Start drilling the ACP from lateral to medial part; having plenty of saline irrigation is needed to avoid heat injury. Open the optic canal at medial part of ACP by using

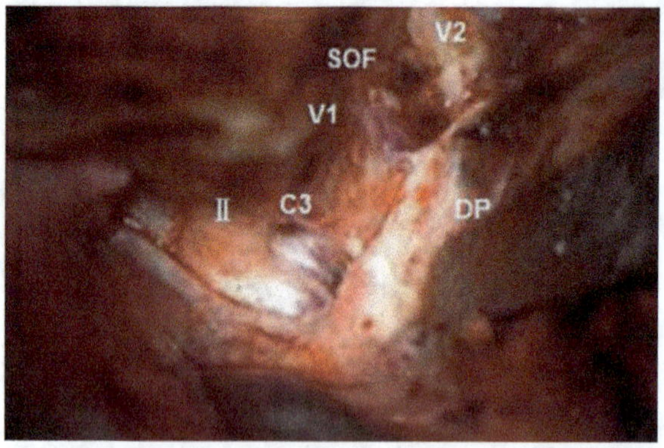

Fig. 13.13 Completion of epidural procedures after removal of the anterior clinoid process and opening of the optic canal. *II* optic nerve, *V1* ophthalmic branch of the trigeminal nerve, *V2* maxillary branch of the trigeminal nerve, *C3* clinoid segment of the internal carotid artery, *DP* dura propria, *SOF* superior orbital fissure

micro-punch, with thinning of the bone along the medial and anterior surfaces of the clinoid process. Drill the core of ACP by using 2-mm coarse diamond, and then it's dissected away from carotid-oculomotor membrane. At the end, we may gently remove ACP, and it usually will be followed with cavernous sinus bleeding and easily be managed with cottonoid and fibrin glue (Fig. 13.13).

13.4.5 Removing Optic Strut to Insert the Clip Blades

The half opening of optic canal can be enlarged by a micro-punch, and the rest of the optic strut (between the opened clinoid space and optic canal) can be taken by small diamond drill or using a fine micro-punch to get a space for clip blade insertion.

13.4.6 Open the Dura and Sylvian Fissure Dissection

The dura is opened following the Sylvian fissure and then extended inferiorly and medially to reach the optic nerve level. Wide dissection of Sylvian fissure helps to minimize brain retraction when we need to expose the optic nerve and ICA. During the dissection, it is necessary to identify the PCoA and anterior choroidal artery. In addition, horizontal portion of anterior cerebral artery must be dissected.

13.4.7 Cutting Falciform Ligament and DDR

Sharp cut of falciform ligament to the optic nerve is made with microscissors in order to be able to move the optic nerve (Fig. 13.14). Another cut is made across the DDR; the purpose is to find ophthalmic artery origin and to get more room to mobilize the ICA (Fig. 13.15).

13.4.8 Clip Application

The dome projection and the relationships between the parent artery and aneurysm dome

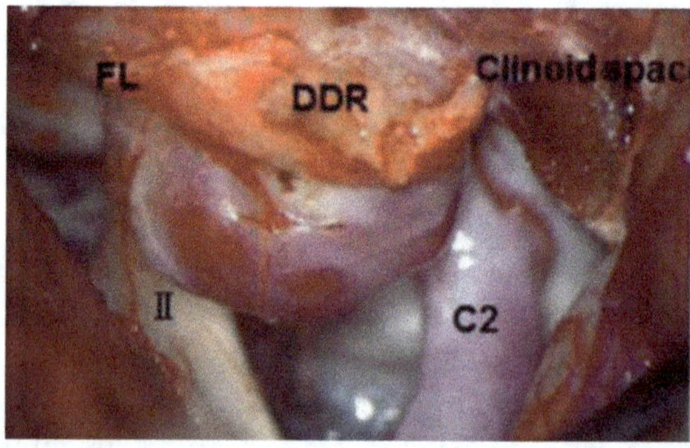

Fig. 13.14 The falciform ligament (FL) and the distal dural ring (DDR) are incised. *II* optic nerve, *C2* ophthalmic segment of the internal carotid artery

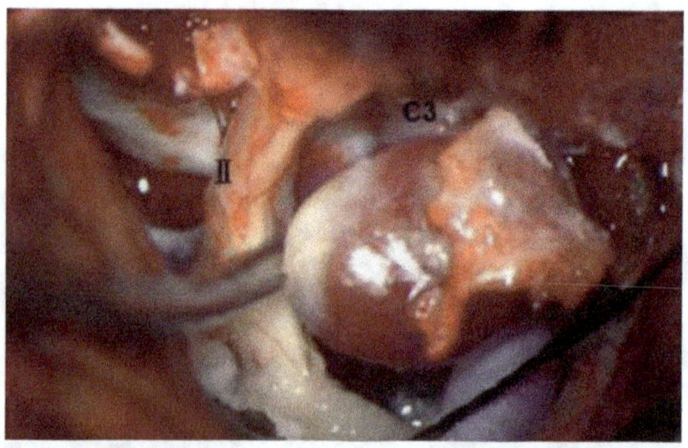

Fig. 13.15 Additional incision is made across the distal dural ring to expose and identify the origin of the ophthalmic artery and to mobilize the internal carotid artery (ICA). *II* optic nerve, *C3* clinoid segment of the ICA

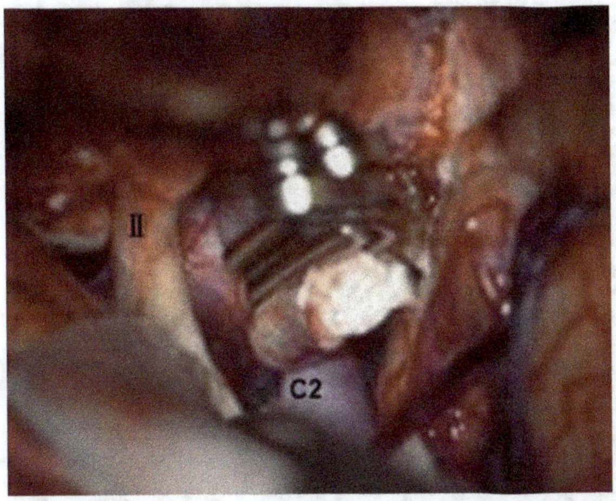

Fig. 13.16 After neck clipping of the paraclinoid aneurysm. *II* optic nerve, *C2* ophthalmic segment of the internal carotid artery

depend on the clip selection [1, 6, 7]. In most situation, the supra-clinoid-type or small ophthalmic artery aneurysms just require a simple straight or slightly curve clip (Fig. 13.16). Side-curved clips also can be used for its configuration. In contrast, angled fenestrated clips are typically required for infra-clinoid-type aneurysms such as superior hypophyseal artery aneurysms or carotid cave aneurysms, particularly large or giant aneurysms.

13.4.9 Suction Decompression (If Necessary)

Suction decompression is useful for detachment of aneurysm dome from the adjacent neurovascular structure such as optic nerve (Fig. 13.17).

13.4.10 Hemostasis and Closure

If during the clinoid drilling we get in to the ethmoidal cells, the chance of CSF leakage is high. It is necessary to pack the ethmoidal cells with periosteum or fat and then sealed with fibrin glue. Skull is fixed with titanium plates, a subcutaneous drain is placed, and the wound is closed as usual.

13.5 Expert Opinion/Suggestion to Avoid Complication

13.5.1 Avoiding Visual Disturbance (Optic Nerve Injury)

Continuous irrigation with cold water is mandatory during drilling procedures to avoid heat injury. While dissecting the aneurysm from optic nerve, meticulous manipulation and minimal use of bipolar coagulation are extremely important to spare the microvessels of the optic nerve. Suction decompression is also useful to perform complete dissection safely without optic nerve injury.

13.5.2 Avoiding CSF Leakage (Rhinorrhea)

The presence of sphenoidal sinus extension into the ACP (pneumatization) should be assessed preoperatively. During drilling of the ACP, avoid going in to optic recess of sphenoid sinus or even ethmoid air cells. The dural ring needs to be sealed with temporal fascia and fibrin glue. Spinal drainage is useful to prevent CSF leakage postoperatively, and it should be maintained for several day.

13.5.3 Intraoperative Rupture of the Aneurysm

The cervical ICA is secured for proximal control.

13.5.4 Occlusion and Injury of Ophthalmic Artery or ICA

The course of ophthalmic artery must be confirmed just before cutting the DDR and after clip placement. Intraoperative angiography or indocyanine green videoangiography is useful to check preservation of the parent artery and complete clipping.

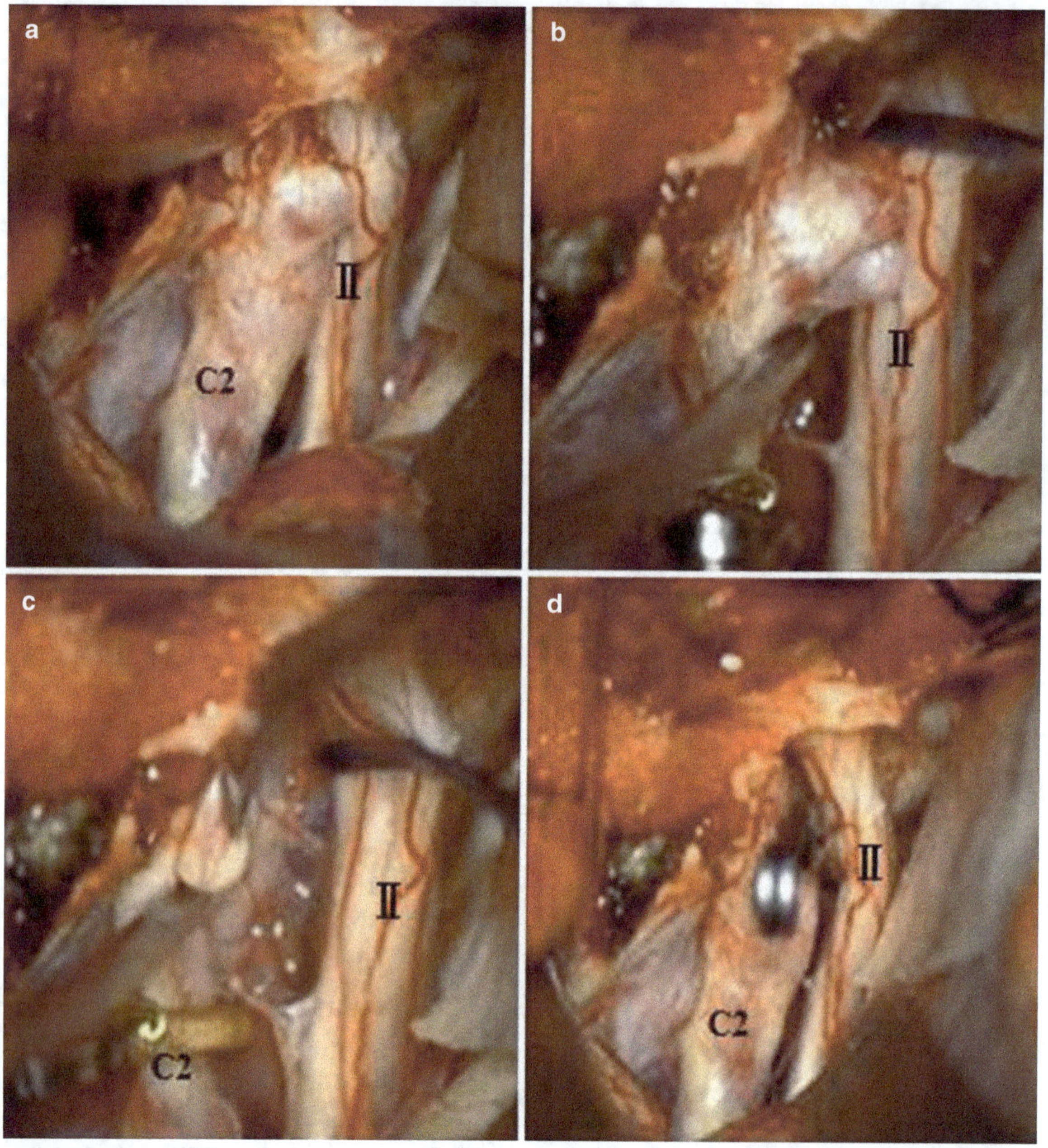

Fig. 13.17 Suction decompression (**b** and **c**) is useful for detachment of the aneurysm dome from the surrounding anatomical structures such as the optic nerve (II) (**a**) and for complete clipping (**d**). *C2* ophthalmic segment of the internal carotid artery

13.6 Things to Be Observed and Postoperative Care/Follow-Up

3D-CT angiography or MR angiography is for postoperative confirmation of complete aneurysm occlusion and ensures patency of parent artery. Close observation and treatment are needed if vasospasm occurs in patients with ruptured aneurysm. CSF leakage and visual disturbance should be closely monitored postoperatively.

References

1. Day AL. Aneurysms of the ophthalmic segment. A clinical and anatomical analysis. J Neurosurg. 1990;72:677–91.

2. Erturk M, Kayalioglu G, Gousa F. Anatomy of the clinoidal region with special emphasis on the caroticoclinoid foramen and interclinoid osseous bridge in a recent Turkish population. Neurosurg Rev. 2004;27:22–6.
3. Dolenc VV. A combined epi- and subdural direct approach to carotid-ophthalmic artery aneurysms. J Neurosurg. 1985;62:667–72.
4. Day JD, Giannotta SL, Fukushima T. Extradural temporopolar approach to lesions of the upper basilar artery and infrachiasmatic region. J Neurosurg. 1994;81:230–5.
5. Mori K, Yamamoto T, Nakao Y, Esaki T. Surgical simulation of extradural anterior clinoidectomy through the trans-superior orbital fissure approach using a dissectable three-dimensional skull base model with artificial cavernous sinus. Skull Base. 2010;20:229–36.
6. Giannota SL. Ophthalmic segment aneurysm surgery. Neurosurgery. 2002;50:558–62.
7. Heros RC, Nelson PB, Ojemann RG, Crowell RM, DeBrun G. Large and giant paraclinoid aneurysms: surgical techniques, complications and results. Neurosurgery. 1983;12:153–63.

14 Surgery of Anterior Communicating Artery Aneurysms

Yoko Kato, Mohsen Nouri, and Guowei Shu

14.1 Sign and Symptoms

Anterior communicating artery (AComA) aneurysms are among the most common aneurysms in different case series. They compose 36 of 175 cases (20.6%) in our latest case series of unruptured aneurysms coming second only after middle cerebral artery aneurysms (69 cases) [1]. In case series of ruptured aneurysms, the incidence is higher, and around 30–40% of all intracranial aneurysms are located in the AcomA region. Their presentation with subarachnoid hemorrhage (SAH) is not essentially different from other aneurysms and will not be repeated in this chapter again. Here, we do not intend to make an exhaustive review of different aspects of medical, interventional, or surgical management of these aneurysms. Instead, we will explain the most important pre-, intra-, and postoperative aspects observed in our institute.

Y. Kato (✉)
Department of Neurosurgery, Fujita Health University, Toyoake, Aichi, Japan
e-mail: kyoko@fujita-hu.ac.jp

M. Nouri
Gundishapour Academy of Neuroscience, Ahvaz, Iran
e-mail: nouri@gan-ac.ir

G. Shu
Department of Neurosurgery, Shuguang Hospital, Shanghai University of Traditional Chinese Medicine, Shanghai, China

14.2 Investigation

To evaluate any patient with subarachnoid hemorrhage or any candidate for aneurysm screening, we request 3D CT angiography (CTA), and digital subtraction angiography is performed only when 3D-CTA is negative for any aneurysm in spite of high clinical suspicion for one [2].

There are important anatomical points which should be paid attention on CTA that may affect our decision-making before or during the operation. Aneurysm projection, the location of neck and dome of aneurysm, its height and distance from the planum sphenoidale, and most condition of A2 fork are the factors affecting our surgical planning. Here, we describe the most important factors and explain how they are pivotal for decision-making.

14.2.1 Aneurysm Projections

Figure 14.1 demonstrates four types of projections of AComA aneurysms.

Each of these projections may obscure some portions of the contralateral A1, A2, or optic nerve which is dependent on the side of the approach.

Posterior projecting aneurysms require special attention: very important tiny perforators are stretched over the posterior wall of these aneu-

J. July, E. J. Wahjoepramono (eds.), *Neurovascular Surgery*,
https://doi.org/10.1007/978-981-10-8950-3_14

rysms. When approached from the side with A2 posterior to the aneurysm, the neck or the posterior stretched perforating arteries cannot be reached and dissected efficiently.

14.2.2 A2 Fork

Bilateral A2s and the AComA are named A2 fork. At the level of AComA, one A2 is usually anterior to the other making the AComA run obliquely instead of in the coronal plane.

When the complex is approached from the side with the anteriorly located A2, the AComA is hidden behind it, and so, the complex is called closed A2 fork. In contrary, when the same complex is approached from the side with the A2 located posteriorly, the AComA is very well visible, and the complex is named open A2 fork (Fig. 14.1).

We approach the AComA aneurysms from the side with open A2 fork because the neck of the aneurysm is usually anterior or superior to the AComA and visible from this side. Posterior-looking aneurysms are exception to this rule, as their neck is

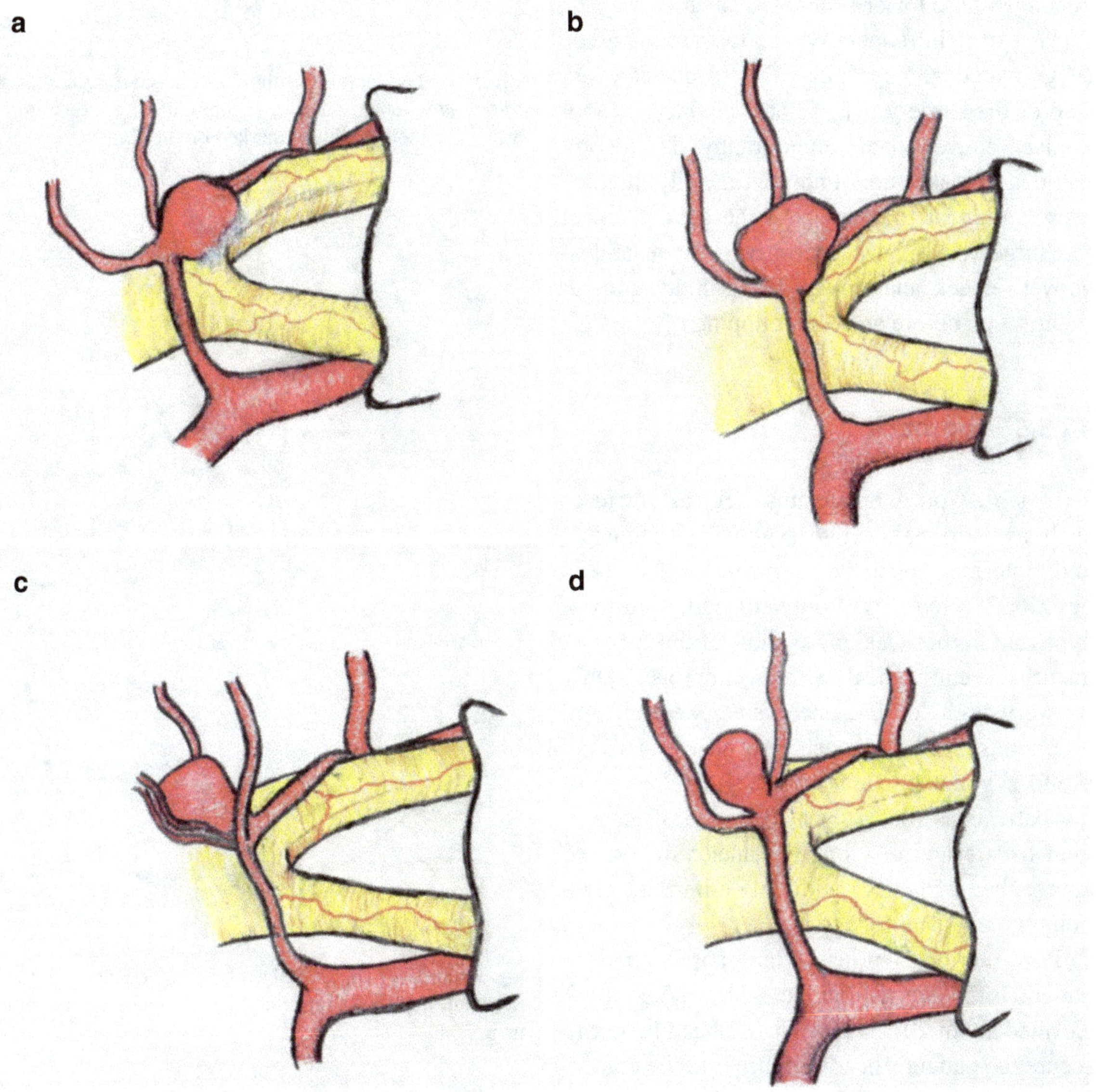

Fig. 14.1 Different projections of anterior communicating artery aneurysms. (**a**) Inferior-, (**b**) anterior-, (**c**) posterior-, and (**d**) superior-looking aneurysms. All the views are from open A2 fork except for the posterior-looking aneurysm (**d**) which is viewed from the close A2 angle (i.e., the ipsilateral A2 is anterior to the contralateral one). Anterior- and inferior-looking aneurysms (**a** and **b**) may conceal the contralateral A1

located posterior to the AComA and should be approached from the side with the closed fork.

14.3 Preoperative Preparation

Although recommended by some authors, inserting a lumbar drain to relax the brain is not necessary in our idea. We administer a dosage of mannitol (1 g/kg) just before the incision, and if blood pressure is not too low, we inject furosemide (20–40 mg) as well. Routine precautions for patient positioning (e.g., padding and elastic bandage of the lower limbs) are taken.

We use intraoperative indocyanine green (ICG) video angiography (VA) to check every step of the surgery [3]. If not available, intraoperative conventional angiography is recommended to make sure of appropriate clipping and preservation of the vessels at the conclusion of the surgery. Also, we use intraoperative endoscopy to check anatomical details hidden under microscope before and after clipping [4].

14.3.1 Approach

To reach AComA aneurysms, several corridors such as pterional, orbito-zygomatic extension, and interhemispheric approaches have been described. Here, we only explain pterional approach to these lesions as most of the AComA aneurysms can be dealt with this approach. Only for very high located aneurysms, we may use interhemispheric approach. We have not found orbito-zygomatic extension necessary for any of our patients as with proper dissection of the sylvian fissure and cisterns; the aneurysm can be approached without or with only minimal retraction on the frontal lobe.

For pterional transsylvian approach, the patient is positioned supine with his/her trunk elevated about 20°. We use Sugita head holder to secure the patient's head and turn it to the contralateral side between 30° and 45° (Fig. 14.2).

Incision is made 5 mm anterior to the tragus and superior to the zygomatic arc toward the midline (Fig. 14.2). A submuscular or interfascial temporalis flap is turned to expose the bony anatomy.

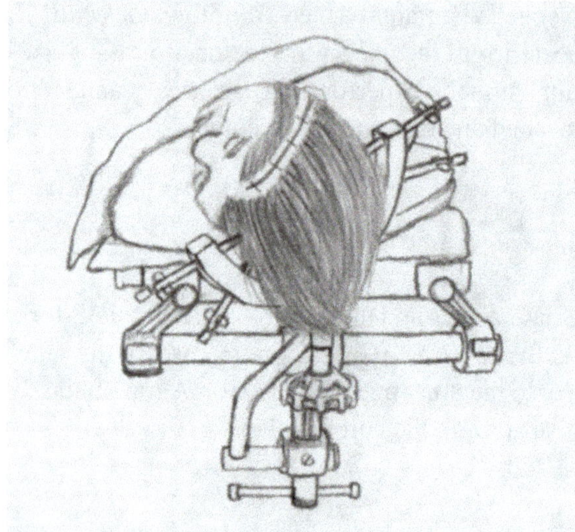

Fig. 14.2 Patient positioning for a classic frontotemporal craniotomy for an anterior communicating artery aneurysm. The incision line is marked on the skin

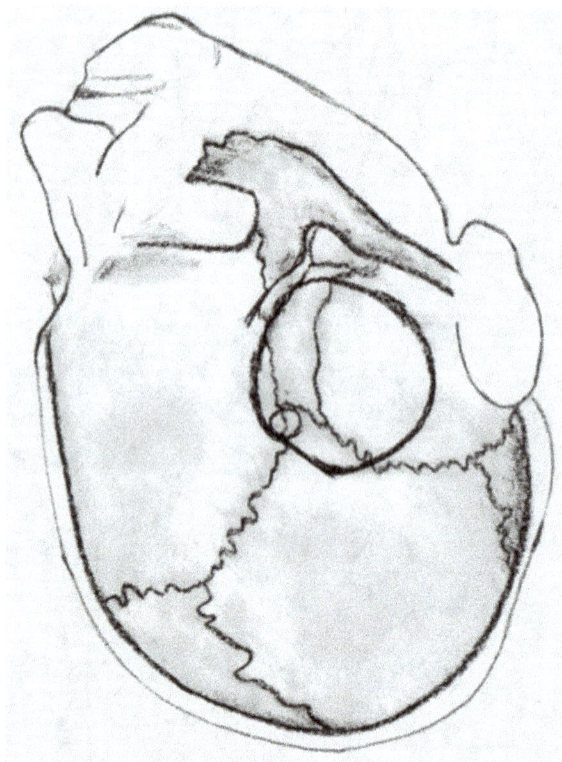

Fig. 14.3 The location of burr hole and craniotomy for a pterional approach for anterior communicating artery aneurysm

One burr hole above the pterion is made, and a fronto-temporo-sphenoidal bone flap is removed with the help of craniotome (Fig. 14.3). The sphenoid ridge is removed with a bone rongeur or high-speed drill. This step helps the surgeon to reach the aneurysm with less retraction on the frontal lobe as this bony structure may obscure the field of view. If required, the orbital roof can also be drilled and flattened for a better view of the aneurysm complex.

14.4 Steps of the Surgery

The dura is incised with its base toward the pterion (Fig. 14.4). Then, under microscopic magnification, the sylvian fissure is incised with a needle or arachnoid knife. This is important to open the arachnoid layer on the frontal side of the sylvian vein(s) to keep them safe on the temporal side while inserting retraction on the frontal lobe (Fig. 14.5). To have an appropriate view of the aneurysm complex, one should perform a wide sylvian fissure dissection to expose the complex with minimal retraction on the frontal lobe. Surgeon should keep it in mind to release the retractor every now and then to prevent ischemic injury to the frontal lobe.

While opening the sylvian arachnoid layers, a slight retraction on the frontal lobe should be exercised to keep the arachnoid membranes under tension: this makes the dissection with microscissors easier and safer as one can see behind the arachnoid layers. You can use a self-retraining retractor on the frontal lobe or may use a blunt suction with your non-dominant hand to retract the frontal lobe. The latter requires more experience but is more desirable as less retraction is exerted on the brain parenchyma. Copious or water jet irrigation helps with better sylvian fissure dissection especially in patients with ruptured aneurysms whose arachnoid layers are extremely adhesive. While dissecting the deep sylvian cistern, no artery should be cut, and extreme care should be exercised to preserve all the veins as much as possible. Fine arachnoid trabecula are separated and cut with sharp dissection or occasionally by gentle maneuvers of bipolar tips.

After reaching into the parasellar cisterns, we may require to change the trajectory of the microscope. There is an arachnoid layer connecting the optic nerve to the frontal lobe which we name "white line" or "Sano's line" (Fig. 14.6). This arachnoid is the first to be dissected after opening the sylvian fissure and should be cut 1 mm away from the frontal lobe to prevent any vascular injury to the brain which may result in cognitive symptoms. Dissecting this line allows the surgeon to mobilize the frontal lobe without retracting the optic complex. By opening the carotid cistern and cerebrospinal fluid (CSF) drainage, we will make the brain even more relax. Arachnoid layer between the ICA and the optic nerve should be dissected until reaching the ICA bifurcation. Dissection of the chiasmatic cistern helps with

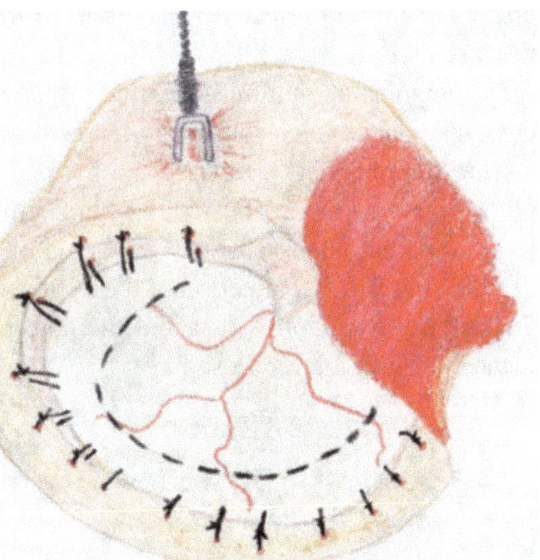

Fig. 14.4 A frontotemporal craniotomy after removing the bone flap. The sphenoid wing and the orbital roof will be flattened with a high-speed drill or bone rongeur. Base of the dura incision is toward the sphenoid wing

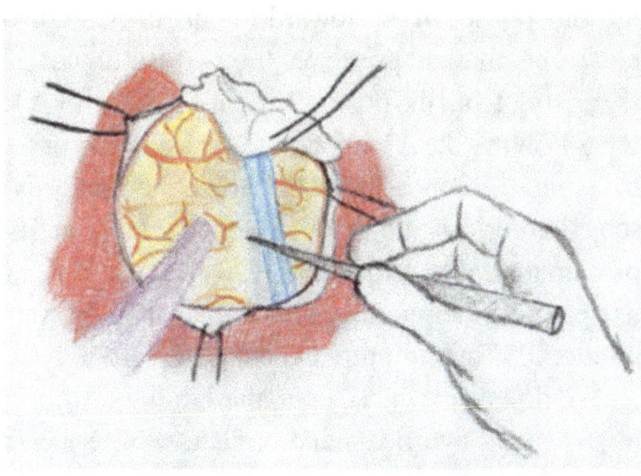

Fig. 14.5 The arachnoid layer between the superficial sylvian vein(s) and the frontal lobe is incised to dissect the sylvian fissure. Slight retraction is put on the frontal lobe to keep the arachnoid layer under constant tension to ease the dissection

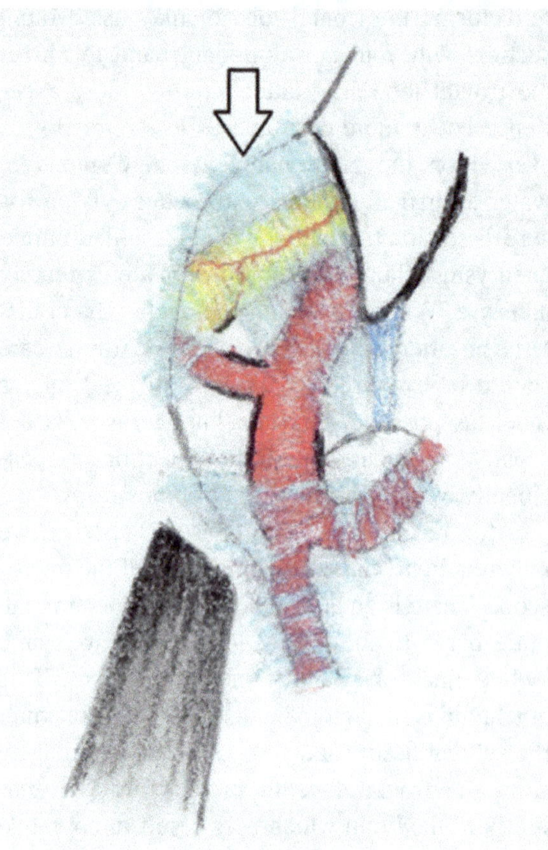

Fig. 14.6 Anterior basal cisterns around the carotid artery, its branches, and the optic nerve. The arrow is referring to the white line or "Sano's line": the arachnoid layer attaching the frontal lobe to the optic nerve

more CSF drainage and easier frontal lobe detachment from the optic apparatus. The cistern of the lamina terminalis should be opened along the inferior border of A1 toward the aneurysm complex. This method preserves the perforating arteries arising from the posterosuperior surface of A1. By following the A1 artery and crossing the optic chiasma, the contralateral A1 is reached and dissected inferiorly to be sure of the contralateral proximal control if needed. However, we do not use proximal temporary clips (either ipsi- or contralaterally) in unruptured aneurysms routinely.

We do not routinely open the lamina terminalis except in hydrocephalic patients where it has been shown to reduce the chance of shunt dependency in the future. When the surgeon decides to open the lamina terminalis, he/she should be careful not to injure optic chiasma inferiorly or anterior commissure superiorly.

14.4.1 Proximal Control Clipping

As mentioned above, we do not recommend routine application of proximal control clipping in all cases. In ruptured aneurysms and in large unruptured cases, we advocate proximal clipping to soften the aneurysm and keep on the safe side in case of any premature rupture. The best place for inserting the temporary clip is the middle third of the A1. A more proximally placed clip may injure the perforating arteries arising from the proximal half of A1, and a more distally placed clip may obscure the surgical view and interfere with proper dissection of the aneurysm neck.

14.4.2 Gyrus Rectus Resection

Dissecting and separating the interhemispheric fissure to expose an unruptured aneurysm are usually all needed. But for ruptured aneurysms where the interhemispheric fissure is adhesive and for large, high riding or posterior-looking unruptured aneurysms, resection of the adjacent gyrus rectus is recommended. For gyrus rectus resection, place the tip of blade just lateral to the A1 where it disappears in the fissure and medial to the olfactory nerve. Two arteries, namely, recurrent artery of Heubner and fronto-orbital artery should be protected and preserved during the resection.

Set bipolar at minimal possible voltage and coagulate the pia meter of the gyrus rectus. After cutting the pia, start removing the gyrus with a blunt-tipped suction. The medial pia should be left over the aneurysm to avoid inadvertent rupture (Fig. 14.7). Resection of the gyrus is safe as posterior as AComA to avoid the posteriorly located perforating arteries.

14.4.3 Aneurysm Dissection and Clipping

Before dissecting the aneurysm, bilateral A1 arteries should be dissected, and with a blunt dissector, check for the probable place of temporary blades. However, exposing the contralateral A1 may not

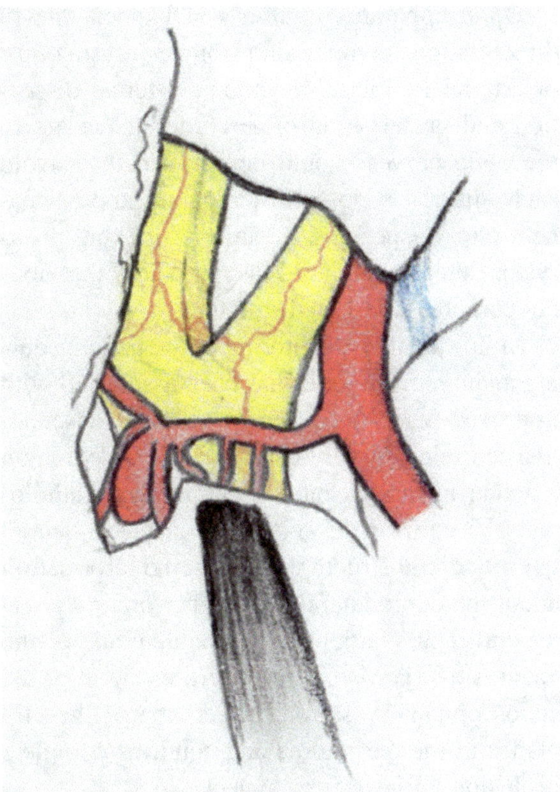

Fig. 14.7 After resecting the gyrus rectus, ipsi- and contralateral A2s should be dissected apart from the aneurysm neck to prepare it for the final clipping

be possible or safe in case of inferior or anterior-looking aneurysms. In this step of surgery, the ICG-VA and endoscope are helpful to localize tiny perforating arteries which should be dissected off the aneurysm. The neck of the aneurysm should be dissected before the dome as it is likely to rupture. Any time during dissection if the chance of rupture is felt, insert proximal temporary clips.

There are some general precautions for clipping these aneurysms. The clip should be applied as parallel as possible to the parent artery. Tips of the clip should not be too long to injure the perforators/structures behind the aneurysm. To check for this, one can use endoscope, ICG-VA, or Doppler ultrasound.

14.4.4 Superior Projecting Aneurysms

The aneurysm neck might be attached to the proximal A2 bilaterally. So, enough space for the blades of the clip should be cleared on proximal A2s and around the aneurysm neck. Before clipping, we usually check the contralateral proximal A2 with endoscope. Most AComA aneurysms can be obliterated with a straight aneurysm clip 1.5 times as much as the neck and parallel to the AComA. After clipping, contralateral A1–A2 complex and perforators should be checked with endoscope and ICG-VA.

14.4.5 Anterior Projecting Aneurysms

In these aneurysms, contralateral A1 and A1–A2 junction are usually obscured by the aneurysm. As dissection of the contralateral A1 is not possible before clipping the aneurysm, these aneurysms are usually approached from the side with dominant A1. A straight clip is usually applied parallel to the AComA to secure the aneurysm, and then, the patency of the contralateral A1 and A2 is checked with ICG-VA and endoscopy.

14.4.6 Inferior Projecting Aneurysms

The aneurysm dome is usually attached inferiorly to the optic chiasm, so, the frontal lobe should be retracted very gently to avoid premature rupture of these aneurysms. Again, as they cover the contralateral A1 artery, they should be approached from the side with dominant A1. A straight clip is usually needed to secure the neck. After clipping, the aneurysm should be dissected off the chiasma to release its pressure on optic system and check the patency of the contralateral A1 artery.

14.4.7 Posterior Projecting Aneurysms

As discussed earlier, these aneurysms are approached from the close A2 fork side. After dissecting behind the ipsilateral A2, the aneurysm is encountered with perforators stretched over its posterior wall. Hypothalamic artery that arises at the junction of A1–A2 is the most important perforator, though it is not present in all cases. Perforating arteries do not need to be entirely dissected off the aneurysm, and enough space for clip passage is all needed. A straight clip parallel to the AComA usually obliterates the aneurysm, but if the ipsilateral A2 is not mobilized anteriorly, a fenestrated clip to incorporate the A2 artery might be used. Again, check the integrity of the perforators and contralateral A2 at the conclusion of clipping.

14.5 Surgeon Plan to Handle the Complication

Immediate postoperative neurological deficits or incomplete recovery from anesthesia should be promptly worked up by a plain brain CT scan, and any major complication (e.g., surgical site hematoma) should be dealt with accordingly. As the normal brain CT scan does not rule out early cerebral ischemia, a vascular study and brain MRI might be indicated for further evaluation of the patient. Vasospasm after surgical treatment of ruptured aneurysms usually happens in distal anterior cerebral artery territories presenting with lower limb weakness. Though there is no strong evidence to support triple-H therapy, we keep the patient slightly hypertensive as soon as securing the aneurysm [5]. Nimodipine is administered prophylactically in all ruptured cases, and in case of symptomatic vasospasm, endovascular intra-arterial Papaverine is injected.

14.6 Expert Opinion/Suggestion to Avoid Complication

Venous infarction can happen due to prolonged brain retraction or coagulation of the veins during sylvian fissure dissection. Appropriate head and trunk positioning, wide sylvian fissure dissection with preserving the veins, extensive cisternal dissection and copious CSF drainage, and judicious gyrus rectus resection help the surgeon with exposing the aneurysm with minimal brain retraction. Intermittent release of the retractor should become a common practice to avoid venous drainage impairment and its consequences.

Optic apparatus injuries can happen due to direct trauma, compression from aneurysm clips, or arterial injuries. Meticulous cisternal dissection and preservation of tiny arterial feeders to the optic nerves should be performed to avoid such injuries. Also, both temporary and permanent clips (especially for inferior-looking aneurysms) should be placed in a trajectory that does not compress the visual structures.

Multimodality monitoring of the patients during aneurysm surgeries has been associated with improved outcome in recent years. Endoscope-assisted microsurgery of aneurysm is a common practice in many centers treating such pathologies. Visualizing the corners concealed behind the superficial structures gives some information about the contralateral A2 and perforating arteries and their relations to the hidden side of the aneurysm [4]. Also, after inserting the clip, the endoscopic view shows the relation of the clip blades to the perforators and confirms complete occlusion of the aneurysm neck.

Another monitoring modality is ICG-VA: it confirms appropriate occlusion of the aneurysm and the patency of the bilateral A2 and perforating arteries [3]. Though there are emerging data considering a role for FLOW 800 software of ICG-VA to quantify blood flow before and after clipping, we still do not rely on such semiquantitative data. Instead, whenever we want to measure blood flow and its changes before and after clipping (e.g., in aneurysms with severely atherosclerotic parent arteries), Doppler ultrasound (20 MHz probe) is used. Although recommended by some, we do not advocate routine intraoperative monitoring of somatosensory or motor-evoked potentials for these patients.

14.7 Things to Be Observed and Postoperative Care/Follow-Up

If the postoperative course is uneventful, we routinely perform 3D CT angiography and perfusion CT scan on the 7th postoperative day to check appropriate closure of the aneurysm neck and subclinical vasospasm on perfusion CT. However, if the patient develops neurological symptoms, an earlier CT angiography and brain MRI are performed, and if not conclusive, a digital subtraction angiography is requested. For patients presenting with SAH, nimodipine will be continued for at least 2 weeks from the attack and tapered in case of normal perfusion CT scan.

References

1. Yamada Y, Kato Y, Ishihara K, Ito K, Kaito T, Nouri M, Ohede M, Inamasu J, Hirose Y. Role of endoscopy in multi-modality monitoring during aneurysm surgery: a single centre experience with 175 consecutive unruptured aneurysms. Asian J Neurosurg. 2015;10(1):52.
2. Kumar A, Kato Y, Motoharu H, Sifang C, Junpei O, Takeya W, Shuei I, Daikichi O, Yuichi H. An update on three-dimensional CT angiography in aneurysms: a useful modality for a neurosurgeon. Turk Neurosurg. 2013;23(3):304–11.
3. Oda J, Kato Y, Chen SF, Sodhiya P, Watabe T, Imizu S, Oguri D, Sano H, Hirose Y. Intraoperative near-infrared indocyanine green-video angiography (ICG-VA) and graphic analysis of fluorescence intensity in cerebral aneurysm surgery. J Clin Neurosci. 2011;18(8):1097–100.
4. Kato Y, Sano H, Nagahisa S, Iwata S, Yoshida K, Yamamoto K, Kanno T. Endoscope-assisted microsurgery for cerebral aneurysms. Minim Invasive Neurosurg. 2000;43(2):91–7.
5. Dabus G, Nogueira RG. Current options for the management of aneurysmal subarachnoid hemorrhage-induced cerebral vasospasm: a comprehensive review of the literature. Intervent Neurol. 2013;2:30–51.

15 Surgery of Middle Cerebral Artery (MCA) Aneurysm

Fusao Ikawa

15.1 Sign and Symptoms

Middle cerebral artery (MCA) aneurysm is one of the most popular cerebral aneurysm. The incidence of ruptured MCA aneurysm is about 21% (which is the third incident). The first incident is anterior communicating artery (AcomA) aneurysm about 40%, and the second is internal carotid artery (ICA) aneurysm about 30% [1]. The most popular portion of MCA aneurysm is M1–M2 bifurcation, and the incidence is 80–85%. MCA aneurysms occasionally arise at the origin of the anterior temporal branch or at the origin of the lenticulostriate arteries. In the rare event that an MCA aneurysm occurs distally in the sylvian fissure, it may become a giant, heavily thrombosed aneurysm so-called giant serpentine aneurysm (Fig. 15.1) [2]. However, small aneurysm that arises far distally in the MCA is usually mycotic. MCA aneurysm can be bilateral and in patient with mirror aneurysms is sometimes difficult to determine which one has bled.

In the report according to the anatomical relationship of ruptured and unruptured MCA aneurysm, the factors of rupture by multivariate analysis were first perpendicular to the height/neck diameter, second flow angle, and third M1–M2 angle. MCA aneurysm is located relative superficial in sylvian fissure. It is relatively easy to find MCA aneurysm than other aneurysms. However, the neck dome ratio is larger than other aneurysms. Branches of the MCA may emerge from the sac or neck of MCA aneurysms, making their treatment quite complicated. Therefore, surgical clipping is preferable to coil embolization in treating MCA aneurysm even now. So, we neurosurgeons must learn harder about the feature, specificity, the method of simulation, intraoperative monitoring, and surgical technique of MCA aneurysm.

Overall patient outcomes are mostly determined by preoperative state, and the surgical-related morbidity is actually low. The preoperative poor Hunt-Hess grade is a strong indication endovascular coiling, except if they have a big temporal hematoma that needs to be evacuated. Also, some patient may benefit from hemicraniectomy. Open surgery may provide the chance to do reconstruction clipping of the majority MCA aneurysms; additional to that at the same time, surgeon may be able to do thrombectomy, bypass, or even entrapment of the aneurysm.

On the other hand, about unruptured MCA aneurysm, the number of registered unruptured MCA aneurysm has the most number in record, and the rate is 36%; however, rupture rate is half of AcomA and ICA aneurysm according to UCAS Japan [3]. In our experience, there is no permanent neurological deficit of 78 cases of unruptured MCA aneurysms [4].

F. Ikawa
Department of Neurosurgery, Shimane Prefectural Central Hospital, Izumo, Japan
e-mail: fikawa-nsu@umin.ac.jp

J. July, E. J. Wahjoepramono (eds.), *Neurovascular Surgery*,
https://doi.org/10.1007/978-981-10-8950-3_15

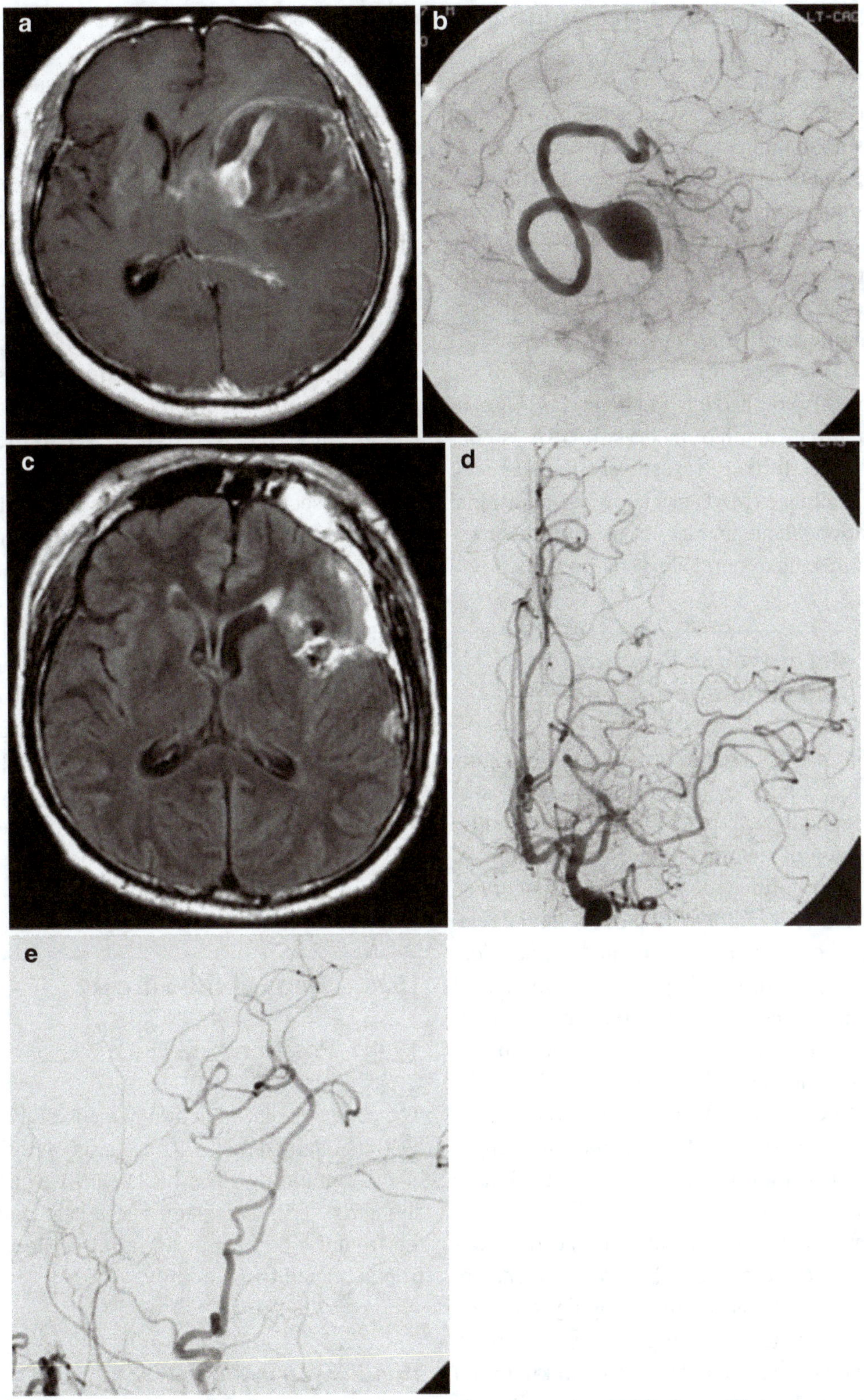

Fig. 15.1 Giant serpentine aneurysm. (**a**) Gd-enhanced MRI T1-wighted image revealed partial thrombosed giant aneurysm in left hemisphere. (**b**) Digital subtraction angiography(DSA) showed giant serpentine aneurysm in capillary phase. (**c**) Postoperative FLAIR image demonstrated disappearance of mass effect. (**d**) AP view of left internal carotid angiography showed no aneurysm. (**e**) Lateral view of left external carotid angiography showed middle cerebral artery from superficial temporal artery

15.2 Investigation and Imaging

Recently, the quality of computed tomography angiography (CTA) was improving. The first diagnostic imaging modality after subarachnoid hemorrhage (SAH) is CT scan, second diagnostic imaging modality about information of ruptured aneurysm is not digital subtraction angiography (DSA) but CTA now in almost institutes in Japan. Actually, we can operate surgical clipping only information by CTA without DSA. CTA have the information not only of the artery but also of the vein and bone. If CTA cannot reveal the ruptured aneurysm, DSA is considered for further investigation. Magnetic resonance image (MRI) can show the additional information about aneurysm of intra-aneurysmal thrombosis or perianeurysmal edema.

15.3 Preoperative Preparation and Simulation

Important preoperative informations by imaging are the following [5]: first the length of M1 segment, second the curvature of M1 segment, third the direction of aneurysm, fourth the location of rupture point, fifth the length between aneurysm and sylvian vein and/or skull base, sixth the relationship between aneurysm and sphenoidal ridge, and seventh the shape and the number of superficial sylvian vein. The preoperative simulation by 3D CTA is more useful because of the information not only of the artery but also of the vein and skull bone. We can decide the dissection point of sylvian fissure and the length between aneurysm and sylvian vein or skull base preoperatively.

In few straightforward cases, no need to routinely expose the entire M1 prior to aneurysm dissection. To translate the imaging information to the surgical planning is very important. The surgeon needs to address few thinking such as: how does he want to start the sylvian fissure dissection? How he should avoid premature rupture either by his retractor placement of his surgical maneuver? And where approximately the aneurysm located and where he will prepare for the proximal control?

On the anteroposterior (AP) view of the CTA, DSA, and MRA, it is important to evaluate the curvatures and length of the M1 to establish proximal control. Namely, when the M1 is straight and long, it is easy to expose the proximal M1 to the aneurysm by distal transsylvian approach. Regardless of the length of M1, if the M1 can curve downward toward the skull base, it is easier to just expose the M1 segment to the aneurysm by distal transsylvian approach. If the segment of M1 is long, we can capture more easily proximal M1 to the aneurysm by distal transsylvian approach, because direct dissection of sylvian fissure reaches the proximal M1 segment. However, aneurysms may be located superficially and within the temporal lobe. It is more dangerous to dissect the superficial sylvian fissure near the skull base, and distal and deep sylvian fissure are safer portion to dissect. When the M1 can be short and curve upward toward the anterior perforated substance and limen insula, it is difficult to expose the M1 segment only by distal transsylvian approach because M1 segment may be hidden by the anterior perforated substance and limen insula.

15.4 Steps of the Surgery

15.4.1 Position (Fig. 15.2)

The patient is placed in a supine position with the head maintained at 20–40° rotation opposite side of the craniotomy. The backboard was tilted up about 20°. With extension of the head and neck, the frontal lobe falls away from the floor of the frontal cranial fossa slightly.

15.4.2 Skin Incision (Fig. 15.3)

The hair is shaved partially even in the case of SAH, and cork screw electrodes for transcranial motor-evoked potential (MEP) are placed in both

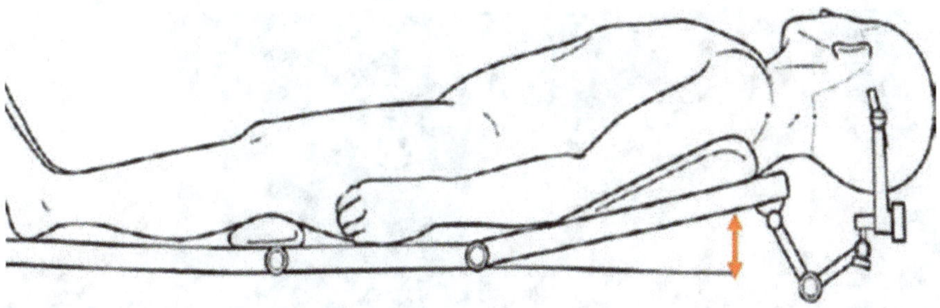

Fig. 15.2 Positioning. The patient is placed in a supine position with the head maintained at 20–40° rotation opposite side of the craniotomy. The back plate was tilted up about 20° (*arrow*). With extension of the head and neck, the frontal lobe falls away from the floor of the frontal cranial fossa slightly

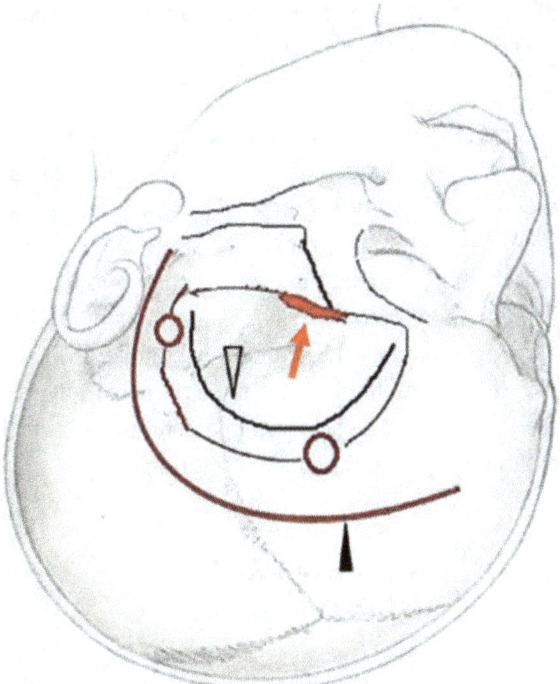

Fig. 15.3 Skin incision, craniotomy incision, and dural incision. Skin incision (*arrow head*) is from the front of ear to midline of forehead. With two burr hole, cosmetic osteotomy is performed by electric craniotomy. The pterion is cut by chisel and hammer with minimum bone defect (*arrow*). Superficial temporal artery (STA) should be preserved during skin incision. Semicircular dural incision (*open arrow*)

sides of the head (Fig. 15.4). Skin incision is from the front of ear to midline of forehead. Superficial temporal artery (STA) should be preserved during skin incision, because STA will be necessary in case of large or giant MCA aneurysm or troublesome cases.

15.4.3 Craniotomy (Fig. 15.3)

With two burr holes, cosmetic osteotomy is performed by electric craniotomy. The pterion is cut by chisel and hammer with minimum bone defect as much as possible. After removing the bone flap, the outer sphenoid wing is removed down to the meningo-orbital band. The outer sphenoid wing is removed with a rongeur. However, if a patient has a large or giant aneurysm or has a tight brain following SAH, the surgeon may also perform wide osteotomy, which entirely removes the pterion from the surgical field and thus increases the workspace. In the case of severe brain swelling due to SAH and sylvian hematoma, external decompression is performed.

15.4.4 Dural Incision (Fig. 15.3)

The dura mater is tacked to the bone margins. After the semicircular dural incision, dura is opened and reflected over the sphenoid wing and temporal muscle to prevent blood from running into the operative field.

15.4.5 Dissection of Sylvian Fissure

To expose an MCA aneurysm, the surgeon must open the sylvian fissure widely. First, we start by splitting the sylvian fissure from distal side, beginning approximately 4–5 cm posterior to the

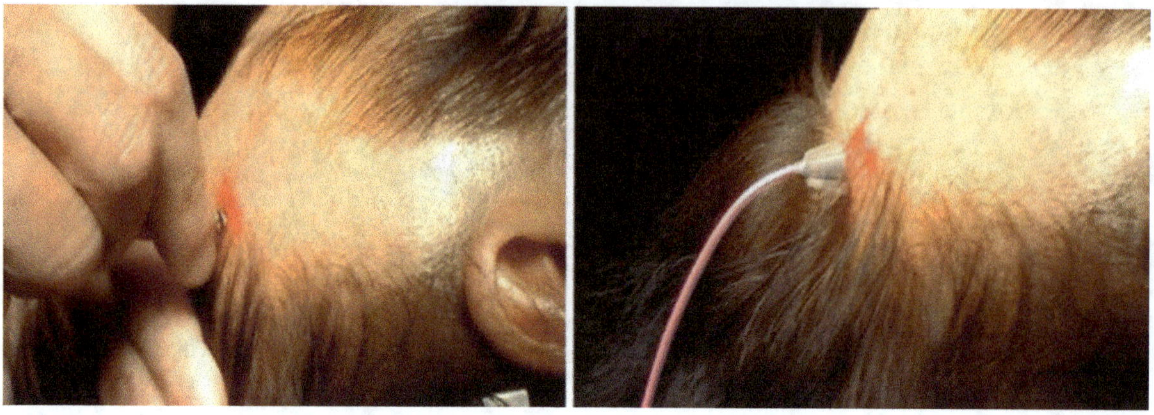

Fig. 15.4 Transcranial motor-evoked potential. Hair is shaved partially even in the case of SAH, and cork screw electrodes for transcranial motor-evoked potential (MEP) are placed in both sides of the head

pterion. We cut the arachnoid membrane with proper tension using fine tip forceps and microscissors. Usually the arachnoid is opened between the large sylvian veins. We can avoid cutting the vein and bleeding by only cutting the arachnoid membrane above the veins. We can preserve any small veins by only cutting the arachnoid membrane even in the case of SAH. The surgeon can begin gradually by separating the frontal and temporal lobes with microforceps and microscissors, achieving gentle retraction with the suction tip and, occasionally, a self-retaining retractor. The proximal aspect of the fissure is opened from the inside out and the outside in to avoid damage to the interdigitated frontal and temporal operculae. This technique is useful principle for neurosurgeon because it is difficult for the surgeon to open the adhesive opercula. Therefore, it is important for us to reach the deep sylvian fissure of insula with perivascular cistern and less adherent area.

From dissecting the distal sylvian fissure, M3 segment is easily caught and confirmed and following M3 segment reached M2 segment. This visible M2 segment in front of you is expected to be superior or inferior trunk by simulating preoperatively; however, especially in SAH case, its confirmation is sometimes difficult because of subarachnoid clot. It is important to irrigate the subarachnoid clot enough, and we can confirm this visible M2 segment is superior or inferior trunk by careful observation. For patients who undergo acute surgery for large temporal hematoma, we usually make a small incision in the middle temporal gyrus, decompressing the hematoma partially. The surgeon can facilitate brain relaxation by further aspirating cerebrospinal fluid from the ventricle drainage. The surgeon separates the frontal and temporal lobes, usually, the arachnoid membrane is opened superomedial to the superficial middle cerebral vein, and the opening is extended to the pterion.

15.4.6 Selection of Proximal and Distal Approach

A principle of aneurysm surgery is capturing the proximal artery to the aneurysm. Whichever approach you select, you must catch the proximal artery to the aneurysm. In some MCA aneurysms, the widely careless dissection of sylvian fissure to reach the internal carotid artery is dangerous, because the aneurysm is located near beneath the sylvian vein which is very superficially than we expected. Thus, from distal M2 to proximal, M1 approach is safer to capture the proximal M1 segment to the aneurysm. We should decide which approach is better preoperatively, proximal or distal approach, for safer clipping of the aneurysms. Therefore, we should simulate preoperatively using CTA, MRA, and/or DSA.

15.4.7 Proximal Approach (From ICA to M1 Approach)

To expose aneurysms located very proximally to so-called M1 aneurysm (i.e., those found at the origin of the anterior temporal artery or lenticulostriate vessels), the fissure must be opened from a proximal IC to M1 direction. The surgeon first opens the lateral sylvian fissure to M1–M2 junction, after that point, stops dissecting from distal side and moves proximal ICA, opens the carotid cistern, and follows the carotid artery toward the bifurcation and further laterally, following the M1 segment. If we select distal approach especially in upward direction M1 aneurysm, we cannot capture proximal M1 safely prior to aneurysm. Even if the aneurysm ruptures during distal approach, proximal control is impossible. Therefore, we should dissect the carotid cistern right after confirming the MCA bifurcation. We should dissect from IC bifurcation to proximal M1 segment to apply temporary clip to proximal M1. While dissecting the MCA and its branches, the surgeon should stay along the anterior and anterolateral surface of the vessel because the lenticulostriate perforators arise from the posterior and medial surfaces.

In case 1 (Fig. 15.5), we operated by proximal approach for M1 aneurysm.

15.4.8 Distal Approach (From M2 to M1 Approach)

To obtain proximal control of the M1 segment, open the sylvian fissure proximally before actually exposing the aneurysm. In most patients with small or large MCA aneurysms, the sylvian fissure

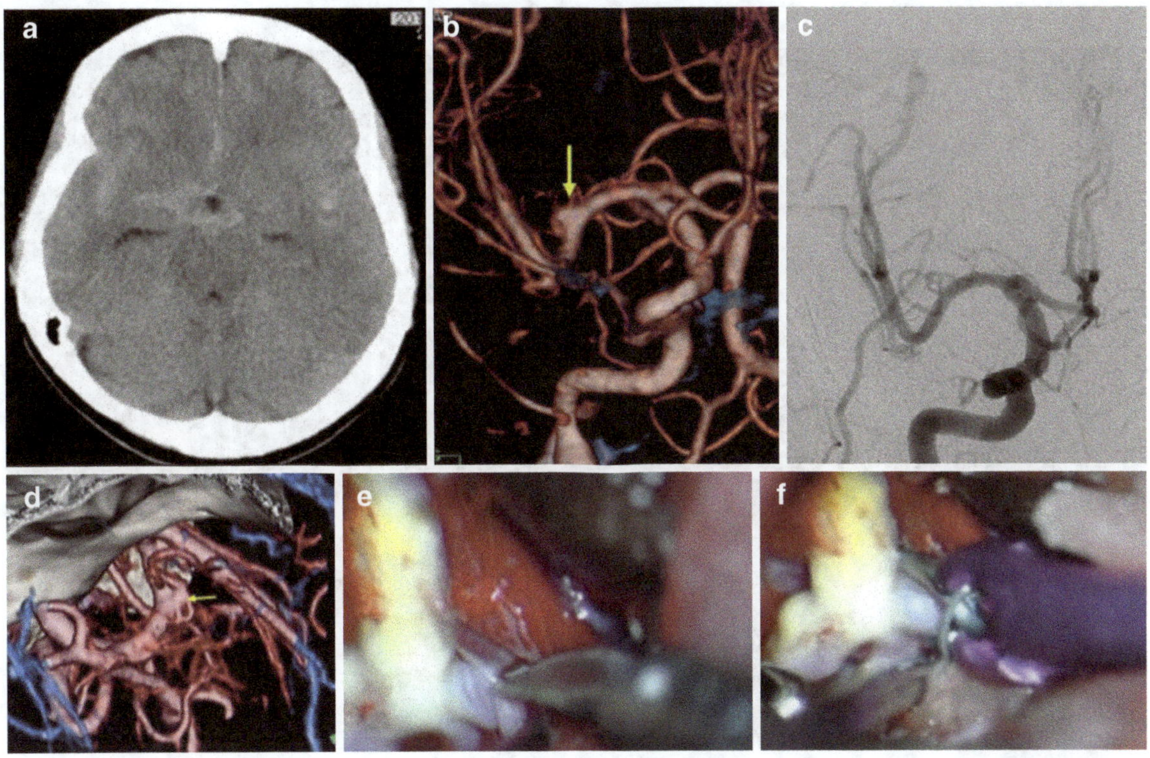

Fig. 15.5 Case1. M1 aneurysm 67-year-old female with subarachnoid hemorrhage. (**a**) CT scan revealed SAH with Fisher group 3. (**b**) CTA on admission showed ruptured M1 aneurysm (*arrow*), which is located at the origin of the lenticulostriate artery. (**c**) Postoperative DSA showed disappearance of aneurysm. (**d**) Simulation image by preoperative CTA showed anatomical relationship between the artery and skull base. You can understand the relationship of aneurysm and lenticulostriate artery. (**e**) Dissection between aneurysm and lenticulostriate artery by microscissors because of severe adhesion. (**f**) After appliance the temporary clip to proximal M1, neck clipping by mini clip is applied

can be adequately opened from a lateral to medial direction starting in its middle portion, even though proximal control is not achieved. In such cases, if the aneurysm will be exposed partially during opening of the sylvian fissure, the surgeon should move further proximally to obtain control of the proximal M1 segment. In the standard transsylvian approach, it is important to remember that the aneurysm usually is located more superficially. Regardless of the length of M1, if the M1 can curve downward toward the skull base, it is easier to just expose the M1 segment to the aneurysm by distal transsylvian approach. In these cases, if we select the conventional transsylvian approach, we may seize the aneurysm before internal carotid artery. So we need not see the internal carotid artery. In the case of long M1 segment, the aneurysm is usually within the temporal lobe. We can catch the proximal M1 by dissection of frontal side of a sylvian fissure.

Distal MCA aneurysms can be approached through an opening of the lateral sylvian fissure. The surgeon usually begins such opening in the middle portion of the fissure and proceeds distally. It is easy to mistake one of the deeper sulci for the sylvian fissure distally. To confirm that the sylvian fissure is actually being entered, the surgeon should trace one of the branches of the MCA proximally. The opening of the distal sylvian fissure must be done meticulously to avoid damaging adjacent areas of the brain, which have great functional importance. If severe intratemporal hemorrhage or brain swelling makes the opening of the fissure impossible, the surgeon can make an incision through the middle temporal gyrus and perfonn brain resection with a suction until the sylvian fissure is exposed.

In case 2 (Fig. 15.6), we operated by distal approach for usual MCA aneurysm.

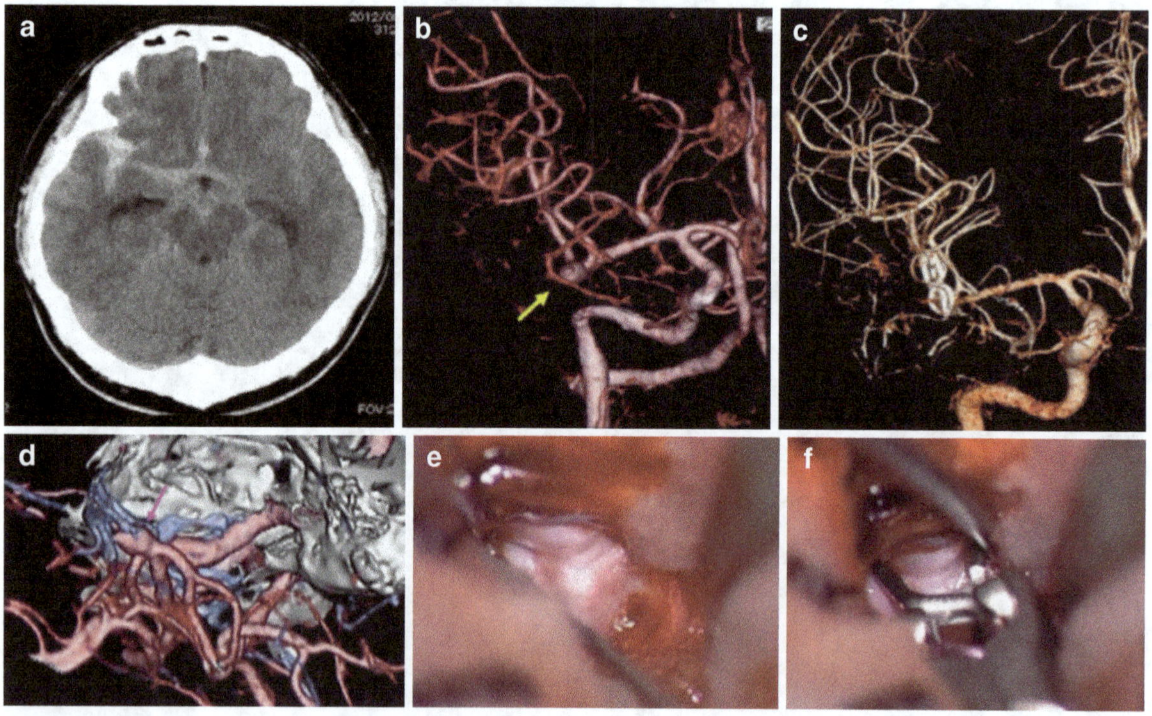

Fig. 15.6 Case 2. Ruptured MCA aneurysm with long and curved downward toward skull base M1, 36-year-old male. (**a**) CT scan revealed SAH with Fisher group 3. (**b**) CTA on admission showed ruptured MCA aneurysm (arrow). M1 segment curve downward toward the skull base. (**c**) Postoperative DSA showed disappearance of aneurysm. (**d**) Simulation image by preoperative CTA showed anatomical relationship of M1, M2, aneurysm, sylvian vein, and skull bone. You can understand the relationship of aneurysm and M1–M2 junction in operative field. (**e**) Dissection of aneurysmal neck by microdissector. (**f**) After appliance of the temporary clip to proximal M1, neck clipping by mini clip is applied

15.4.9 Dissection of the Aneurysm and Neck Clipping

After the proximal and distal vessels have been exposed, dissection of the aneurysm can begin. During this stage of the operation, we usually employ temporary clipping of the proximal vessel, with keeping normotension over 100 mmHg of systolic blood pressure, normothermia under 36.5 °C, and brain protective drugs. The aneurysm must be dissected in its neck, with no perforating vessels remaining adherent to the posterior surface of the aneurysm. It is sometimes useful to place a tentative clip across the dome of the aneurysm and then to dissect it from around the structure further before placing the final clip. MCA aneurysms often have a wide-based neck that involves 180° or more of the circumference of the bifurcation point. Optimal occlusion of such aneurysms requires the use of the application of multiple clips (Fig. 15.7). In some of these cases, it may also be necessary to use wrapping with some material to reinforce any unclipped areas of the neck. Perforators arising from the MCA must be handled with care. Most lenticulostriate vessels arise from the posteromedial surface of the M1 segment and enter the anterior perforated substance to supply the internal capsule and the basal ganglia.

Often, pan of the neck or dome is adherent to the vein and small artery. A fine micro dissector and microscissors are useful in the dissection from their vessels (Figs. 15.8 and 15.9). After the neck has been identified, selection and appliance of optimal clip help protect these vessels. Usually, multiple clips are needed for proper clipping of the MCA aneurysm.

15.4.10 Dural Closure

Primary tight dural closure by nylon suture with fibrin glue can prevent liquorrhea postoperatively.

15.5 Surgeon Plan to Handle the Complication

Many MCA aneurysms have a wide-based neck. Accordingly, placement of the clip may compromise the origin of one of these vessels, especially if the base of the aneurysm is partially calcified or atherosclerosis. A lenticulostriate artery originates from the deep side of the MCA distally along the M1 segment close to the bifurcation. This vessel may be occluded inadvertently by the tips of the aneurysm clip.

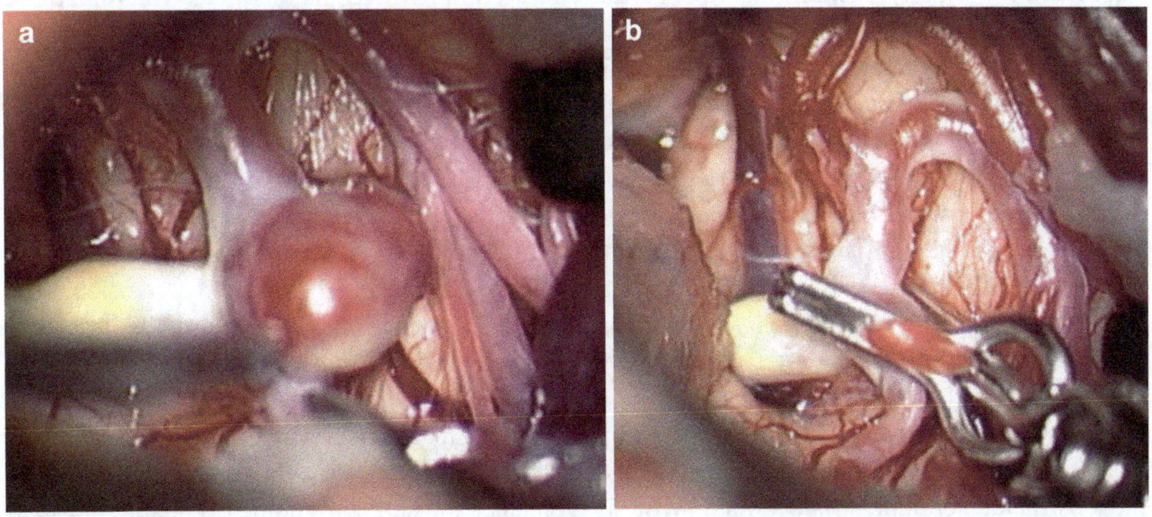

Fig. 15.7 Multiple clipping method for broad neck MCA aneurysm. (**a**) Broad neck MCA aneurysm. (**b**) Multiple clipping methods for MCA aneurysm using ring clip

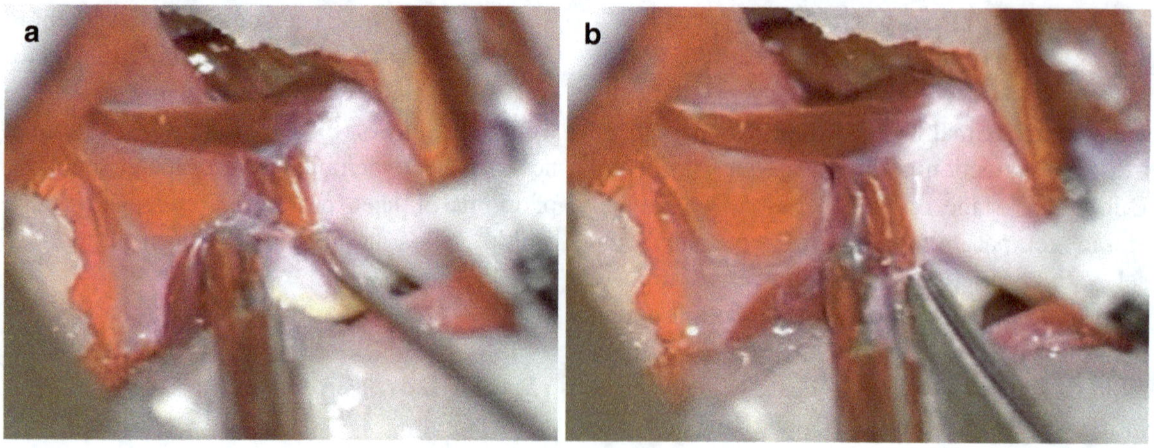

Fig. 15.8 Dissection between vein and aneurysm. (**a**) Dissection between vein and aneurysm by micro dissector. (**b**) Dissection between vein and aneurysm by microscissors

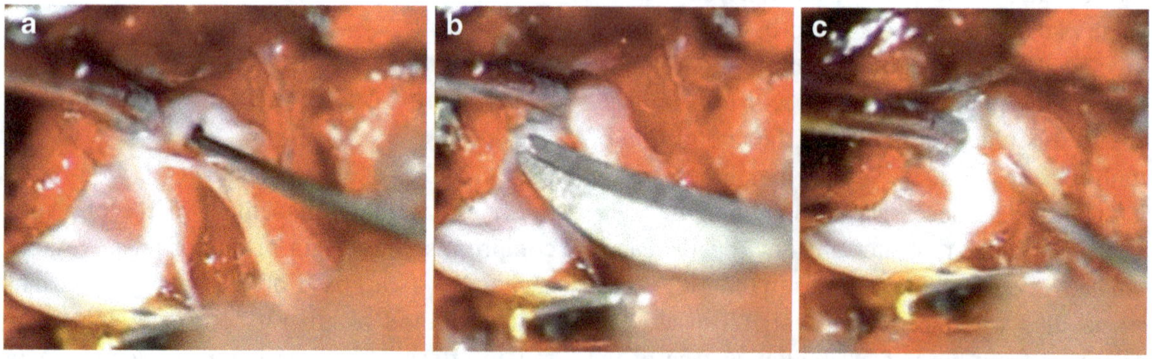

Fig. 15.9 Dissection between small artery and aneurysm. (**a**, **c**) Dissection between small artery and aneurysm by micro dissector. (**b**) Dissection between vein and aneurysm by microscissors

Thus, after the aneurysm clip is placed, it is important to visually inspect the tips of the aneurysm clip and to auscultate the M1 branches with a micro-Doppler probe. To inspect the all arteries around aneurysm, we must check them by using indocyanine green (ICG) video angiography. There are rare cases of postoperative small infarction of perforating area in spite of checking these modalities completely. So, MEP is the most useful intraoperative monitoring especially in M1 aneurysm in relation with lenticulostriate artery. If the wave of MEP reduced in its amplitude under 50% after neck clipping, we should release the clip and investigate all around aneurysm and find the obstructed lenticulostriate artery. MEP is very sensitive regarding with the damage of corticospinal tract, so we can trust MEP monitoring. If the patient has postoperative small infarction by MRI, he (she) is asymptomatic as long as MEP is normal.

It is important to reduce the pressure of parent artery and aneurysm using temporary arterial occlusion during the neck clipping of broad-based MCA aneurysm. In all cases, the brain must be protected during temporary arterial occlusion by brain protected drug, avoiding not only hyperthermia but also hypotension. The temporary occlusion time is usually less than 5 min per once. At the conclusion of the clipping process, papaverine is applied over the vessels to relax the mechanical spasm.

Preoperative three-dimensional CTA can enhance the surgeon's ability to picture the anatomy of the aneurysm before surgery to plan the optimal clipping.

15.6 Expert Opinion/Suggestion to Avoid Complication

In patients with giant MCA aneurysms, the surgeon must often completely trap the MCA and its branches and empty the aneurysm before final clipping. However, even with this technique, it is impossible to achieve optimal clipping of some heavily thrombosed or calcified aneurysms. Such cases often require a bypass procedure. Options include the STA to MCA bypass, the saphenous vein graft, and radial artery graft bypass to the major branches of MCA, transposition of some MCA branches.

Large sylvian veins should be left intact and displaced laterally with the temporal lobe or medially with frontal lobe. We can preserve almost all sylvian vein by careful finding the anastomosis between sylvian veins. Extremely small bridging veins across the sylvian fissure call can be safely cauterized and divided; however, we should understand that careful dissection of small veins can lead us expert microsurgeon.

15.7 Things to Be Observed and Postoperative Care/Follow-Up

In case of SAH, the prevention and treatment of delayed cerebral ischemia (DCI) are essential. We use intraoperative irrigation by artificial cerebrospinal fluid (CSF) (Artcereb) and postoperatively statin, cilostazol for prevention of DCI. Especially in severe cases of MCA aneurysm with sylvian hematoma, external decompressive craniotomy is performed for better circulation of CSF to prevent the DCI.

References

1. Kassel NF, et al. The International Cooperative Study on the timing of aneurysm part 1: overall management results. J Neurosurg. 1990;73:18–36.
2. Abiko M, Ikawa F, et al. Giant serpentine aneurysm arising from the middle cerebral artery successfully treated with trapping and anastomosis—case report. Neural Med Chir (Tokyo). 2009;49:77–80.
3. Morita A, et al. The natural course of unruptured cerebral aneurysms in a Japanese cohort. N Engl J Med. 2012;366:2474–82.
4. Ikawa F, et al. Indication of surgery for unruptured cerebral aneurysm and role of Japan: feature of Japanese medical system and according to the data of ruptured aneurysm. Surg Cereb Stroke (Jpn). 2012;40:381–6.
5. Ikawa F, Miyachi S. MCA aneurysm. Tokyo: Medicus Shuppan; 2014.

16 Surgery of Posterior Cerebral Artery Aneurysm

Joseph C. Serrone, Ryan D. Tackla, and Mario Zuccarello

16.1 Sign and Symptoms

This case illustration was a 62-year-old male presenting with the acute onset of worst headache of life symptoms (Hunt and Hess grade 2). Head computed tomography (CT) revealed Fisher grade 3 subarachnoid hemorrhage (SAH).

16.2 Investigation

As in most centers, CT angiography is the preferred imaging modality for the identification and evaluation of intracranial aneurysms at our institution. In this case, the CT angiogram revealed a 3.5-mm saccular aneurysm arising from P1 segment of right posterior cerebral artery (PCA) (Figs. 16.1 and 16.2).

16.3 Preoperative Preparation

Procurement of proximal control must be considered first when preparing to approach any ruptured aneurysm. For PCA aneurysms, we obtain proximal control at the distal part of basilar artery

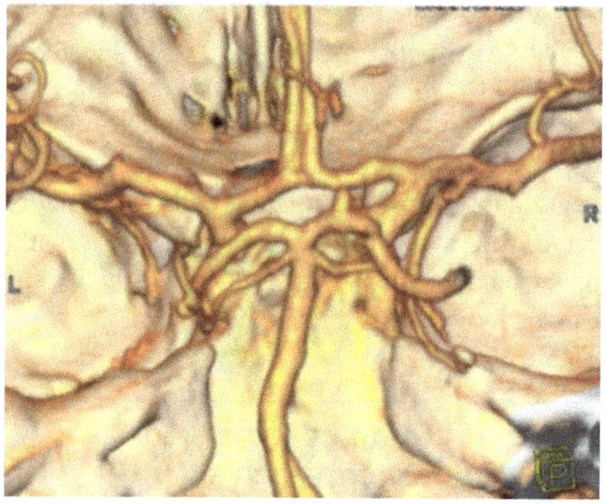

Fig. 16.1 A superiorly projecting right P1 segment PCA aneurysm is seen from this CT angiogram. Also of note, the basilar apex is well above the posterior clinoidal process allowing easy exposure of the basilar artery from an anterolateral approach for proximal control

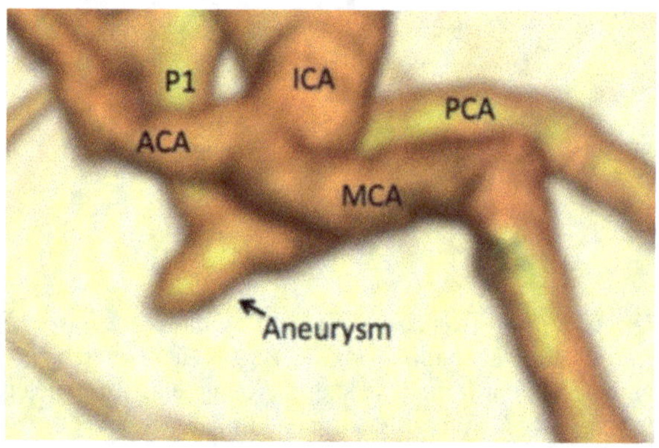

Fig. 16.2 Using CT angiography to create a surgical view of the aneurysm, neurosurgeons can study the vascular anatomy as it will be encountered intraoperatively. This view, through the supracarotid window, exposes the aneurysm well for clip application

J. C. Serrone · R. D. Tackla
Department of Neurosurgery, Virginia Mason Medical Center, Seattle, WA, USA

M. Zuccarello (✉)
Department of Neurosurgery, University of Cincinnati, Cincinnati, OH, USA
e-mail: zuccarm@ucmail.uc.edu

J. July, E. J. Wahjoepramono (eds.), *Neurovascular Surgery*, https://doi.org/10.1007/978-981-10-8950-3_16

just proximal to the origins of the superior cerebellar arteries. This area of the basilar artery is usually devoid of brainstem perforating arteries. The anatomical obstruction when approaching the posterior circulation through a pterional craniotomy is the posterior clinoid process (PCP). The relationship of the PCP to the basilar apex is assessed through sagittal or coronal reconstruction of the CT angiogram, which best demonstrates vascular and bone anatomy. If the basilar apex is above the PCP, it is possible to obtain proximal control of the basilar artery prior to clipping the posterior cerebral artery aneurysm. If the basilar apex is at the level of the PCP, removal of the PCP with a drill or ultrasonic bone curette may be required to achieve proximal control. If the basilar apex is below the PCP, proximal control cannot be achieved with a pterional approach, and a subtemporal approach is usually preferred.

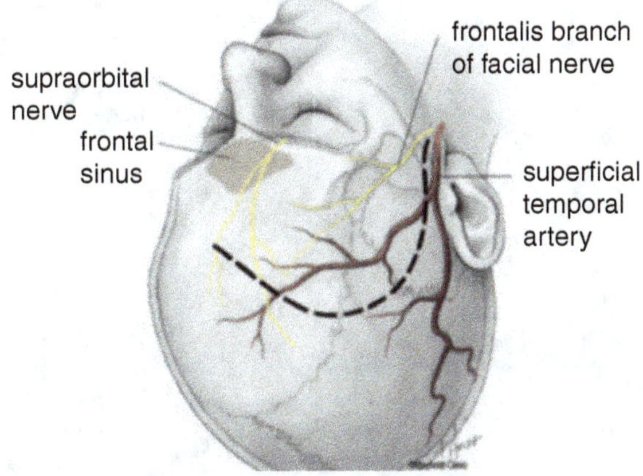

Fig. 16.3 The patient is positioned supine with the head extended and rotated 15° contralaterally. Relevant anatomy when using the pterional approach is seen with this schematic. Commonly the frontal branch of the superficial temporal artery is under the skin incision and must be ligated. The skin incision is kept posterior to the frontalis branch of the facial nerve to prevent its injury. There is wide variation in the pneumatization of the frontal sinus, and this must be studied preoperatively to prevent entering the sinus and causing a cerebrospinal fluid leak (Printed with permission from Mayfield Clinic)

16.3.1 Approach

Dealing with most aneurysm near basilar apex (including P1 segment aneurysms), we prefer an anterolateral approach based upon the pterional approach popularized by Dr. Yasargil [1]. As an extension of this approach, the pterional approach via the extended lateral (PAVEL) corridor is helpful [2]. The patient position is supine, with the head extended and rotated 15° contralaterally (Fig. 16.3). Relevant anatomy to consider when planning the craniotomy includes the superficial temporal artery, frontalis branch of facial nerve, and frontal sinus (Fig. 16.4) [3]. A branch of superficial temporal artery is often encountered during the skin incision and must be ligated. The skin incision must remain posterior to the frontalis branch of the facial nerve for prevention of postoperative frontalis palsy. The extent of pneumatization of the frontal sinus should be assessed preoperatively to prevent encountering the frontal sinus during craniotomy. In the event that the craniotomy is exposing the frontal sinus, cranialization of frontal sinus should ensue.

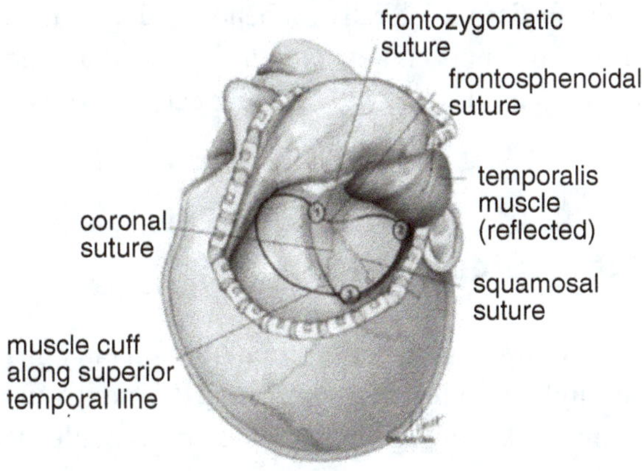

Fig. 16.4 The skin incision has been made with the myocutaneous flap retracted anteriorly. A frontal, temporal, and posterior burr hole is made to aid in dissection of the dura from the inner skull cortex and prevents a durotomy by the craniotome (Printed with permission from Mayfield Clinic)

After minimal shaving of the hair, a skin incision is made behind the hairline. The incision starts 1 cm anterior to tragus at zygoma root, and curve extends to midline. Then myocutaneous flap is detached in one single layer and retracted with spring hooks toward the anterior to expose the orbital rim. We prefer a one layer myocutaneous flap as opposed to an inter- or subfascial dissection that is associated with more jaw pain and temporal wasting [4]. Three burr holes are made to allow adequate dissection of the dura

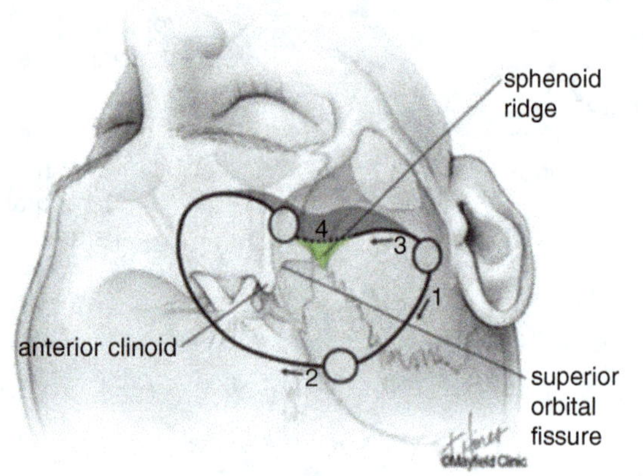

Fig. 16.5 Using a craniotome, cuts 1–3 are made until the sphenoid ridge is encountered. Cut #4 is made with a high-speed drill. Green-shaded area represents the thickened bone of the sphenoid ridge, which will subsequently be drilled off (Printed with permission from Mayfield Clinic)

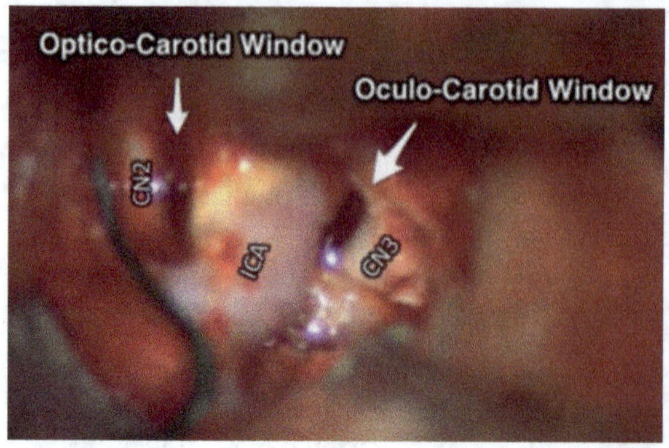

Fig. 16.6 After opening of the proximal Sylvian fissure, wide exposure of the optic nerve (CN2), supraclinoidal internal carotid artery (ICA), and oculomotor nerve (CN3) are demonstrated. The opticocarotid and oculocarotid windows are visualized

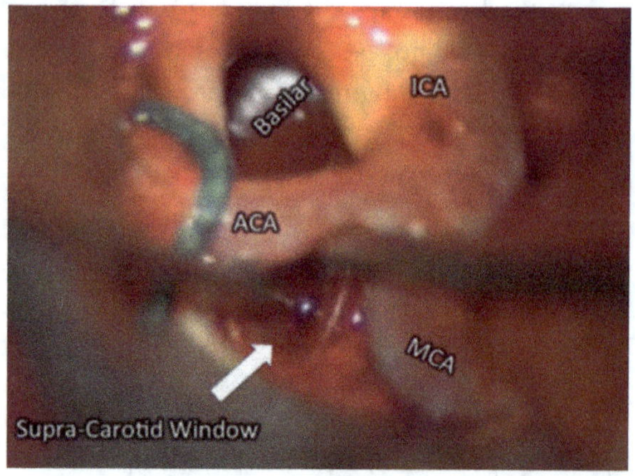

Fig. 16.7 Further dissection allows utilization of the supracarotid window above the carotid terminus, which will eventually be used for clipping of the PCA aneurysm. Exposure of the basilar artery within the opticocarotid window is well seen from this image. The opticocarotid window will be used for temporary clipping of the basilar artery for proximal control

away from the inner skull cortex (Fig. 16.5). A side-cutting craniotome with footplate is used to create a bone flap from the supraorbital notch, medially, to the mid-temporal lobe, exposing Sylvian fissure laterally. Sphenoid ridge is then drilled off in its entirety with the coarse diamond drill. Dura is cut with curvilinear shape and reflected anterolaterally.

16.4 Steps of the Surgery

When clipping posterior circulation aneurysms through the pterional approach, the neurosurgeon works through the opticocarotid, oculocarotid, and supracarotid windows (Figs. 16.6 and 16.7). To safely access these corridors, mobilization of the temporal lobe is required [2]. This is accomplished with several key steps. It is important to split the sylvian fissure widely, and expose the supraclinoidal ICA (internal carotid artery) and MCA (middle cerebral artery). This is a crucial step, as retracting the temporal lobe without detethering the ICA and MCA can result in a vascular injury and stroke [5]. The middle Sylvian vein at its entrance into the sphenoparietal sinus must be coagulated and cut to allow for retraction of the anterior temporal lobe. Subsequent dissection is done to mobilize the anterior choroidal artery from the uncus, making it possible to retract the temporal lobe laterally. Lastly, third cranial nerve is followed posteriorly, and Liliequist membrane is opened to get to PCA (posterior cerebral artery). These steps comprise the PAVEL extension of the pterional approach and are described in detail elsewhere [2].

After extensive subarachnoid dissection in this case, the opticocarotid corridor was used to obtain proximal control at basilar artery (Fig. 16.8). With the proximal control achieved, attention was directed toward the P1 segment aneurysm through the supracarotid window (Fig. 16.9). Given that this was a simple, small aneurysm, a straight clip was used to occlude the

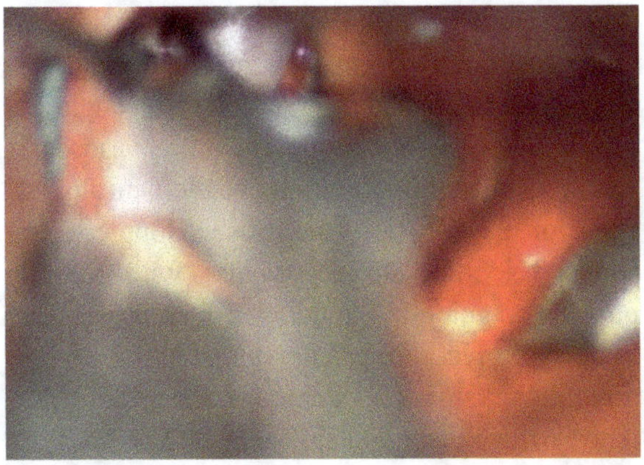

Fig. 16.8 A temporary clip is being placed on the basilar artery through the opticocarotid window

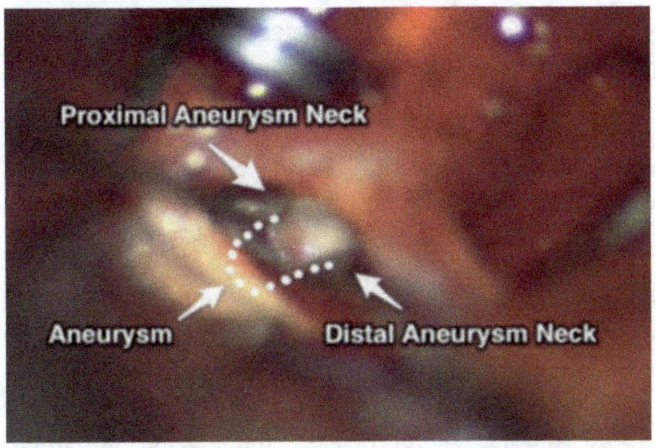

Fig. 16.9 The temporary clip has been placed on the basilar artery through the opticocarotid window. Looking above the carotid terminus (through the supracarotid window), the aneurysm is well exposed for clipping

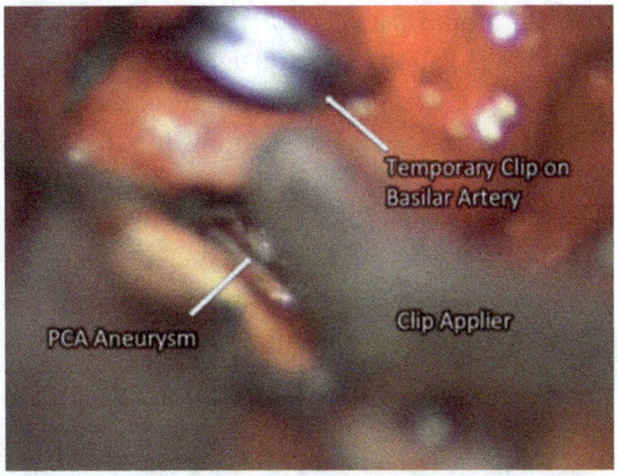

Fig. 16.10 A temporary clip has been placed on the basilar artery through the opticocarotid window. The PCA aneurysm is being clipped through the supracarotid window with a straight aneurysm clip

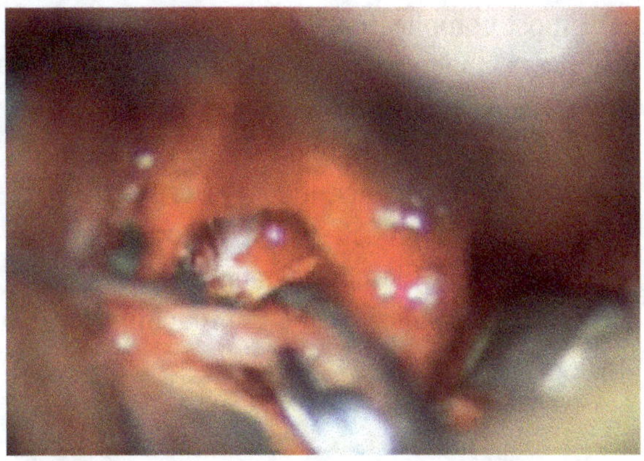

Fig. 16.11 After permanent clip placement through the supracarotid window and removal of the temporary clip, the tips of the permanent clip are inspected through the opticocarotid window to ensure complete occlusion of the aneurysm without incorporation of thalamoperforator arteries within the clip blades

aneurysm (Fig. 16.10). Lastly, the tips of the clip were inspected through the opticocarotid window to ensure the aneurysm was completely occluded and that no thalamoperforator arteries were incorporated within the clip (Fig. 16.11).

16.5 Surgeon Plans to Handle the Complication

A dreaded complication when using the pterional approach for posterior circulation aneurysms is vascular dissection of the middle cerebral artery [5]. Management of this complication depends on the presence of collaterals and the time from ictus. If the complication is identified intraoperatively by loss of somatosensory-evoked potentials or motor-evoked potentials, surgical revascularization by middle cerebral artery thrombectomy or bypass between the external carotid artery and the middle cerebral artery should be considered. However, the dissection commonly occurs during surgery, but occlusion of MCA occurs in a delayed fashion, with the acute onset of hemiparesis occurring postoperatively. At this time, cerebral angiography should be performed.

With good collaterals, postoperative augmentation of blood pressure is the preferred treatment. If poor collaterals are seen and the ictus of the patient's stroke is within 6 h, endovascular or surgical revascularization can be considered. Endovascular therapy is approached with caution, as the patient will require some form of anticoagulation or antiplatelet therapy after thrombectomy to prevent recurrent occlusion. If there is any uncertainty regarding the timing of ictus, revascularization should be avoided, as this will likely result in the conversion of a morbid ischemic complication into a fatal hemorrhagic complication. The size of the stroke should be assessed radiographically for consideration of a prophylactic decompressive hemicraniectomy in order to prevent cerebral herniation due to malignant middle cerebral artery infarction.

16.6 Expert Opinion/Suggestion to Avoid Complication

Like most complications, they are better to prevent than manage. This complication is prevented by extensive mobilization of the temporal lobe and detethering of the middle cerebral artery as described above. In fact, the PAVEL extension of the pterional approach was developed specifically to prevent the complication of the middle cerebral artery injury while approaching basilar aneurysms [2, 5].

16.7 Things to Be Observed and Postoperative Care/Follow-Up

This is a ruptured cerebral aneurysm case that will have the clinical sequelae of SAH, including posthemorrhagic cerebral vasospasm. Prophylactic treatment of vasospasm should include maintenance of a euvolemic state and administration oral nimodipine. Monitoring of posthemorrhagic cerebral vasospasm with frequent neurological exams and transcranial Doppler ultrasound should be performed. Consideration of cerebral angiography with endovascular treatment of vasospasm should occur with alterations of the neurological exam or elevation in transcranial Doppler ultrasound velocities. In accordance with recently published guidelines, delayed cerebrovascular imaging is recommended after clipping of ruptured aneurysms to evaluate for aneurysm recurrence (which occurs in approximately 4%) [6].

References

1. Yasargil MG, Antic J, Laciga R, Jain KK, Hodosh RM, Smith RD. Microsurgical pterional approach to aneurysms of the basilar bifurcation. Surg Neurol. 1976;6(2):83–91.
2. Bendok BR, Getch CC, Parkinson R, O'Shaughnessy BA, Batjer HH. Extended lateral transsylvian approach for basilar bifurcation aneurysms. Neurosurgery. 2004;55(1):174–8; discussion 178.
3. Moss CJ, Mendelson BC, Taylor GI. Surgical anatomy of the ligamentous attachments in the temple and periorbital regions. Plast Reconstr Surg. 2000;105(4):1475–90; discussion 1491–1478.
4. de Andrade Junior FC, de Andrade FC, de Araujo Filho CM, Carcagnolo Filho J. Dysfunction of the temporalis muscle after pterional craniotomy for intracranial aneurysms. Comparative, prospective and randomized study of one flap versus two flaps dieresis. Arq Neuropsiquiatr. 1998;56(2):200–5.
5. Hua SE, Gluckman TJ, Batjer HH. Middle cerebral artery occlusion after pterional approach to basilar bifurcation aneurysm: technical case report. Neurosurgery. 1996;39(5):1050–3; discussion 1053–1054.
6. Connolly ES Jr, Rabinstein AA, Carhuapoma JR, et al. Guidelines for the management of aneurysmal subarachnoid hemorrhage: a guideline for healthcare professionals from the American Heart Association/American Stroke Association. Stroke. 2012;43(6):1711–37.

17 Surgery of Upper Basilar Artery Aneurysm

Kentaro Mori, Terushige Toyooka, and Naoki Otani

17.1 Signs and Symptoms

Aneurysms of the basilar artery (BA) may occur at several locations including the BA-vertebral artery junction, BA-anterior inferior cerebellar artery junction, BA-superior cerebellar artery junction, and BA tip. Upper BA aneurysm is usually considered to include BA tip aneurysm and BA-superior cerebellar artery junction aneurysm. BA aneurysm seldom manifests as neurological problems before rupture. Partially thrombosed BA aneurysm may manifest as progressive neurological deficits due to compression of the brain stem and cranial nerves caused by aneurysm growth. Unruptured BA tip aneurysm has a higher tendency to rupture compared to other types of cerebral aneurysm. Therefore, the surgical indications for unruptured BA aneurysm should consider this fact as well as the age, size, and shape of the aneurysm.

17.2 Investigation

Upper BA aneurysms are surrounded by many important osseous and neurovascular structures such as the anterior (ACP) and posterior clinoid processes (PCP), optic nerve, oculomotor nerve, internal carotid artery (ICA), posterior communicating artery and its perforators (anterior thalamoperforating arteries), and posterior cerebral artery and its perforators (posterior thalamoperforating arteries: PTPAs) (Fig. 17.1). The PTPAs arise from the superior or posterosuperior surface of the P1 segment of the posterior cerebral artery and at a distance of 0.41–4.71 mm (mean 1.93 mm) from the BA apex. The PTPAs number 1–8 (mean 3.6) with diameter of 0.24–1.18 mm (mean 0.7 mm) [1]. Dissection of the PTPAs from the BA tip aneurysm is the key step to successful clipping surgery.

17.3 Preoperative Preparation

Three-dimensional computed tomography angiography and/or digital subtraction angiography are mandatory to investigate the BA complex with the aneurysm (Fig. 17.2). The distance of the aneurysm neck from the clinoid line (the line between the tips of the ACP and PCP) is particularly important to determine the operative approach. Anterolateral approaches such as the pterional transsylvian approach and extradural temporopolar approach (ETA) are suitable for the treatment of BA aneurysms located between 15 mm above and 5 mm below the clinoid line. The subtemporal transtentorial approach or

K. Mori (✉) · T. Toyooka · N. Otani
Department of Neurosurgery, National Defense Medical College, Tokorozawa, Saitama, Japan
e-mail: kmori@ndmc.ac.jp; toyo@ndmc.ac.jp; naotani@ndmc.ac.jp

J. July, E. J. Wahjoepramono (eds.), *Neurovascular Surgery*,
https://doi.org/10.1007/978-981-10-8950-3_17

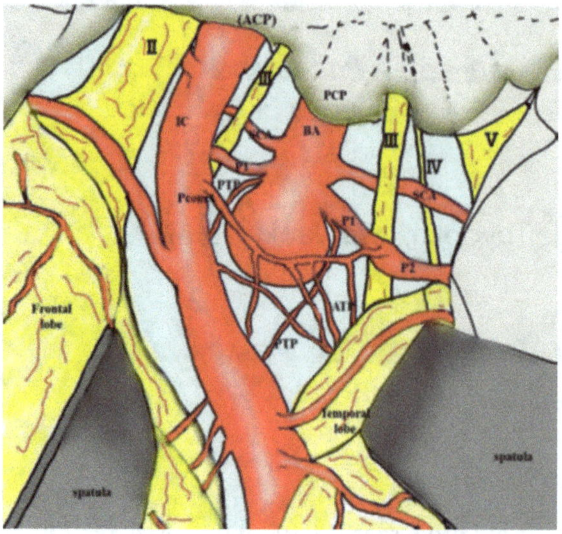

Fig. 17.1 Illustration of the basilar artery (BA) complex with BA tip aneurysm via the anterolateral approach. Note the anterior thalamoperforating arteries from the posterior communicating artery (p-com) and the posterior thalamoperforating arteries from the posterior cerebral artery (P1 and P2). *II* optic nerve, *III* oculomotor nerve, *IV* trochlear nerve, *V* first branch of trigeminal nerve, *ACP* anterior clinoid process(resected), *PCP* posterior clinoid process, *IC* internal carotid artery, *SCA* superior cerebellar artery

anterior petrosal approach should be considered for aneurysms located more than 5 mm below the clinoid line.

17.3.1 Approach

17.3.1.1 Extradural Temporopolar Approach ETA

The pterional transsylvian approach and subtemporal transtentorial approach are usually used to treat upper BA aneurysms, but both have advantages and disadvantages. The anterior temporal approach, which retracts the temporal tip posteriorly, combines the advantages of both these approaches and facilitates the surgical trajectory from the anterolateral direction. The anterior temporal approach is a pure intradural approach based on dissecting the superficial middle vein and anterior temporal artery from the temporal lobe. The ETA is an epidural approach involving posterior displacement of the temporal lobe with

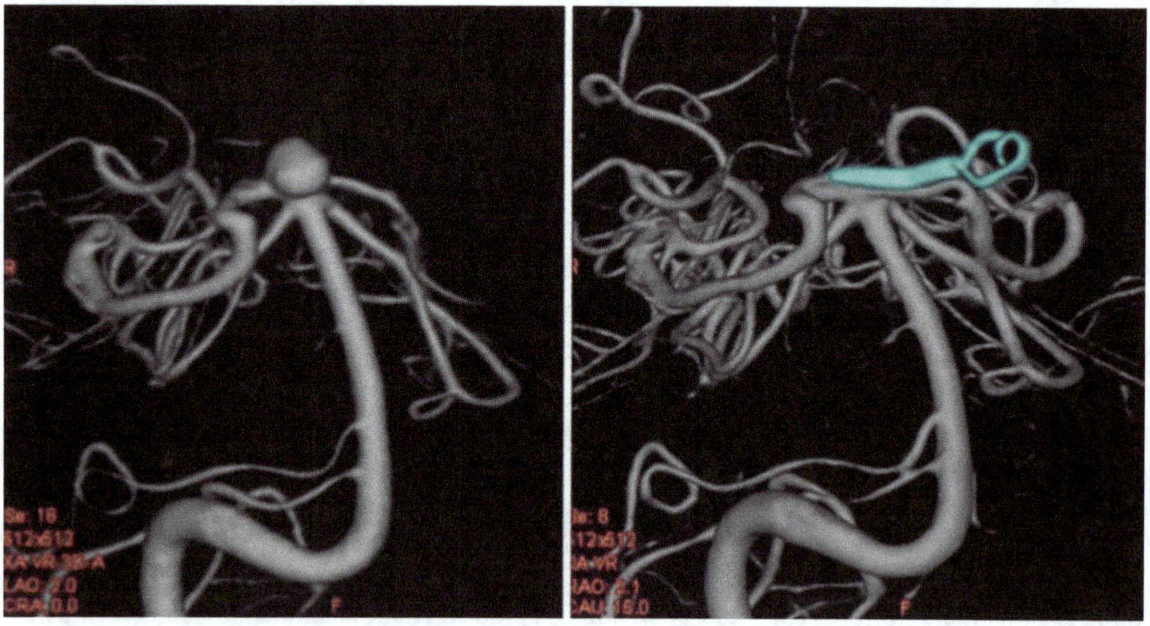

Fig. 17.2 Three-dimensional computed tomography angiograms of a case of basilar tip aneurysm. *Left* preoperative, *Right* postoperative

the dura mater [2, 3] and includes extradural anterior clinoidectomy, optic canal opening, peeling the lateral wall of the cavernous sinus, and retraction of the temporal lobe over the dura mater. The ETA enables the neurosurgeon to pass through the open anterior part of the cavernous sinus to the retrocarotid space and interpeduncular cistern. Such epidural temporal lobe retraction is less likely to cause contusion. Furthermore, opening the oculomotor foramen and drilling the PCP provide space for securing the proximal BA. The use of the ETA for treatment of BA top aneurysm is discussed below.

17.3.1.2 Patient Position, Skin Incision, and Craniotomy

After induction of general anesthesia, lumbar spinal drainage is placed for cerebrospinal fluid (CSF) aspiration to relax the dural tension during the epidural procedures. The patient is placed in the supine position, and the head is rotated away from the operative side at about 30° (Fig. 17.3). Semi-coronal skin incision and interfascial dissection of the temporal muscle fascia are then performed. The temporal muscle is detached from the superior temporal line but not incised. The temporal muscle is dissected subperiosteally

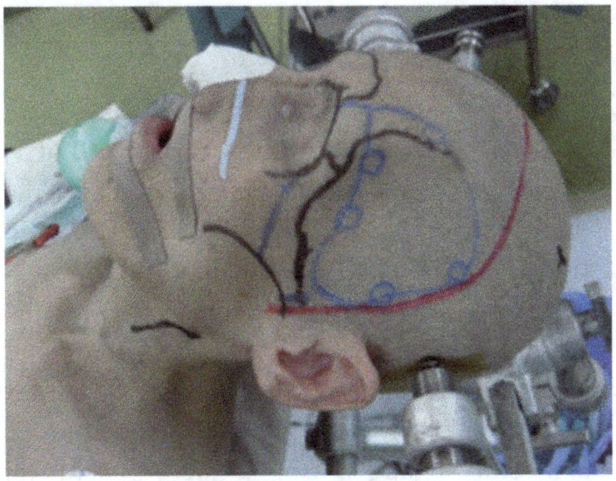

Fig. 17.3 Scheduled skin incision, frontotemporal craniotomy with orbitozygomatic osteotomy

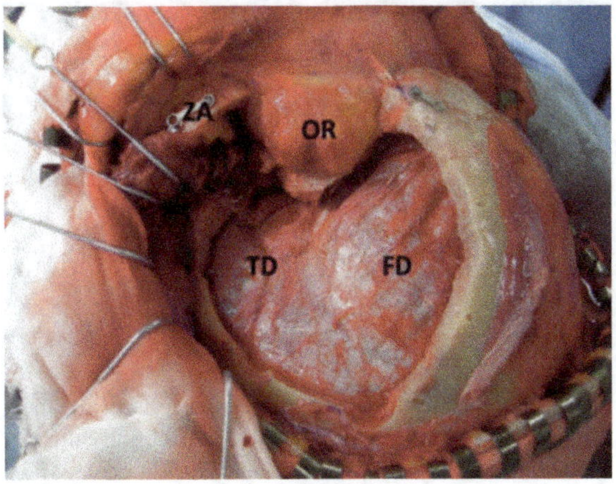

Fig. 17.4 After frontotemporal craniotomy with orbitozygomatic osteotomy. *ZA* zygomatic arch, *OR* orbit (opened), *FD* frontal dura mater, *TD* temporal dura mater

and retracted posteroinferiorly using fish hooks. Standard frontotemporal craniotomy is performed with the anterior border at the midpoint of the orbit, and the temporal squama is rongeured out until the floor of the middle cranial fossa is exposed. If the orbitozygomatic approach is needed for specific cases such as high position BA tip aneurysm, the orbitozygomatic bar is removed as in the two-piece method (Fig. 17.4).

17.4 Steps of the Surgery

The frontal dura and the temporal dura are dissected subperiosteally until flush with the frontal and middle fossae. The lesser wing of the sphenoid and the orbital apex is drilled away until the meningo-orbital band is exposed. Dissection of the middle fossa dura is continued until the orifices of the superior orbital fissure (SOF) and foramen rotundum are exposed (Fig. 17.5). The roof of the SOF is opened to a width of 2 mm to expose the junction between the dura propria of the temporal lobe and the periosteal dura (Fig. 17.5 arrowhead). The meningo-orbital band is pulled proximally using forceps or a

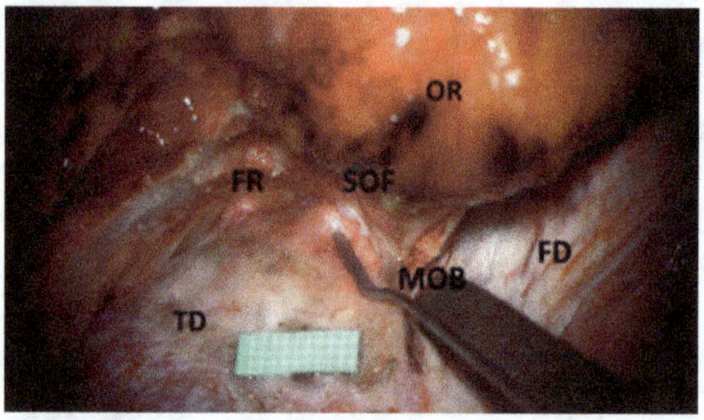

Fig. 17.5 Junction between the dura propria of the temporal dura mater (TD) and periosteum at the superior orbital fissure (SOF). *FD* frontal dura mater, *MOB* meningo-orbital band, *OR* orbit. Arrowhead indicates the junction

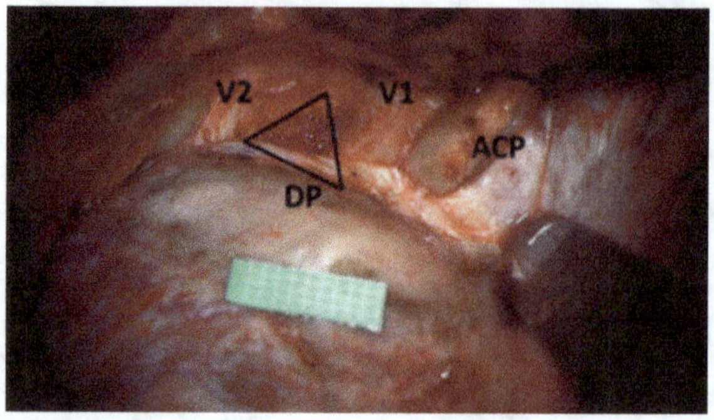

Fig. 17.7 After peeling of the dura propria (DP) of the temporal dura mater and exposure epidurally of the anterior clinoid process (ACP). *V1* ophthalmic branch of the trigeminal nerve, *V2* maxillary branch of the trigeminal nerve. Open triangle shows Mullan's anterolateral triangle

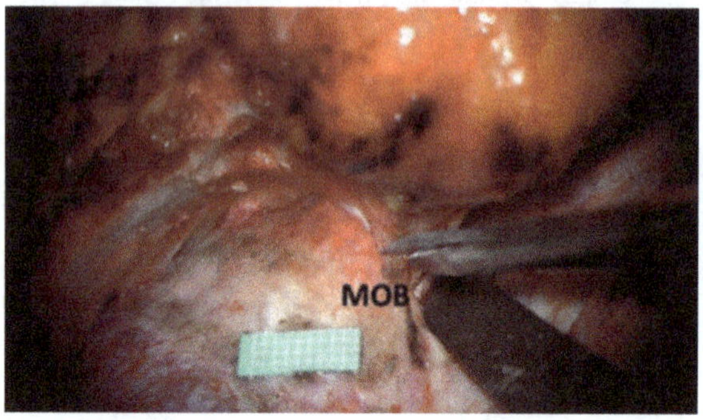

Fig. 17.6 Cutting the meningo-orbital band (MOB)

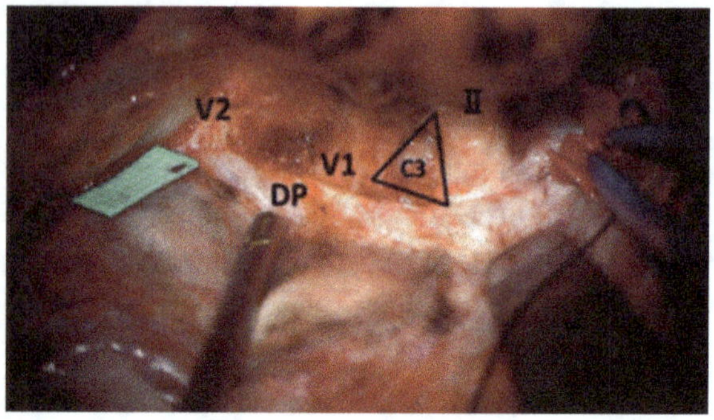

Fig. 17.8 Completion of epidural procedures after removal of the anterior clinoid process and opening of the optic canal. *II* optic nerve, *III* oculomotor nerve, *V1* ophthalmic branch of the trigeminal nerve, *V2* maxillary branch of the trigeminal nerve, *C3* clinoid segment of the internal carotid artery, *DP* dura propria. Open triangle shows Dolenc's anteromedial triangle

stitch and cut with micro-scissors for about 4 mm. The tip of the micro-scissors should be pointed toward the exposed junction at the SOF (Fig. 17.6). Any bleeding from the meningo-orbital artery should be coagulated and divided. Peeling of the dura propria from the inner membrane can be started anywhere, with the easiest point between the SOF and foramen rotundum, using a micro-dissector with a sharp edge. If the dura propria and inner membrane are tightly attached, sharp dissection using micro-scissors is recommended. The peeling is continued until the entire ACP is exposed epidurally. The trochlear nerve and first and second branches of the trigeminal nerve can be seen though the semi-transparent inner membrane (Fig. 17.7). Care should be taken to maintain the sphenoparietal sinus at the dura propria side and to stop the peeling at the point where the sphenoparietal sinus drains into the cavernous sinus to prevent problems with venous congestion. Drilling of the ACP with a high-speed drill using saline irrigation is started from the lateral part of the ACP, and the optic canal is then opened partially in the medial part of the ACP. The ACP is hollowed like an egg shell, and the remainder of the ACP can be removed en bloc. The anterior loop of the ICA (clinoid segment, C3) in the opened clinoid space can be seen through the thin carotid oculomotor membrane. The partially opened optic canal can be enlarged using a micro-punch, and the remainder of the optic strut between the opened clinoid space and optic canal can be removed with either a small diamond drill or a micro-punch (Fig. 17.8). During the skull base drilling, if the posterior ethmoid sinus is opened and the mucous membrane is injured, a muscle piece should be inserted and sealed with fibrin glue to avoid CSF leakage. At this point, the temporal lobe with the temporal dura mater can be displaced posteriorly by 25–30 mm from the tip of the middle cranial fossa. The dura mater is cut along the sylvian fissure as far as the optic nerve, the falciform ligament is cut, and then the dural cutting is continued to the inferior frontal dura mater in an L-shaped fashion over the distal dural ring. Incision of the falciform ligament and distal dural ring will facilitate movement of the optic nerve and ICA. Before tentorial incision, the sylvian fissure should be opened widely, and the arachnoid membrane around the oculomotor nerve should be incised to free the nerve from the medial temporal lobe. By observing at the cisternal and extradural parts of the oculomotor nerve, the medial tentorial edge is cut for separation from the cavernous sinus around the oculomotor nerve. Following these procedures, the temporal lobe can be retracted posteriorly with the temporal dura mater to complete the ETA with the surgical corridor of the opened anterior part of the middle fossa and the cavernous sinus (Fig. 17.9). Opening of the oculomotor foramen facilitates mobilization of the oculomotor nerve. If the target pathology is located beneath the PCP, the latter can be drilled away to expose the pontine cistern to secure the proximal BA. The ICA is retracted medially to expose the BA complex with the BA tip aneurysm (Figs. 17.10 and 17.11). After temporary clips are applied to the

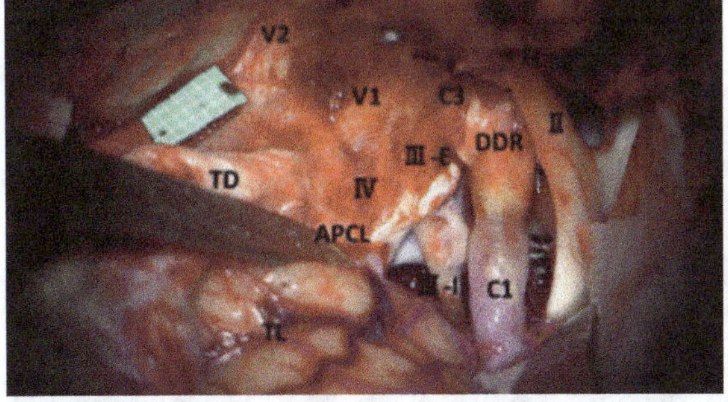

Fig. 17.9 After dural opening and tentorial incision. The falciform ligament (FL) and the distal dural ring (DDR) are incised. The tentorium is incised along the anterior petroclinoid ligament (APCL). The temporal dura is retracted posteriorly with the temporal dura mater (TD). *II* optic nerve, *III-I* intradural oculomotor nerve, *III-E* extradural oculomotor nerve, *IV* trochlear nerve, *V1* ophthalmic branch of the trigeminal nerve, *V2* maxillary branch of the trigeminal nerve, *C3* clinoid segment of the internal carotid artery

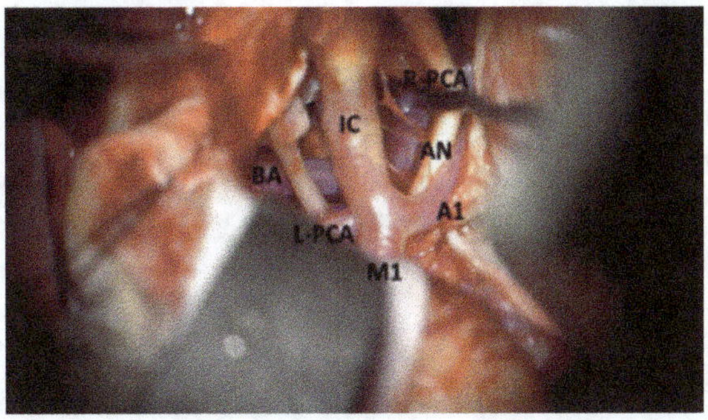

Fig. 17.10 Basilar artery (BA) complex and BA tip aneurysm. Note the small thalamoperforating arteries around the aneurysm (AN). *IC* internal carotid artery, *A1* anterior cerebral artery, *M1* middle cerebral artery, *R-PCA* right posterior cerebral artery, *L-PCA* left posterior cerebral artery

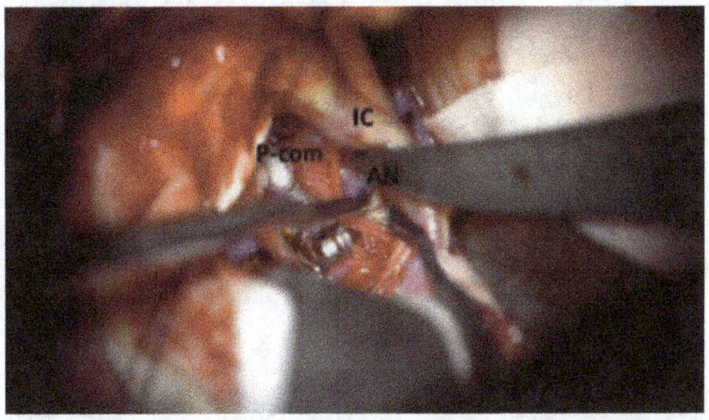

Fig. 17.11 Dissection of the basilar tip aneurysm (AN) via the retrocarotid space. *p-com* posterior communicating artery, *IC* internal carotid artery

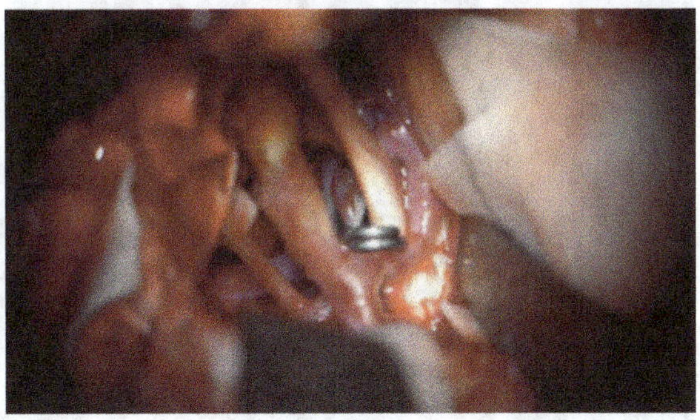

Fig. 17.12 After neck clipping of the basilar tip aneurysm

BA and bilateral posterior cerebral arteries, aneurysm dissection is started. If the posterior communicating artery obstructs the operative view, this vessel can be ligated and divided except for the fetal type. Great care is required to dissect the PTPAs in the vicinity of the aneurysm before neck clipping is performed (Fig. 17.12).

After clipping of the aneurysm, the dural defect around the dural ring can be approximated with a small piece of harvested temporal fascia and fibrin glue. The skull is fixed with titanium plates, a subcutaneous drain is placed, and the wound is closed as usual.

17.5 Specific Plans to Handle Complications and Expert Opinion

17.5.1 How to Avoid Heat Injury During Skull Base Drilling

Constant cooling with saline irrigation is extremely important to avoid heat injury to the neurovascular structures. Before drilling the ACP, the ACP should be carefully dissected from the surrounding tissue because the oculomotor nerve passes along the inferolateral face of the ACP. The optic canal is partially opened with a drill and should be enlarged using a micro-punch. Opening the optic canal using a micro-punch can avoid heat injury.

17.5.2 How to Control Bleeding from the Cavernous Sinus

There are two major points of bleeding from the cavernous sinus, Dolenc's anteromedial triangle and Mullan's anterolateral triangle. Bleeding from the cavernous sinus can be controlled by packing with Surgicel® cotton soaked with fibrin glue or direct injection of fibrin glue into the sinus (Fig. 17.13).

17.6 Important Observations and Postoperative Care

CSF drainage (about 150 cm^3/day) from the lumbar spinal tube should be continued for several

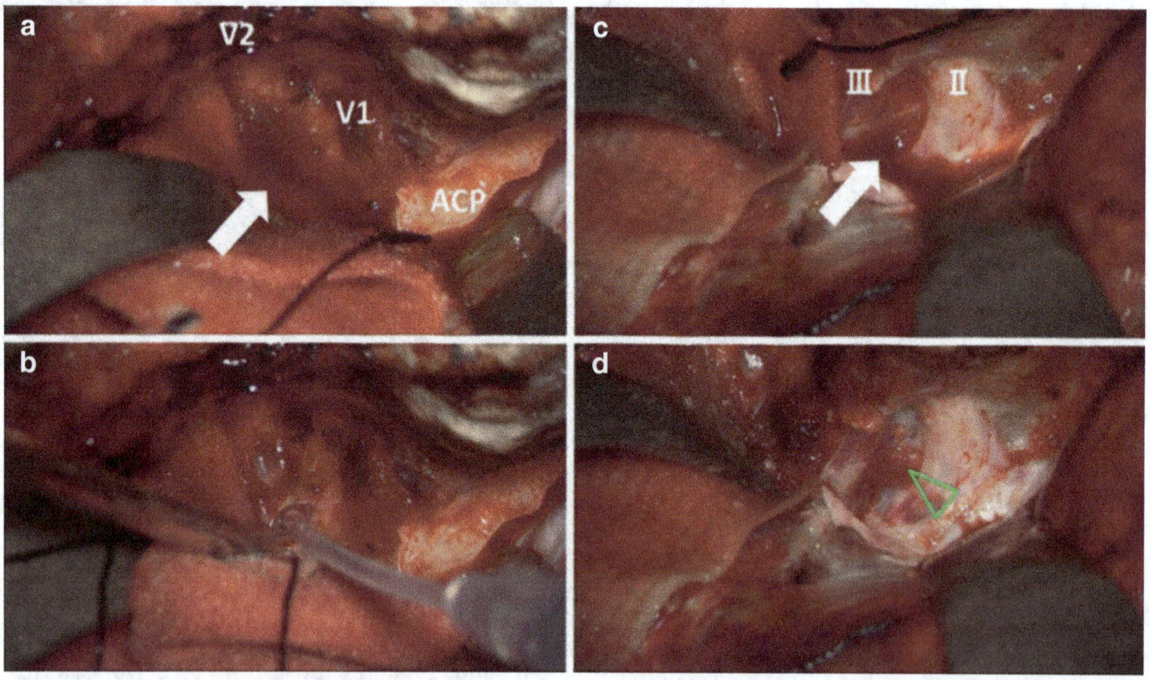

Fig. 17.13 How to control bleeding from the cavernous sinus. (**a**) Bleeding from Mullan's anterolateral triangle (*arrow*). (**b**) Direct injection of fibrin glue into Mullan's triangle. (**c**) Bleeding from Dolenc's anteromedial triangle (*arrow*). (**d**) Application of Surgicel® soaked with fibrin glue (*open triangle*). *ACP* anterior clinoid process, *II* optic nerve, *III* oculomotor nerve, *V1* ophthalmic branch of the trigeminal nerve, *V2* maxillary branch of the trigeminal nerve

days (3–7 days) after the operation to prevent CSF rhinorrhea, especially if the ethmoid sinus is opened during surgery.

References

1. Park SQ, Bae HG, Yoon SM, Shim JJ, Yun IG, Choi SK. Morphological characteristics of the thalamoperforating arteries. J Korean Neurosurg Soc. 2010;47:36–41.
2. Day JD, Giannotta SL, Fukushima T. Extradural temporopolar approach to lesions of the upper basilar artery and infrachiasmatic region. J Neurosurg. 1994;81:230–5.
3. Day JD, Fukushima T, Giannotta SL. Cranial base approaches to posterior circulation aneurysms. J Neurosurg. 1997;87:544–54.

18 Surgery of Superior Cerebellar Artery Aneurysm (SCA)

Miguel A. Arraez, Miguel Dominguez, Cristina Sanchez-Viguera, Bienvenido Ros, and Guillermo Ibañez

18.1 Signs and Symptoms

Patient a 57 years old male, a persistent headache was evaluated by neurologists. MRI was done, and incidental superior cerebellar artery (SCA) aneurysm was discovered after assessment of abnormal image at the lateral aspect of the mesencephalon. CT-angio and angiography (Fig. 18.1) showed an aneurysm with saccular form at proximal portion of right SCA. Endovascular treatment was precluded by neuroradiologist due to the morphological characteristics of the aneurysm's neck [1–3].

18.2 Investigation

The most striking neuroradiological examination was angiography and CT-angio. The superior cerebellar and posterior cerebral arteries were seen arising from a common origin ("N" type according to the McCullough classification of the anatomical variations of the circle of Willis) [4]. The aneurysm was close to the origin of the artery from basilar trunk at the anterior pontomesencephalic segment. The relation neck/dome suggested a good indication for surgery.

M. A. Arraez (✉) · M. Dominguez · C. Sanchez-Viguera · B. Ros · G. Ibañez
Department of Neurosurgery, Carlos Haya University Hospital, Malaga, Spain
e-mail: marraezs@uma.es

One of the important points before surgery is the appropriate anatomical characterization of the origin and location and morphology of the aneurysm. Among the segments of the SCA (prepontine, ambient, and quadrigeminal), the aneurysm was seen at the prepontine portion of the artery. It is noteworthy that in this segment, the SCA is giving off perforating branches to the pons before the origin of the lateral (marginal) branch. It is also interesting to mention that SCA aneurysms usually arise at the 2 mm proximal to the artery of origin (usually the basilar trunk). SCA aneurysms are not frequent (1.7% of the total), but 42% of the cases are found in the context of multiple aneurysms. Unlike our patient, the most common presentation is SAH (60%) followed by compression of III, IV, or V cranial nerve. The hemorrhagic presentation is frequently seen in lesions smaller than 7 mm.

18.3 Preoperative Preparation

Preoperative preparation is crucial in aneurysm surgery. Relaxation of the brain is of outstanding importance. The timing for surgery is decided in accordance to the clinical presentation (SAH, incidental aneurysm), morphology and size of the aneurysm, Hunt and Hunt scale, and choice of the surgical approach. Not infrequently posterior fossa lesions require significant brain retraction making advisable delayed procedure. In our

J. July, E. J. Wahjoepramono (eds.), *Neurovascular Surgery*,
https://doi.org/10.1007/978-981-10-8950-3_18

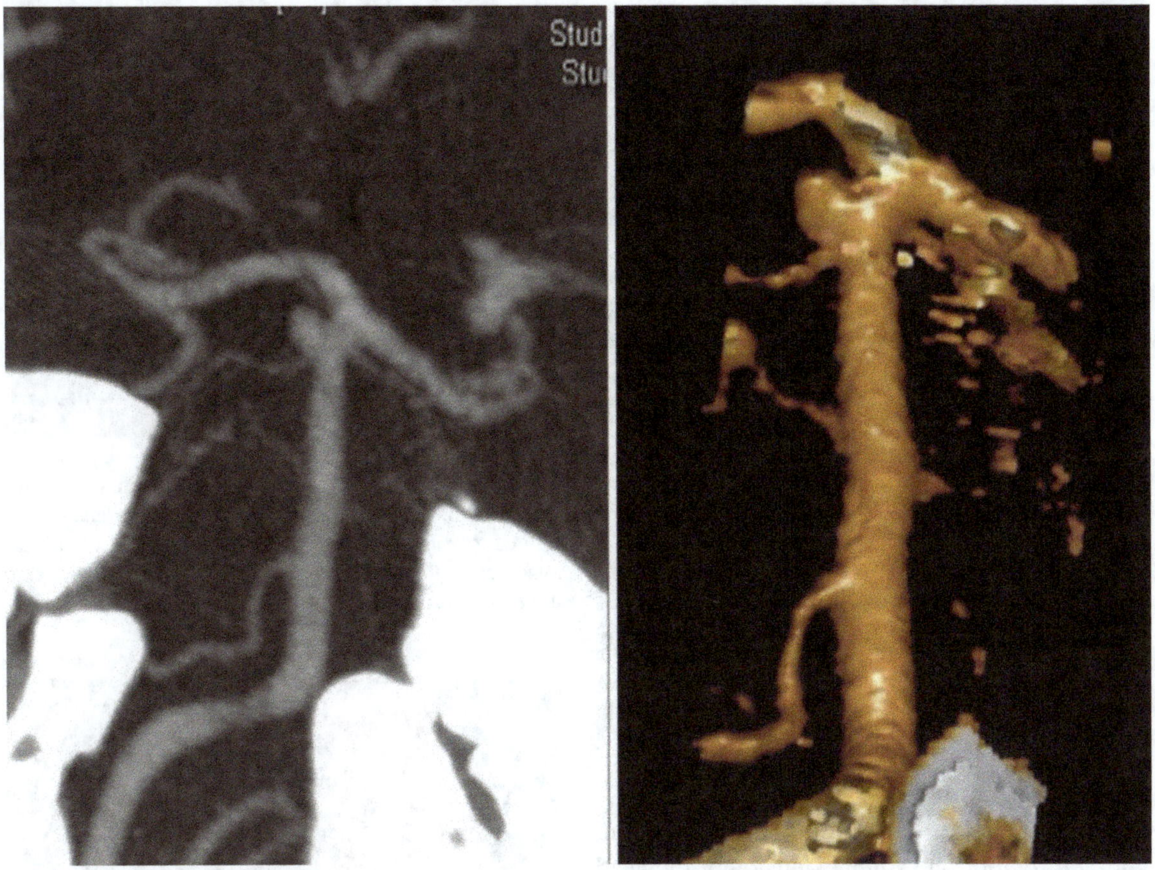

Fig. 18.1 Aneurysm of the right superior cerebellar artery in a 57-year-old male. Incidental finding. Angiography and CT-angio

patient (incidental aneurysm) elective surgery was done with preoperative spinal drainage and osmotic diuretics as perioperative adjunct measures.

18.4 Steps of Surgery

The approach selected for this case was a right frontotemporal craniotomy with limited zygomatic osteotomy (no need for orbito-zygomatic osteotomy in our opinion). The choice of approach for exposure of SCA aneurysm will depend on the segment where the lesion lies. The SCA might be separated into four segments: the pontine segment also called as anterior pontomesencephalic segment, the ambiens segment also called as the lateral pontomesencephalic segment, the quadrigeminal segment also called as the cerebellomesencephalic segment, and then the last one which is called cortical segment. According to location of aneurysm in one of these segments, the following approaches can be used: subtemporal, pretemporal extradural with clinoidectomy, subtemporal with addition of zygomatic or orbito-zygomatic osteotomy, and presigmoid and posterior fossa suboccipital. The latter is used to approach the cortical segment and the former to get access to the tentorial incisura and *perimesencephalic* segments of the SCA [5, 6].

In our patient, the lesion was placed at the pontine segment. This part of SCA is located between dorsum sellae and the upper brainstem [5]. This segment starts at the exit of the SCA from the basilar artery. The aneurysm in the presented case arose in this point (as very frequently seen in SCA aneurysms). In this area, special care must be taken as basilar artery and SCA at its origin show intermingled perforating vessels. Another relevant anatomical structure is the III nerve, constantly

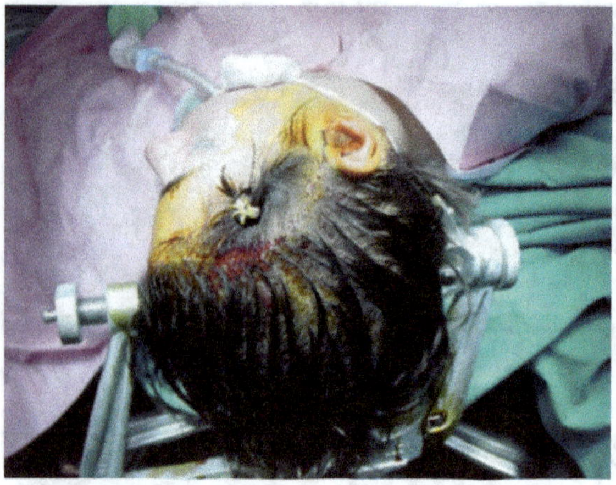

Fig. 18.2 Positioning of the head for the surgical approach to the right tentorial incisura. Left rotation and extension of the head. No hair shaving

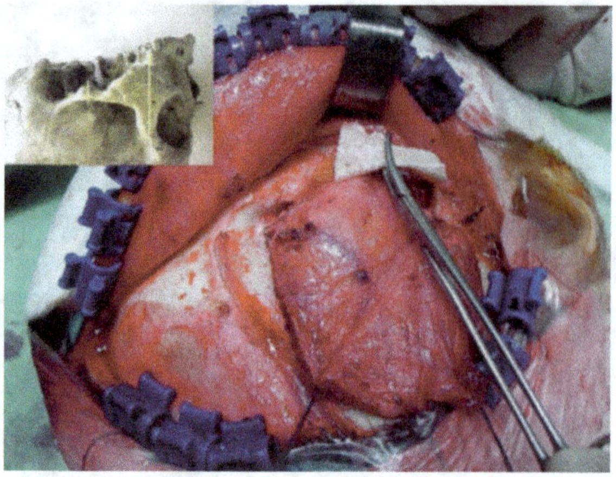

Fig. 18.3 Exposure of the zygomatic bone after careful dissection of the layers of the deep temporal fascia. A very limited zygomatic osteotomy is done instead of orbito-zygomatic osteotomy (see the osteotomy lines depicted in upper left corner)

above SCA and below the PCA (posterior cerebral artery). Due to location of aneurysm at the anterior pontomesencephalic segment, the choice of the approach was a subtemporal-pretemporal transzygomatic approach.

The patient was placed in supine position, with left rotation and slight extension of the head (Fig. 18.2). We usually do not shave the hair (previously prepared with antiseptic solution). A skin incision is made curvilinear from the hairline to anterior of tragus. After skin incision, the identification of the fascia at temporal is very important; there are superficial and deep layer of the fascia and dissection of the fat in between to avoid injury to facial nerve that innervates the frontal side. The zygomatic bone needs to be exposed. In our opinion, only a limited osteotomy is necessary to increase the reflection of the temporal muscle after detachment from the temporal bone (Figs. 18.3 and 18.4) instead of the more time-consuming orbito-zygomatic osteotomy that adds unnecessary morbidity. This maneuver diminishes the retraction of the temporal lobe increasing also the view of the tentorial incisura region. A frontotemporal craniotomy is done and dura is opened (Fig. 18.5). The brain is relaxed after mannitol and CSF release through spinal drainage or through opening the arachnoid layer at the basal cisterns in the context of the microsurgical approach. The intradural part of the operation starts with a very minimal retraction just to hold the temporal lobe. The tentorial incisura is exposed with the relevant structures. The exposure will allow the recognition of the anterolateral mesencephalon, carotid artery, posterior communicating artery and its perforating arteries, PCA, SCA, and oculomotor nerve, typically running below PCA and above SCA (Fig. 18.6). Also, IV nerve can be seen in its typical course along tentorium [7].

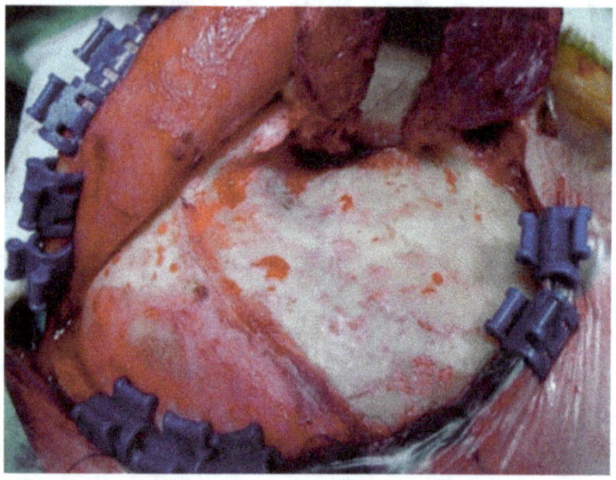

Fig. 18.4 Reflection downward of the temporal muscle exposes adequately the temporal bone to increase the temporal component of the craniotomy

All these steps were done in our patient. The III nerve was right in the direction of our sight,

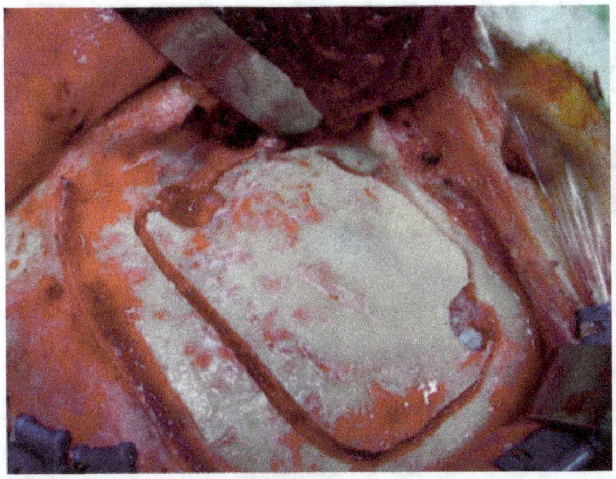

Fig. 18.5 Right frontotemporal craniotomy. The frontal component is small. The temporal flap almost reaches the level of the middle fossa floor to diminish the intradural retraction of the temporal lobe

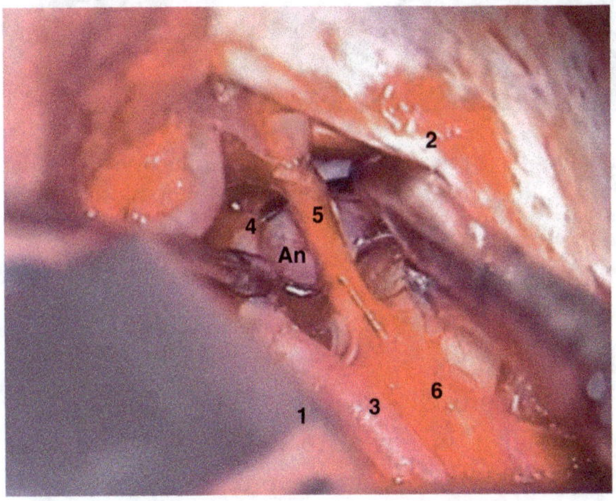

Fig. 18.6 Exposure of the right tentorial incisura and pontomesencephalic segment of the SCA. Temporal lobe retracted (1), tentorium (2), posterior cerebral artery (3), basilar artery (4), III nerve interposed in the direction of the sight of the surgeon (5), right mesencephalon (6), and aneurysm dome right before clipping

making slightly difficult in the identification and clipping of the neck. A Sugita clip was use to exclude the aneurysm from the circulation (Fig. 18.7). The effectiveness of the procedure was confirmed by means of ICG intraoperative angiography (Fig. 18.8).

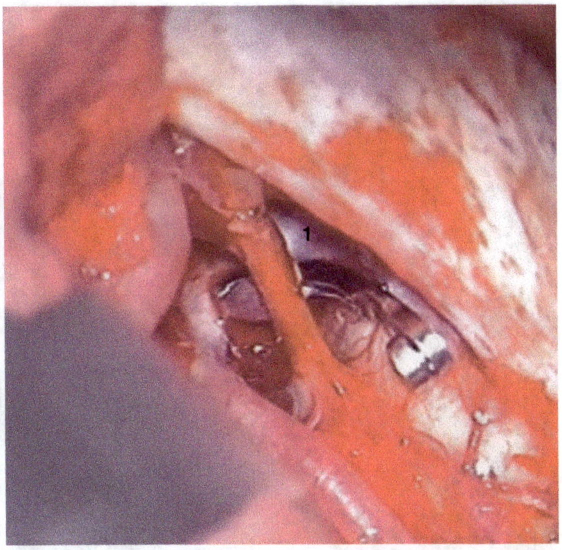

Fig. 18.7 SCA aneurysm clipped. The SCA main trunk has been preserved (1)

18.5 Expert Opinion/Suggestion to Avoid Complication

One of the possible complications would come from bad exposure due to wrong choice of the surgical approach [8, 9]. Wrong approaches very seldom happen, at the anterior circle of Willis, but the posterior circle offers many more possibilities and difficulty to reach appropriately the aneurysm neck. The anatomy of the vessels and their variations along with morphology of the aneurysm, its neck, and relation with perforating vessels are of course of paramount importance. Thus, preoperative assessment (angiography, CT-angio) is absolutely crucial to establish the choice of the approach [10, 11]. The segment in which the aneurysm is located and the relation of the aneurysm and posterior clinoid must be carefully evaluated. The segment harboring the lesion will suggest anterior, lateral, or posterior approach. In regard to the relation of the aneurysm and posterior clinoid, a very low origin would preclude the use of anterior intradural approaches.

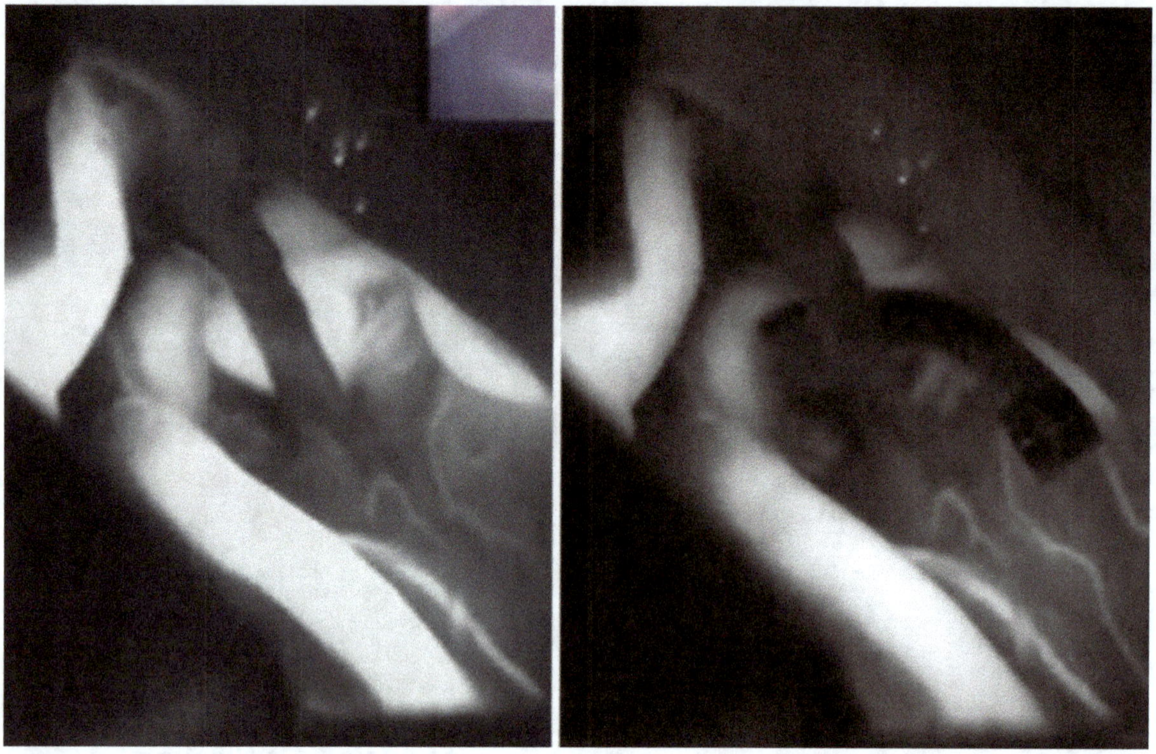

Fig. 18.8 ICG intraoperative angiography before (**a**) and after clipping (**b**) showing exclusion of the aneurysm. Basilar artery (1), posterior cerebral artery (2), superior cerebral artery (3), SCA aneurysm (4), and III nerve interposed (5)

Another frequent source of complications in *para-temporal* approaches is the improper management of the temporal lobe (contusion, infarction, hemorrhage). In our selected approach (anterolateral), a very gentle retraction of the temporal lobe must be done lifting the tip not subtemporally but anteriorly. No veins are encountered in a long avenue from the sylvian fissure (anterior and medial) to the Labbé area (posterior and lateral). This lifting of the temporal lobe is very well tolerated unlike some other forms of compression or distortion. Sylvian fissure usually doesn't need to be opened. Care must be taken not to tear sylvian veins during the exposure. The proper extension of the head and gravity can help diminish any harmful effect of the retractors over the temporal lobe.

18.6 Postoperative Measures

This approach doesn't differ from other approaches in regard to the general care after other aneurysm surgery procedures or craniotomy. We administer postoperative calcium antagonist, antiepileptic drugs, and low weight subcutaneous heparin along with early mobilization. The external lumbar drainage is removed 24 h after surgery.

References

1. Chaloupka JC, Putman CM, Award IA. Endovascular therapeutic approach to peripheral aneurysms of the superior cerebellar artery. AJNR Am J Neuroradiol. 1996;17:1338–42.

2. Jin SC, Park ES, Kwon do H, Ahn JS, Kwun BD, Kim CJ, et al. Endovascular and microsurgical treatment of superior cerebellar artery aneurysms. J Cerebrovasc Endovasc Neurosurg. 2012;14:29–36.
3. Peluso JP, van Rooij WJ, Sluzewski M, Beute GN. Superior cerebellar artery aneurysms: incidence, clinical presentation and midterm outcome of endovascular treatment. Neuroradiology. 2007;49:747–51.
4. McCullough AN. (Rewritten posthumously for the author by Howard K. Suzuki). Some anomalies of the arterial circle (of Willis) and related vessels. Anat Rec. 1952;142:537–43.
5. Bozboga M, Canbolat A, Savas A, Türker K. Aneurysms arising from the medial branch of the superior cerebellar artery. Acta Neurochir. 1996;138:1013–4.
6. Hardy DG, Peace DA, Rhoton AL Jr. Microsurgical anatomy of the superior cerebellar artery. Neurosurgery. 1980;6:10–28.
7. Collins TE, Mehalic TF, White TK, Pezzuti RT. Trochlear nerve palsy as the sole initial sign of an aneurysm of the superior cerebellar artery. Neurosurgery. 1992;30:258–61.
8. Gács G, Viñuela F, Fox AJ, Drake CG. Peripheral aneurysms of the cerebellar arteries. Review of 16 cases. J Neurosurg. 1983;58:63–8.
9. Yasargil MG. Microsurgical anatomy of the basal cisterns and vessels of the brain, diagnostic studies, general operative techniques and pathological considerations of the intracranial aneurysms. Stuttgart, Germany: Georg Thieme Verlag; 1984.
10. Day JD, Fukushima T, Giannotta SL. Cranial base approaches to posterior circulation aneurysms. J Neurosurg. 1997;87:544–54.
11. Nair P, Panikar D, Nair AP, Sundar S, Ayiramuthu P, Thomas A. Microsurgical management of aneurysms of the superior cerebellar artery—lessons learnt: an experience of 14 consecutive cases and review of the literatura. Asian J Neurosurg. 2015;10:47.

19 Surgery of Posterior Inferior Cerebellar Artery (PICA) Aneurysm

Ivan Ng and Julian Han

19.1 Sign and Symptoms

Posterior circulation aneurysms account for approximately 10% of all aneurysms, which affect 1–6% of the population [1, 2]. Aneurysms of the posterior inferior cerebellar artery (PICA) are very rare, only 0.5–3% of all aneurysms [3]. Patients with PICA aneurysms usually present with subarachnoid hemorrhage, or they might have symptoms due to compression of the brainstem or lower cranial nerves. Microsurgical clipping of PICA aneurysms is difficult and very challenging due to the limited working space and its surrounding neurovascular structure, the brainstem and lower cranial nerves IX, X, XI, and XII, and very often the aneurysm is located very deep and far from the surgeon's view. Surgical maneuvers require moving around and sometimes in between cranial nerves. PICA aneurysms may vary widely within a range in terms of their complex anatomy, as a result either of their origin, branching out of the vertebral artery (VA), or their course along the lower cranial nerve. The PICA itself is usually of a small caliber, and aneurysms on it with a wide neck create a difficult situation with respect to clipping the aneurysm and preserving the PICA.

I. Ng (✉) · J. Han
National Neuroscience Institute (NNI), Singapore, Singapore
e-mail: ivan.ng.h.b@singhealth.com.sg

19.2 Investigation and Vascular Anatomy

The VA branches out of the subclavian artery, ascends along the lateral aspect of the cervical vertebra through transverse processes, turns posterior of the lateral mass of C1, and enters the subarachnoid space between foramen magnum and ring of C1. The initial part of the intradural VA passes the superior–anterior to the first cervical roots, then crosses in front of the dentate ligament, also in front of the accessory nerve at the spinal part. The VA then ascends in front of the hypoglossal nerve to reach the medulla at its anterior surface, where it meets and unites with the contralateral VA to become the basilar artery at the junction of the medulla and pons.

The PICA is the VA's largest and most clinically significant branch. The PICA is very complex, sometimes long and tortuous, having a variable course and a wide area of supply compared to other branches of the cerebellar arteries. It supplies the medulla, cerebellar tonsil, inferior part of the vermis, and inferior surface of the cerebellar hemisphere. The PICA has five segments: anterior medullary (p1), lateral medullary (p2), tonsillomedullary (p3), telovelotonsillar (p4), and cortical (p5) segments (Fig. 19.1).

The first segment (p1) starts from the PICA's origin just in front of the medulla near the inferior olivary, then turns posteriorly through hypoglossal rootlets and continues on, then

J. July, E. J. Wahjoepramono (eds.), *Neurovascular Surgery*,
https://doi.org/10.1007/978-981-10-8950-3_19

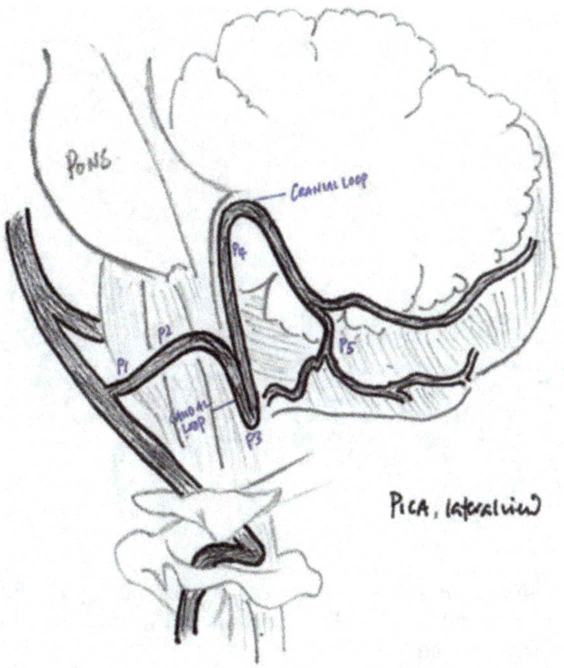

Fig. 19.1 Drawing of PICA and its segments: anterior medullary (p1), lateral medullary (p2), tonsillomedullary (p3), telovelotonsillar (p4), and cortical (p5) segments. It supplies the medulla, cerebellar tonsil, inferior vermis, and suboccipital surface of the cerebellar hemisphere

turning to the lateral surfaces of the medulla. The second segment (p2) starts from the turn at the prominent point of the olivary until the outlet of the lower cranial nerve. The third segment (p3) starts at the outlet of the lower cranial nerve and crosses medially at the posterior aspect of the medulla, making a big loop starting from the lateral surface of the tonsil until it reaches the pole and turning up at the medial surface of the tonsil. The fourth segment (p4) starts at the midpoint of the PICA at the medial surface of the tonsil, moves toward the fourth ventricle roof, then comes out through the fissure to reach the cerebellar surface. There is almost always a cranial loop where the apex usually overlies the inferior part of the medullary velum. The fifth segment (p5) starts where the PICA extends out from the fissure between the tonsil, vermis, and cerebellar hemisphere. It often happens that the bifurcation of the PICA occurs at this fifth segment; the lateral trunk will supply the tonsil and cerebral surface, while the medial trunk will supply the vermis.

CT angiography and 3D reconstruction are usually sufficient for diagnostic purposes and surgical planning. Interventional angiography is rarely required, but for selective cases it still provides additional value for treatment.

19.3 Steps in Surgery

Microsurgical treatment of PICA aneurysms could be done either by clipping the aneurysm or trapping/occluding it with bypass surgery.

PICA aneurysms most commonly occur at the p2 and p3 segments [4]. Common approaches include by the lateral suboccipital or far lateral suboccipital for more proximal PICA aneurysms and paramedian or midline suboccipital for more distal PICA aneurysms. Other more complex skull-base approaches have also been described, such as retro-labyrinthine presigmoid and transsigmoid exposures. A modified far lateral approach, which has been the approach most frequently used by the senior author in dealing with PICA aneurysms, is described here.

The patient may be placed in a true lateral position, with the operative side facing upward (Fig. 19.2). The dependent extremity is hung in a sling. The contralateral shoulder is pushed forward anteriorly, and there is mild inferior traction of the shoulder with tape. The vertex of the head is tilted slightly toward the ground, and there is also a slight lateral rotation of the head toward the ground. This opens up the working space at the lateral suboccipital region. Skin incision is made in the manner of golf club with the descending limb remaining at the midline from inion to C2. The muscles and soft tissue are dissected with monopolar blade then retracted, exposing the occipital, mastoid bones and posterolateral arch of C1; when dissection is done near the foramen magnum, especially 2–3 cm laterally from the midline, where yellowish fat tissue occurs, one must be careful not to injure the extracranial VA. Place a burr hole near the transverse–sigmoid junction, gently detach the dura from the bone, and perform a craniotomy up to 1 cm from the midline and the foramen magnum inferiorly; additional C1 laminectomy is necessary for better

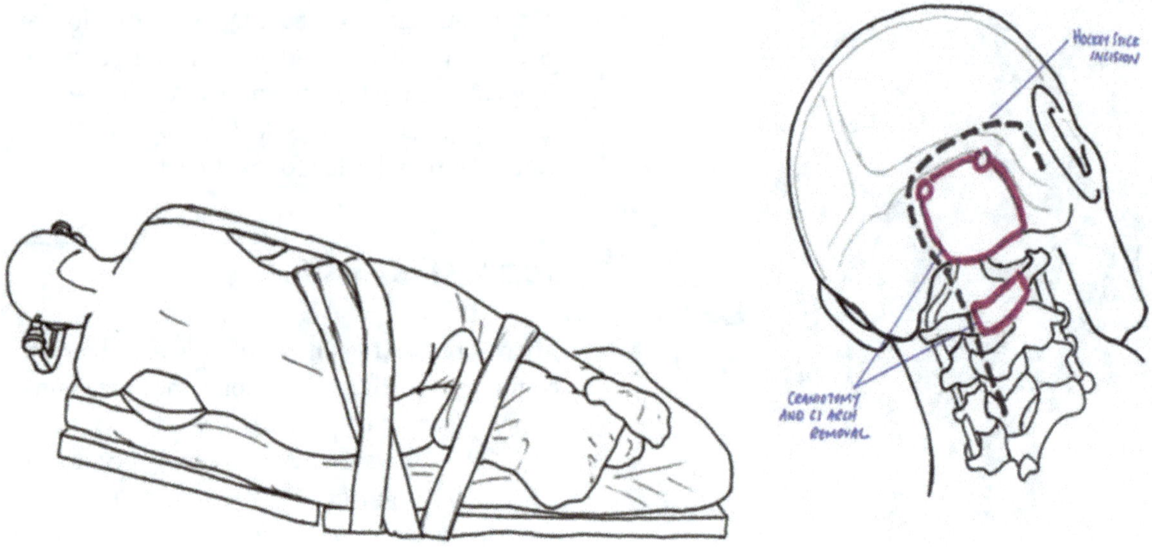

Fig. 19.2 *Left*: Patient is placed in lateral position with operative side upward. The dependent extremity is hung in a sling. The contralateral shoulder is pushed forward anteriorly, and there is mild inferior traction of shoulder with tape. *Right*: Vertex of head is tilted slightly toward ground, and there is also a slight lateral rotation of head toward ground

proximal control. Lateral suboccipital bony exposure should be up to the line where the VA enters the dura. The dura opening is a gentle curve and the edges are holded with silk stiches. The Cerebrospinal fluid needs to be released slowly so the brain is relaxed, and everything must be done under a microscopic view. Preparing the vertebra artery (VA) for the proximal control and usually the VA is under the dentate ligament when it comes to intracranially. The ligament must be cut gently from the foramen magnum and at C1 to enable viewing of the VA anteriorly and to widen the surgical corridor by detaching the upper cervical spinal cord. The proximal VA just after it becomes intracranial should be prepared for temporary clipping. In cases where the PICA originates right at the point where the VA pierces the dura, extradural/extracranial dissection of the VA may be performed. Typically, authors expose the VA at the point where the vessel forms a groove in the upper surface of the C1 lamina, which is marked anatomically by the sulcus limitans. Dissection of the PICA should not be a difficult procedure; in fact, it is relatively simple, and one should be able to locate the aneurysm by simply following the PICA's course. We can start following the PICA just under the tip of the tonsil and tracking it to the cistern. Sharp dissection may be done by opening the arachnoid layer to expose the vagoaccessory triangle, which provides a good natural working space, and many surgeons use this method in a far lateral approach (Fig. 19.3). Superiorly there is the vagus nerve, laterally the accessory nerve, and medially the medulla. One's view of the meeting point of the VA and PICA is usually obstructed by the IX–X–XI complex. Each case may have unique features, such as the shape of the aneurysm, the parent artery anatomy, and the tortuosity of the vessel, so the dissection strategy, including the pathway, should be formulated accordingly.

For more distally positioned aneurysms, surgical access may be achieved using a telovelar approach (Figs. 19.4 and 19.5).

PICA aneurysms are often associated with unusual anatomy, and direct clipping is not always possible. Several factors such as the branch anatomy, the size of the aneurysm, dolicho-ectatic morphology, or even atherosclerotic neck, will contribute to the difficulty. This then requires alternative techniques such as a trapping and

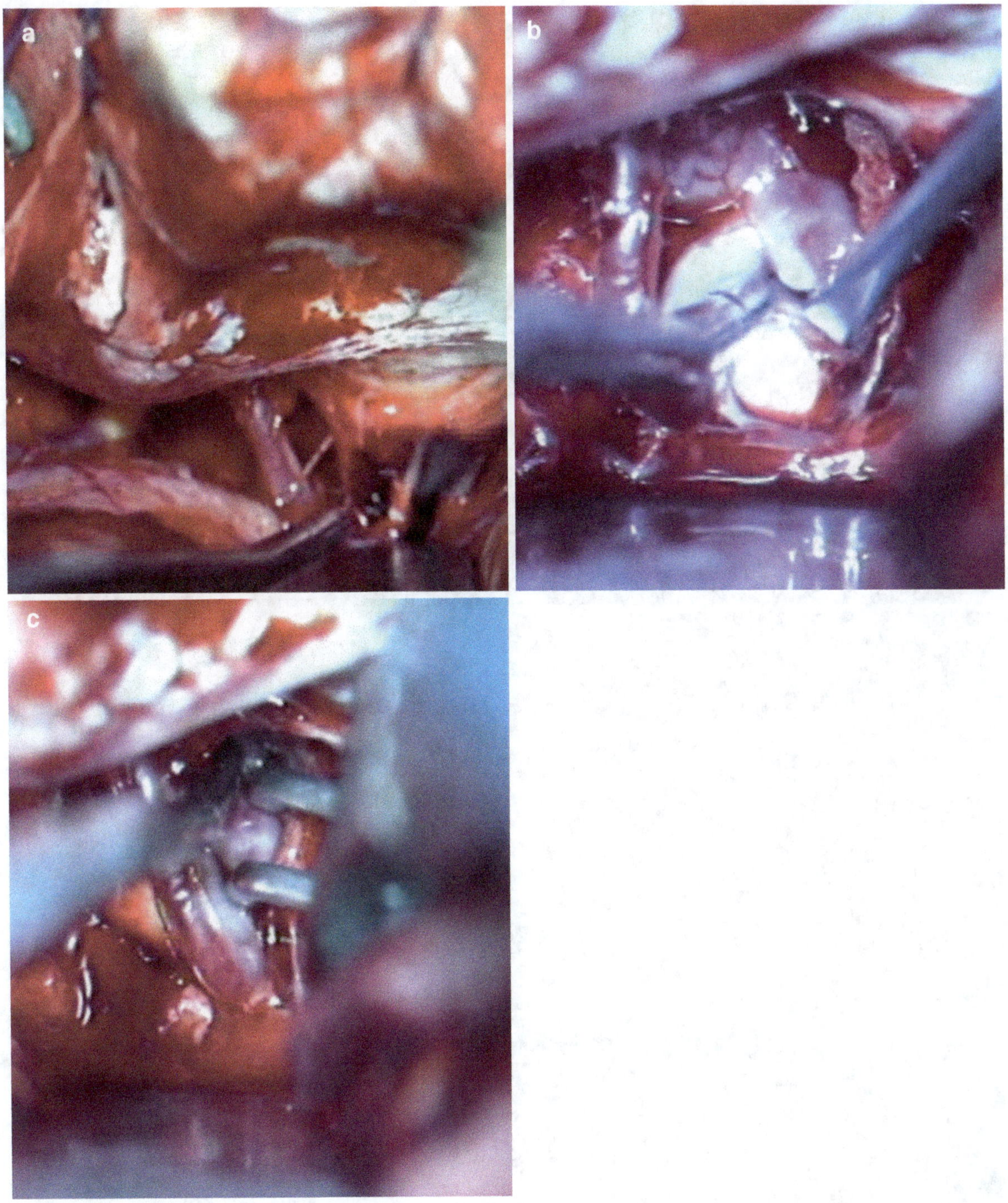

Fig. 19.3 (**a**) This patient has a proximal left PICA aneurysm in lateral medullary zone. The approach is via a modified far lateral approach. (**b**) The dissection is deep to the rootlets of the accessory nerve to expose the aneurysm neck. (**c**) The aneurysm was clipped simply with a bayonet clip

bypass procedure. Preoperative study and planning are very important if revascularization procedures are necessary. This is particularly significant in proximally located aneurysms, particularly at the VA–PICA junction. In scenarios potentially requiring the occlusion of the PICA, bypass procedures may be necessary.

There are various options of extra-intracranial (EC-IC) bypass surgery. However, Authors generally favor an in situ bypass (PICA–PICA) that matches donor and recipient arteries well because it can be performed quickly.

Bypass options include the following (Fig. 19.6):

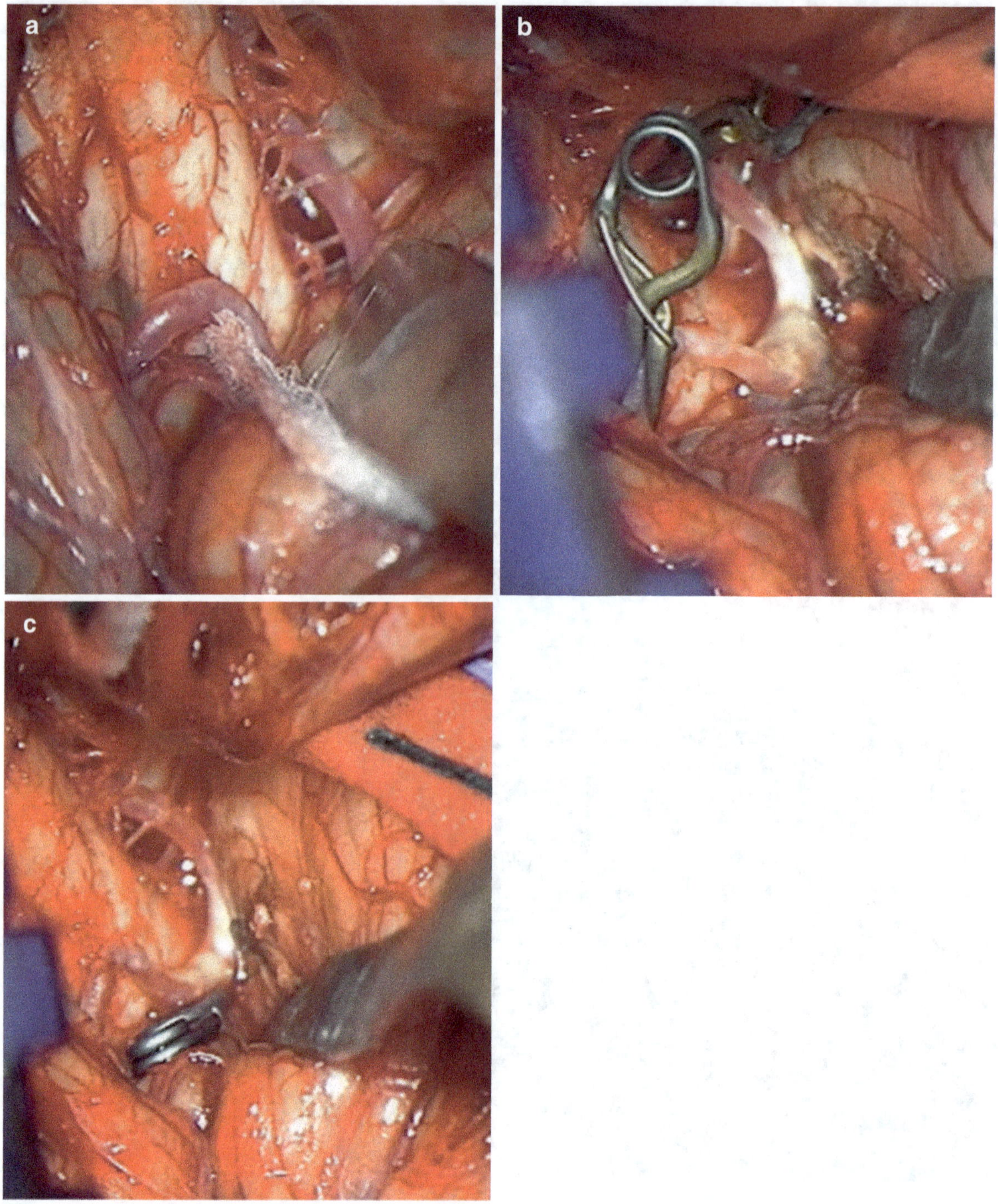

Fig. 19.4 (**a**) Some PICA aneurysms are located more distally, such as this one, at the ascending loop of the p3 segment of the left PICA. This is better accessed via a midline suboccipital approach. (**b**) Proximal and distal control was achieved with temporary clipping, before dissecting out the aneurysm neck. (**c**) The aneurysm was clipped simply with a straight clip

1. PICA-to-PICA bypass,
2. Reimplantation of PICA in VA,
3. Reanastomosis of PICA,
4. High-flow bypass from VA to PICA using radial artery graft,
5. Occipital artery (OA)–PICA bypass.

PICA–PICA bypass involves the using two PICAs that lie close to each other at the midline in the ascending portion of the p3 segment running at the medial surface of the tonsil. The two loops are generously mobilized and their arachnoid trabecula is cut to make the vessel free

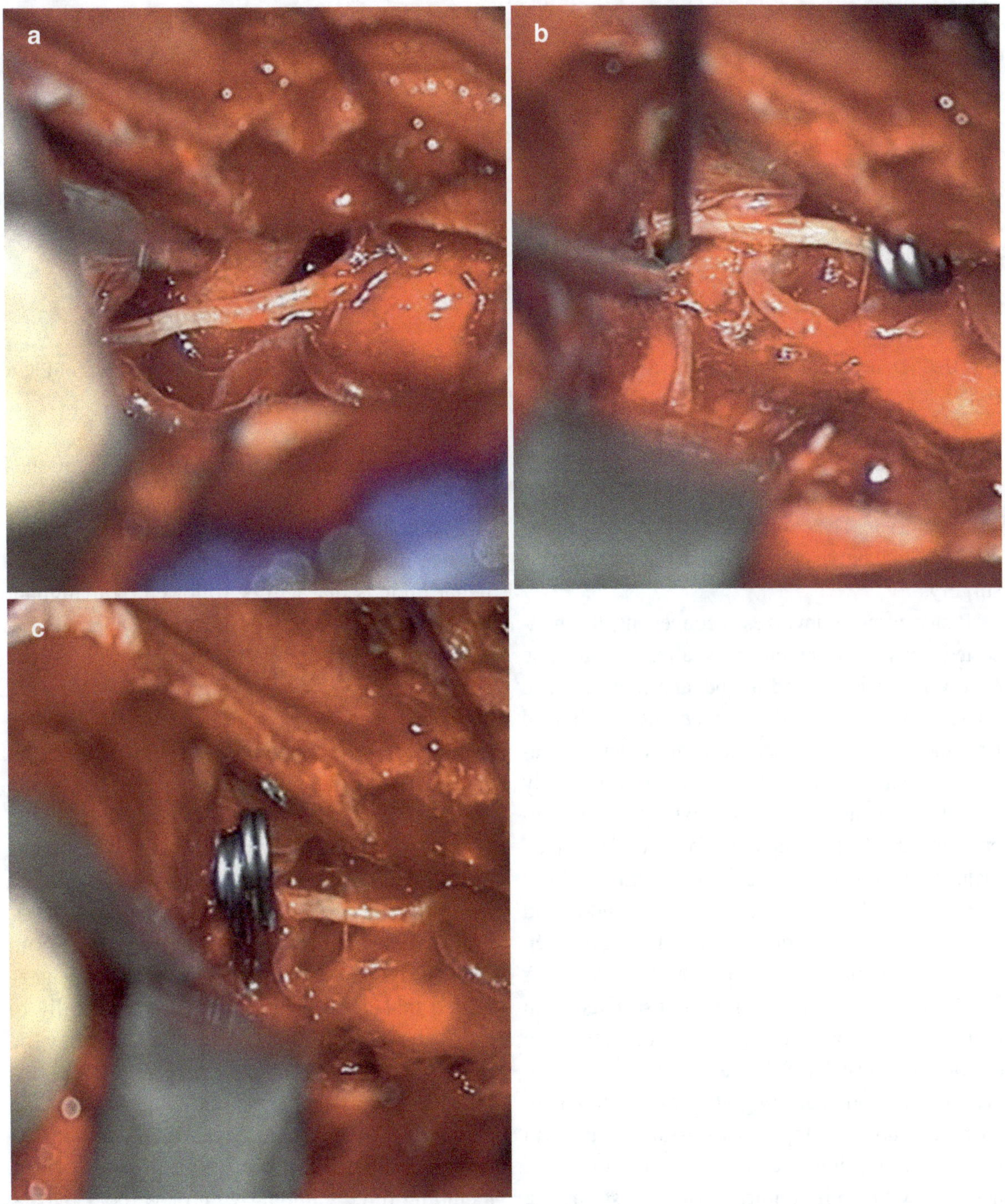

Fig. 19.5 (**a**) This is a case of proximal right PICA aneurysm located at the lateral medullary segment. Dissection was via a modified far lateral approach. Intradural VA was identified for proximal control. (**b**) Aneurysm neck excised just beyond the traversing accessory nerve. (**c**) The aneurysm neck was obliterated with tandem clipping

and to allow for tension-free side-to-side anastomosis. With the temporary clips in place on both PICAs, a longitudinal arteriotomy is made in each artery, ideally two to three times the PICA diameter. Both PICAs should have almost identical diameters, or the donor should be larger than the ipsilateral recipient.

Reimplantation of the PICA can be done if the clip obliteration of the aneurysm also sacrifices the PICA but preserves the VA. The occluded PICA can be revascularized by cutting at its origin, transposing and reimplanting it proximally to the original PICA origin. This is an end-to-side anastomosis. Reimplantation is probably the

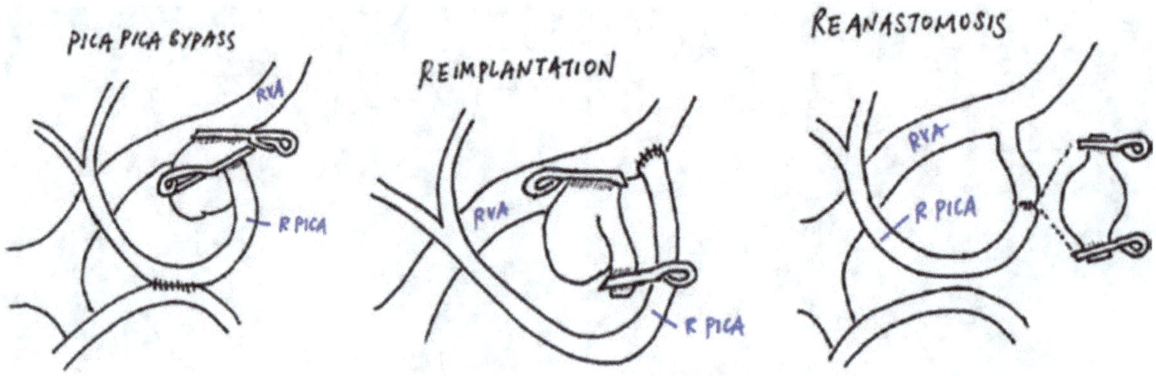

Fig. 19.6 Drawing of PICA–PICA bypass (*left*), reimplantation of PICA to VA (middle), and reanastomosis of PICA (*right*)

hardest of the IC–IC bypasses because the location is deep and it is surrounded by all the lower cranial nerves. The complication of postoperative lower cranial nerve palsy is much higher with this surgery.

Reanastomosis involves reconnecting the transected ends of a parent artery after excising the aneurysm; it is an end-to-end anastomosis. The afferent and efferent ends are generously mobilized from their arachnoid adhesions to allow approximation without tension. A PICA's tortuosity usually provides adequate length to get to the arteries without tension. Ideal situations for such a bypass include aneurysms that are fusiform in their distal portions and have no branches. The end-to-end anastomosis line is shorter, making suturing quicker.

Large complex aneurysms at the VA–PICA junction may be trapped and reconstructed with an interposition graft using the radial artery. The donor site is usually at V3, and the recipient site is a PICA. A radial artery graft is more suitable in terms of caliber compared to a saphenous vein graft. Interposition means that two grafts are needed, with both requiring two anastomoses, either end to end or end to side.

An alternative bypass is an OA–PICA bypass for large complex aneurysms involving the VA–PICA junction. The OA is located at the posteriormost of the eight branches of the External Carotid artery and lies medially and posteriorly of the mastoid process. It is identified preoperatively using a handheld Doppler probe. It is usually densely adhered to its surrounding muscular tissue, making it more difficult to dissect compared to the Superficial Temporal Artery. It is an end-to-side anastomosis.

Parent artery sacrifice of the PICA is a possible treatment, but it may cause medullary and cerebellar infarcts that will be followed by malignant edema, causing acute hydrocephalus or, in the worst case, direct brainstem compression. These complications may be tolerable if the patient's condition deteriorates, in which case urgent decompressive craniectomy may become necessary. Many surgeons might simply sacrifice the parent artery without revascularization if the aneurysm arises at the most distal two segments of the PICA [5]. The more proximally parent PICA should not be sacrificed because of variations in perforating vessels that may arise from more proximal segments. Liew et al. have suggested that if an aneurysm is located distally to the last perforator artery, then a clip may be safely placed on the parent artery after the perforator artery [6]. If there is no evidence that the patient will be able to tolerate PICA sacrifice, the surgeon will need to prepare all alternatives, including direct clipping with or without bypass to preserve the PICA; additional endovascular coiling will likely be required to achieve complete aneurysm occlusion [7].

19.4 Expert Opinion

PICA aneurysms are relatively rare and pose significant challenges to neurosurgeons owing to their proximity to critical structures and their variable complex anatomy. However, they can be successfully managed microsurgically, and the neurosurgeon has a variety of options at her disposal that can be used aside from direct clipping, such as occlusion or trapping, with several bypass possibilities.

References

1. Schievink WI. Intracranial aneurysms. N Engl J Med. 1997;336:28–40.
2. Rinkel GJ, et al. Prevalence and risk of rupture of intracranial aneurysms: a systematic review. Stroke. 1998;29:251–6.
3. Hudgins RJ, et al. Aneurysms of the posterior inferior cerebellar artery. A clinical and anatomical analysis. J Neurosurg. 1983;58:381–7.
4. Rodríguez-Hernández A, et al. Distal aneurysms of intracranial arteries: application of numerical nomenclature, predilection for cerebellar arteries, and results of surgical management. World Neurosurg. 2013;80:103–12.
5. Heros RC. Posterior inferior cerebellar artery. Editorial. J Neurosurg. 2002;97:747–8.
6. Liew D, et al. Surgical management of ruptured and unruptured symptomatic posterior inferior cerebellar artery aneurysms. Br J Neurosurg. 2004;18:608–12.
7. Abla AA, et al. Intracranial-to-intracranial bypass for posterior inferior cerebellar artery aneurysms: options, technical challenges, and results in 35 patients. J Neurosurg. 2016;124(5):1275–86.

20 Surgery of Giant Aneurysm

Petra Wahjoepramono
and Eka J. Wahjoepramono

20.1 Sign and Symptoms

Aneurysm bigger than 25 mm is called giant aneurysm [1], further subdivided by morphology into saccular, fusiform, or dolichoectatic aneurysms [2]. Epidemiologically, they are very rare, comprising only 0.5% of all intracranial aneurysms, while others describe it as 3–5% of all intracranial aneurysms [1, 3, 4]; the epidemiology of intracranial aneurysms among the general population amounts to 0.2–9.9% [5]. In pediatric patients, the incidence of giant aneurysms and aneurysms of the posterior circulation is greater than those in adult patients [6]. The most common type is the saccular giant aneurysm, accounting for 98% of cases [7]. Fusiform types are more commonly found in the posterior circulation and MCA [1]. These lesions have a female preponderance and are diagnosed mostly between 40 and 60 years of age [2]. These lesions are found most often in the anterior circulation, affecting the ICA, MCA, and ACA [1, 2], while in the posterior circulation, they most commonly occur at the basilar artery, vertebrobasilar junction, PCA, and PICA [2]. Multiple giant aneurysms can be found in 7% of patients [2].

The most common presenting symptoms for these lesions are mass effect complaints, seizures caused by irritated neural tissue, or compression of cranial nerves [2, 4], which are very different from the subarachnoid bleed usually found in smaller aneurysms [2, 4]. Additionally, the occurrence of thrombus formation in these aneurysms may produce symptoms of thromboembolic event in the parent vessel or perforator vessels [2]. Thromboembolism may occur in up to 60% of giant aneurysms, and its probability increases along with aneurysm size. Hydrocephalus had been reported due to the compression of giant aneurysms near the cerebral aqueduct, and carotid-cavernous fistulae (CCF) can result from ruptured aneurysms of the ICA cavernous segment [2].

20.2 Investigation

These aneurysms must be thoroughly investigated as to its vascular anatomy, such as the presence of perforators, the size and orientation of the aneurysm neck, and its distal outflow (Fig. 20.1). Giant aneurysms frequently display calcification,

P. Wahjoepramono
Department of Neurosurgery, Medical Faculty of Universitas Padjadjaran, Hasan Sadikin Hospital, Bandung, West Java, Indonesia

Department of Neurosurgery, Faculty of Medicine Universitas Pelita Harapan (UPH), Neuroscience Centre Siloam Hospital Lippo Village, Tangerang, Indonesia

E. J. Wahjoepramono (✉)
Department of Neurosurgery, Faculty of Medicine Universitas Pelita Harapan (UPH), Neuroscience Centre Siloam Hospital Lippo Village, Tangerang, Indonesia

J. July, E. J. Wahjoepramono (eds.), *Neurovascular Surgery*,
https://doi.org/10.1007/978-981-10-8950-3_20

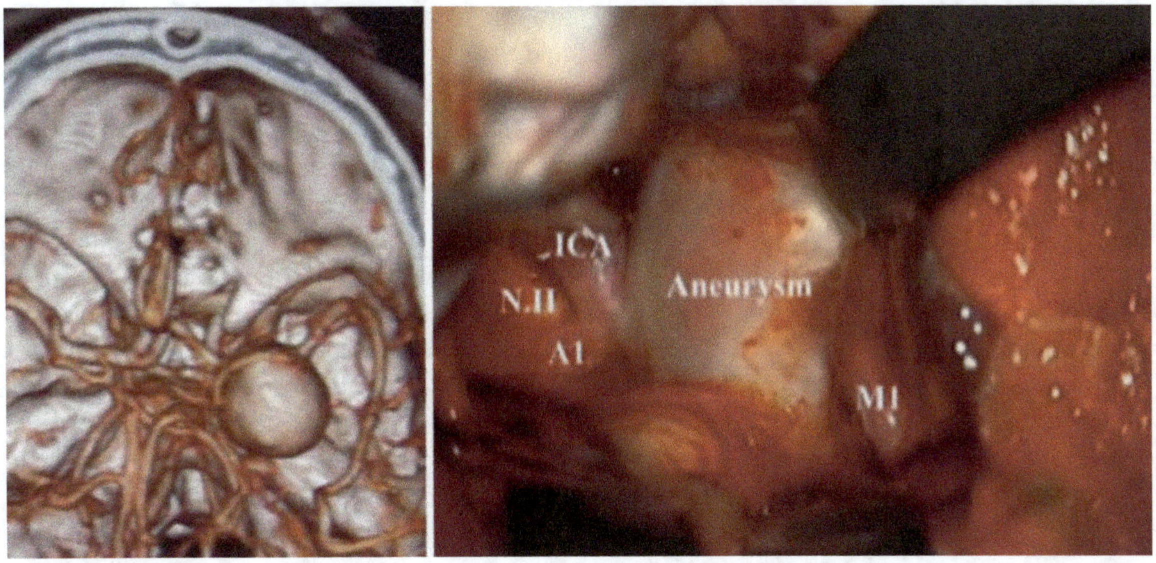

Fig. 20.1 *Left:* Three-dimensional CT scan of a 50-year-old, female with left M1 giant aneurysm. *Right:* Intraoperative finding after a wide sylvian fissure dissection

thrombosis, and wall thickening around the neck, while there may be multiple perforator vessels present from the parent artery or even from the aneurysmal sac in the case of fusiform aneurysms [4]. The gold standard diagnostic procedure would be digital subtraction angiography (DSA), which provides the best picture of cerebrovascular anatomy and provides information about the suitability for vessel bypass. DSA can be combined with CT angiography to provide information about surrounding bony anatomy for surgical approach and monitor the presence of calcified thrombus. CT scan is very useful in evaluating for calcification [1], and MRI may be performed if there is a suspected ischemic event, to investigate peritumoral edema and to evaluate intraluminal thrombus [1]. Preoperative assessment of these patients includes balloon occlusion tests during angiography, if the surgeon plans to sacrifice the ipsilateral ICA [2]. Intraoperatively, patients may be monitored using electroencephalography (EEG) to detect any changes in the electrical activity, as well as continuous transcranial Doppler (CTD) to check the cerebral blood flow [2].

The natural course of giant unruptured aneurysm has been previously reported by Wiebers et al. [8]; in anterior circulation the 5-year cumulative risk is about 40%, while in the posterior circulation including posterior communicating artery, the risk is about 50%. A study by ISUIA (International Study of Unruptured Intracranial Aneurysms) group shows the rupture rate at 6% in the first year after diagnosis alone [5, 9], with a more recent study by the UCAS Japan investigators reporting a rupture risk of giant aneurysms at 76.26% within 3 years [3], with aneurysms at the posterior and anterior communicating arteries being more likely to rupture [3, 5, 9]. The mortality rate of such ruptures reaches 20–70% [10, 11], reaching higher than 60% within 2 years of diagnosis [12]. It is therefore established that such rupture rates were similar or worse to the risks taken when a similar lesion is treated, either through surgery or endovascular treatment. More recent studies on the natural course of aneurysms have not found any other parameters indicative of rupture risk [13].

20.3 Steps of Surgery

20.3.1 Surgical Approach

Microsurgical clipping has the advantage of being able to relieve mass effect associated with nerve compression, especially in aneurysms with thrombus formation or atheroma [14].

The main principles of giant aneurysm surgery are to prepare the proximal and distal control, avoid the blunt dissection, and appreciate all the perforators, and to achieve circumferential dissection of the aneurysm might be very difficult [12]. The goals of surgical management of giant aneurysms are:

1. To isolate the aneurysm from the blood circulation
2. To preserve cerebral blood flow distal to the aneurysm
3. To relieve mass effect on neural structures caused by the aneurysm [1, 2, 15].

Several microsurgical techniques which are used in the management of giant aneurysms include: microsurgical clipping, bypass of parent artery (ICA) using saphenous vein graft or the MCA, temporary ligation of the ICA to help clipping, aneurysm wrapping with muscle or fascia, or combined microsurgical and endovascular treatment [2].

Microsurgical clipping of giant aneurysms can be performed, because all aneurysms must have a "neck." [4] With the use of fenestrated clips, aneurysms with large necks can undergo vessel reconstruction to create an aneurysm neck [4] (Fig. 20.2).

The presence of perianeurysmal edema, which is most often found in the MCA circulation, may complicate the microsurgical clipping [16].

There are several approaches available for microsurgery of giant aneurysms of the carotid artery or the basilar tip; an approach through the middle fossa is recommended. The important surgical anatomy in this region is the cavernous sinus, which includes several natural corridors available to access this region, usually divided into the ten triangular spaces [2]. Skeletonization of the ICA in the carotid canal through Glasscock's triangle [12] is performed to treat intracavernous aneurysms [2]. Orbito-zygomatic approach is used to maximize exposure [12].

Certain location of the posterior circulation aneurysm could be approach through subtemporal such as the upper basilar artery segment [2]. The transpetrosal approach or far-lateral approach may be used for lower lesions [12, 17].

To reduce mass effect of the giant aneurysm after clipping is performed, the aneurysm dome can be directly punctured to exsanguinate the sac when no thrombus is present and perform suction decompression [4, 12] (Fig. 20.3). If there is thrombus, calcification or atheroma is present, thrombectomy may be performed on the aneurysm sac, also called endoaneurysmectomy [4].

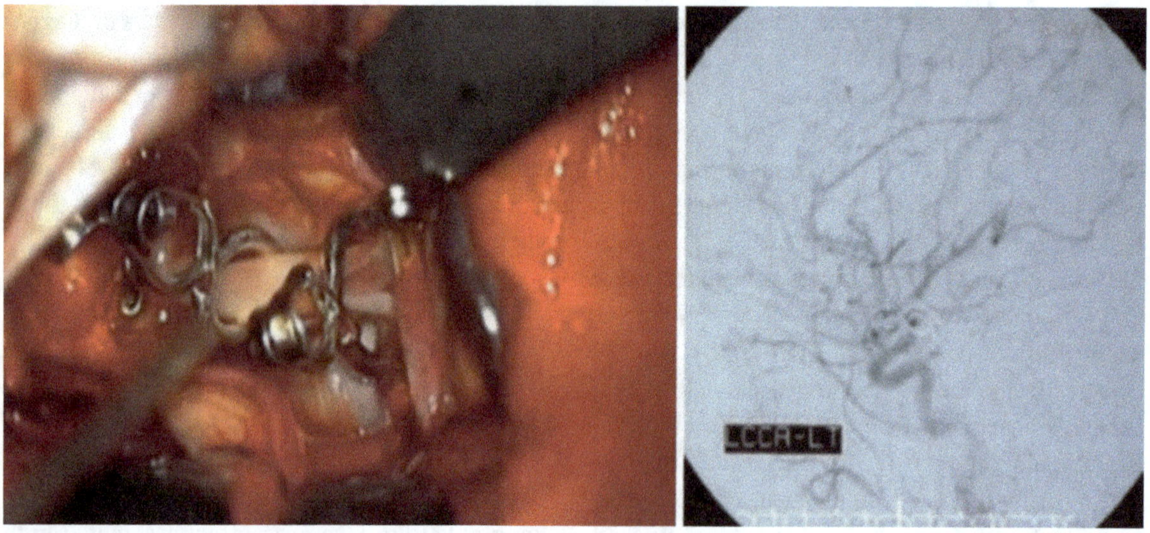

Fig. 20.2 *Left:* Same case of Fig. 20.1 shows intraoperative view of giant aneurysm undergoing vessel reconstruction with multiple fenestrated clips. *Right:* Angiography confirmation of MCA flow

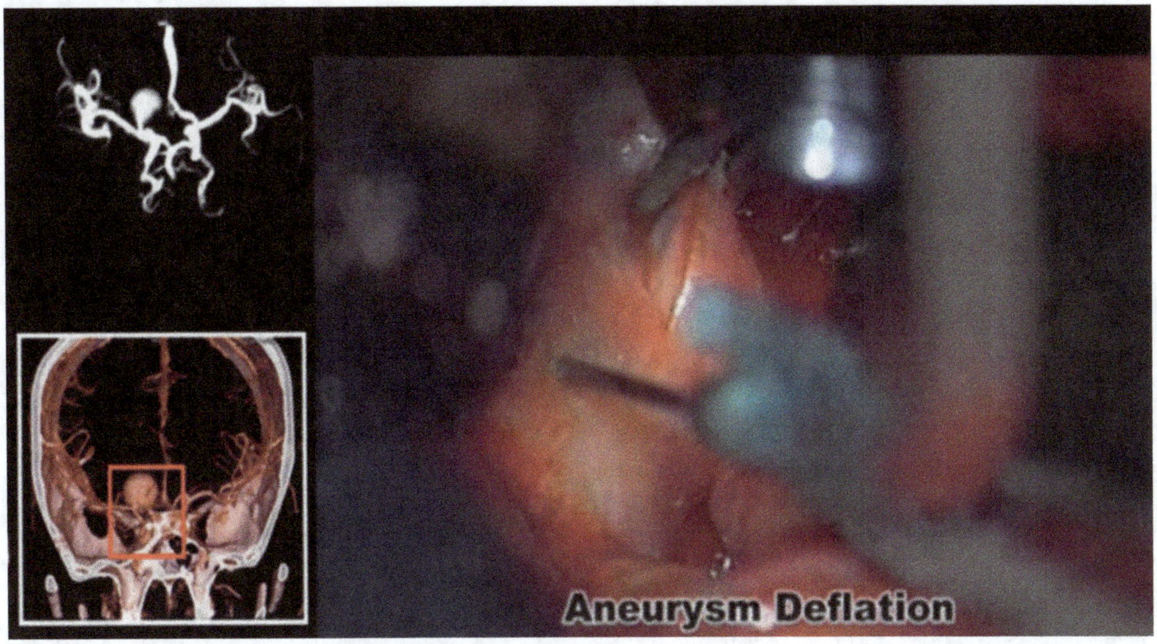

Fig. 20.3 Aneurysm deflation using the wing needle no 25G

Aneurysm repair using wrapping or clip wrapping with the muscle or fascia can be used to maximize outcomes in ruptured aneurysms [12]. Aneurysms which are broad-based, frail, or complex may also be clipped using augmented "cotton-clipping" technique [18]. This technique can also be used to perform emergency repair in the case of ruptured aneurysm.

Low-flow and high-flow bypass techniques have been used to provide revascularization of the distal circulation in the treatment of giant aneurysms [4]. Vessel reconstruction using clips also serve the same function, which is to guarantee CBF distal to the aneurysm [4].

Microsurgical treatment may be advantageous in comparison with endovascular treatment in cases of complex basilar artery aneurysms. Performing surgical clipping of the aneurysm may provide selective occlusion of the basilar artery aneurysm while avoiding damage to the thalamoperforators which may adhere to the posterior aspect of the aneurysm, compared to endovascular treatment where visualization of the perforators cannot be achieved, and the risk of brainstem damage due to ischemia is greater [19].

Adjunctive techniques which can be used in giant aneurysm surgery include deep hypothermic circulatory arrest (DHCA) [4, 20, 21] and the use of excimer laser-assisted nonocclusive anastomosis (ELANA) bypass [22, 23]. DHCA may be performed to temporarily reduce blood flow to the aneurysm, facilitating the surgeon to perform surgical clipping and neck reconstruction. However, it has several drawbacks, including unpredictable recovery after circulatory arrest and possibility of postoperative brain hemorrhage [24]. A study by Ponce et al. also shows significant mortality and morbidity rates for using DHCA, even though most patients had improved neurological function after surgery [21]. Neuroprotective agents may also be used to improve outcome after surgery, especially if DHCA will be used. Barbiturates are traditionally used to reduce cerebral blood volume and metabolism before the ischemic procedure [12].

The ELANA technique enables surgeons to perform a high-flow bypass without utilizing temporary clips, which makes it a reasonable alternative to other methods of direct revascularization, such as direct anastomosis [23]. The elimination of temporary clips from the procedure provides the surgeon with longer safe operating time without cerebral ischemia and eliminates the need of exposing the proximal parent artery before the procedure, which is especially beneficial in the posterior fossa [23].

20.3.2 Endovascular Approach

Endovascular management has the advantage of decreased morbidity, due to its nonsurgical nature [25]; aneurysms at the posterior circulation especially show higher morbidity after microsurgery [26]. The endovascular management of giant aneurysms can be performed as long as the aneurysm does not show signs of intraluminal thrombus; if there is thrombus, then endovascular management will not be able to relieve the mass effect caused by the aneurysm itself, even though it could occlude the aneurysm from the circulation.

The endovascular management for giant aneurysms are [25]:

1. The parent artery could be occluded by using coils or balloons.
2. Coiling of the aneurysm coiling of the aneurysm and spare the parent artery.
3. Balloon-, stent-, or neck-bridging-assisted device for selective coiling [27].
4. Selective occlusion with ethylene vinyl alcohol copolymer (ONYX).
5. Sacrifice the parent artery after bypass surgery.

Parent vessel occlusion is a very simple technique which is guaranteed to exclude the aneurysm from cerebral circulation [4, 25]. This is the endovascular treatment of choice if the patient can tolerate parent vessel occlusion [25]. Multiple tests must be done before this treatment, using balloon occlusion test, to ensure that the cerebral circulation is not compromised by blocking the parent artery [25]. A study by Linskey et al. demonstrated that even without previous BOT, up to 75% of patients can tolerate ICA occlusion [28]. The vertebral artery, however, can be safely occluded, except where the patient only has a single vertebral artery without a patent PCoA [25].

Selective occlusion of giant aneurysms, whether using coils or ONYX embolization device, emphasizes on filling the aneurysm lumen and occluding the aneurysm from the circulation as thrombus forms within the lumen [25]. As most giant aneurysms are formed with large necks, coil-assisted devices such as stents, balloons, or flow diverters are often used [25]. The re-endothelialization of the parent artery after such a procedure is key to preserving a patent lumen and reducing reopening of the aneurysm [29].

Another treatment option is to use flow-diverting stents [4]. These devices have more metal coverage and lower porosity in comparison with standard intracranial stents and have the capability of creating blood flow inside their artificial lumen and induce thrombus formation in the dome of giant aneurysms as blood flow into the dome decreases. These stents are also capable of providing a scaffold for neointimal growth in the vessel. The role of flow diverters against giant aneurysms is effective, with permanent major complication occurring in 3% of patients in a study by Piano et al. [30] and 5–10% of patients in other studies [31]. Previous studies have documented encouraging results when these stents are used against aneurysms of the anterior circulation [32, 33], defined as aneurysms from the ICA below the anterior choroidal artery. However, they are not as effective against aneurysms in the vertebrobasilar system [34]. It is thought that the vertebrobasilar system with its many perforators are not suitable for flow-diverting stents, as these stents also occlude the perforators, in some cases up to 2 years after stent placement [34]. The resulting ischemia of the pons may lead to unacceptable morbidity [34]. These devices may also be used in conjunction with coils to achieve complete occlusion of the aneurysm [35].

The main concern about selective occlusion is that the embolization device may disengage over time, either by coil become compaction, the coil sometimes migrate, degeneration of the thrombus intraluminal or migration of the ONYX clot into the parent artery [25, 26, 36]. This problem is caused by the inherent nature of giant aneurysms, with their large lumen volume, which sometimes cannot be adequately packed with these devices [25, 26]. Stable occlusion of these aneurysms requires at least 25% packing of its volume, which is difficult to achieve with large-volume aneurysms [25]. In a study by van Rooij et al. [25], it is found that nearly all giant aneurysms show reopening after endovascular treatment in the 6-month postoperative period, even up to several years of stable condition. The follow-up strategy for these patients is to schedule additional coiling procedures along with routine follow-up, with decreased patient compliance as a result [25, 37]. MRA has also been suggested as a routine follow-up procedure after endovascular treatment [37].

20.4 Expert Opinion/Suggestion to Avoid Complication

In several cases such as paraclinoid giant aneurysms, combined approach using microsurgical and endovascular management can be performed [38]. Paraclinoid giant aneurysms are often atherosclerotic and calcified, difficult exposure and dissection of the aneurysm dome, and difficulty in exposure and proximal control through temporary clipping [38, 39]. In such cases, temporary occlusion of the parent artery can be achieved through the endovascular method, while microsurgery is used to expose and clip the tumor, followed with suction decompression of the aneurysm dome [4]. Flow alteration using a combined microsurgical and endovascular method may be used to treat fusiform basilar artery aneurysms [40]. Sughrue et al. [18] championed a combined approach using microsurgery and endovascular therapy as an adjunct in the treatment of giant aneurysms.

References

1. Hanel RA, Spetzler RF. Surgical treatment of complex intracranial aneurysms. Neurosurgery. 2008;62(6):11.
2. Aguiar PH, Zicarelli CA, Isolan G, Antunes AC. Giant brain aneurysms of anterior circulation. Surgical anatomy. Revista Chilena de Neurocirugía. 2013;39:6.
3. Investigators TUJ. The natural course of unruptured cerebral aneurysms in a Japanese cohort. N Engl J Med. 2012;366(26):9.
4. Sekhar LN, Tariq F, Mai JC, Kim LJ, Ghodke B, Hallam DK, et al. Unyielding progress: treatment paradigms for giant aneurysms. Clin Neurosurg. 2012;59:16.
5. Investigators TISOUIA. Unruptured intracranial aneurysms—risk of rupture and risks of surgical intervention. N Engl J Med. 1998;339(24):8.
6. Mehrotra A, Nair AP, Das KK, Srivastava A, Sahu RN, Kumar R. Clinical and radiological profiles and outcomes in pediatric patients with intracranial aneurysms. J Neurosurg Pediatr. 2012;10:7.
7. Yasargil M. Microneurosurgery. New York: Georg Thieme Verlag; 1994.
8. Wiebers D, Whisnant J, Huston J, Meissner I, Brown RJ, Piepgras D, et al. Unruptured intracranial aneurysms: natural history, clinical outcome, and risks of surgical and endovascular treatment. Lancet. 2003;12(362):7.
9. Investigators ISoUA. Unruptured intracranial aneurysms—risk of rupture and risks of surgical intervention. N Engl J Med. 1998;3339:8.
10. Barrow DL, Alleyne C. Natural history of giant intracranial aneurysms and indications for intervention. Clin Neurosurg. 1995;42:30.
11. Orz Y, Kobayashi S, Osawa M, Tanaka Y. Aneurysm size: a prognostic factor for rupture. Br J Neurosurg. 1997;11:5.
12. Ramachandran M, Retarekar R, Raghavan ML, Berkowitz B, Dickerhoff B, Correa T, et al. Assessment of image-derived risk factors for natural course of unruptured cerebral aneurysms. J Neurosurg. 2016;124:7.
13. Komotar RJ, Mocco J, Solomon RA. Guidelines for the surgical treatment of unruptured intracranial aneurysms. The 1st annual J Lawrence Pool Memorial Research Symposium, New York; 2008. p. 39.
14. Dengler J, Maldaner N, Bijlenga P, Burkhardt J-K, Graewe A, Guhl S, et al. Perianeurysmal edema in giant intracranial aneurysms in relation to aneurysm location, size, and partial thrombosis. J Neurosurg. 2015;123:7.
15. Rodríguez-Hernández A, Lawton MT. Anatomical triangles defining surgical routes to posterior inferior cerebellar artery aneurysms. J Neurosurg. 2011; 114:7.
16. Safavi-Abbasi S, Moron F, Sun H, Oppenlander ME, Kalani MYS, Mulholland CB, et al. Techniques and long-term outcomes of cotton-clipping and cotton-augmentation strategies for management of cerebral aneurysms. J Neurosurg. 2016;125:720.
17. Kellner CP, Haque RM, Meyers PM, Lavine SD, Connolly ES Jr, Solomon RA. Complex basilar artery aneurysms treated using surgical basilar occlusion: a modern case series. J Neurosurg. 2011;115:9.
18. Sughrue ME, Saloner D, Rayz VL, Lawton MT. Giant intracranial aneurysms: evolution of management in a contemporary surgical series. Neurosurgery. 2011;69(6):10.
19. Wait SD, Killory BD, Nakaji P, Zabramski JM. Cardiac standstill for cerebral aneurysms in 103 patients: an update on the experience at the Barrow Neurological Institute. J Neurosurg. 2011; 114:8.
20. van Doormaal T, van der Zwan A, Verweij B, Regli L, Tulleken C. Giant aneurysm clipping under protection of an excimer laser-assisted non-occlusive anastomosis bypass. Neurosurgery. 2010;66(3):8.

21. Langer DJ, Vajkoczy P. ELANA: excimer laser-assisted nonocclusive anastomosis for extracranial-to-intracranial and intracranial-to-intracranial bypass: a review. Skull Base. 2005;15(3):15.
22. Khandelwal P, Kato Y, Sano H, Yoneda M, Kanno T. Treatment of ruptured intracranial aneurysms: our approach. Minim Invasive Neurosurg. 2005;48(6):4.
23. Rooij WJ, Sluzewski M. Endovascular treatment of large and giant aneurysms. Am J Neuroradiol. 2009;30:6.
24. Sluzewski M, Menovsky T, Rooij WJ, Wijnalda D. Coiling of very large or giant cerebral aneurysms: long-term clinical and serial angiographic results. Am J Neuroradiol. 2003;24:5.
25. Aguilar-Perez M, Kurre W, Fischer S, Bazner H, Henkes H. Coil occlusion of wide-neck bifurcation aneurysms assisted by a novel intra- to extra-aneurysmatic neck-bridging device (pCONus): initial experience. Am J Neuroradiol. 2014;35:965.
26. Linskey ME, Jungreis CA, Yonas H Jr, Hirsch WL, Sekhar LN, Horton JA, et al. Stroke risk after abrupt internal carotid artery sacrifice: accuracy of preoperative assessment with balloon test occlusion and stable xenon-enhanced CT. Am J Neuroradiol. 1994;15:15.
27. Niemela M, Koivisto T, Kivipelto L, Ishii K, Rinne J, Ronkainen A, et al. Microsurgical clipping of cerebral aneurysms after the ISAT study. Acta Neurochir. 2005;94:3.
28. Piano M, Valvassori L, Quilici L, Pero G, Boccardi E. Midterm and long-term follow-up of cerebral aneurysms treated with flow diverter devices: a single-center experience. J Neurosurg. 2013;118:9.
29. Wong GKC, Kwan MCL, Ng RYT, Yu SCH, Poon WS. Flow diverters for treatment of intracranial aneurysms: current status and ongoing. Clin Trials. 2011;18(6):4.
30. Lylyk P, Miranda C, Ceratto R, Ferrario A, Scrivano E, Luna H, et al. Curative endovascular reconstruction of cerebral aneurysms with the pipeline embolization device: the Buenos Aires experience. Neurosurgery. 2009;64(4):10.
31. Nelson PK, Lylyk P, Szikora I, Wetzel S, Wanke I, Fiorella D. The pipeline embolization device for the intracranial treatment of aneurysms trial. Am J Radiol. 2011;32(1):7.
32. Siddiqui AH, Abla AA, Kan P, Dumont TM, Jahshan S, Britz GW, et al. Panacea or problem: flow diverters in the treatment of symptomatic large or giant fusiform vertebrobasilar aneurysms. J Neurosurg. 2012;116:8.
33. Nossek E, Chalif DJ, Chakraborty S, Lombardo K, Black KS, Setton A. Concurrent use of the pipeline embolization device and coils for intracranial aneurysms: technique, safety, and efficacy. J Neurosurg. 2015;122:8.
34. Voormolen MH, Plazier M, Parizel P, Ridder DD, Maas AIR, Hernesniemi JA. Microsurgical removal of Onyx HD-500 from an aneurysm for relief of brainstem compression. J Neurosurg. 2010;113:3.
35. Plowman RS, Clarke A, Clarke M, Byrne JV. Sixteen-year single-surgeon experience with coil embolization for ruptured intracranial aneurysms: recurrence rates and incidence of late rebleeding. J Neurosurg. 2011;114:12.
36. Arnautović K, Al-Mefty O. Angtuaco E. A combined microsurgical skull-base and endovascular approach to giant and large paraclinoid aneurysms. Surg Neurol. 1998;50(6):14.
37. Ota T. The treatment of large and giant paraclinoid internal carotid artery aneurysms. J Vascu Med Surg. 2013;1(2):2.
38. Hoh BL, Putman CM, Budzik RF, Carter BS, Ogilvy CS. Combined surgical and endovascular techniques of flow alteration to treat fusiform and complex wide-necked intracranial aneurysms that are unsuitable for clipping or coil embolization. J Neurosurg. 2001;95:12.
39. Roloff C, Berg P, Bendicks C, Zähringer K, Janiga G, Thévenin D. Flow investigation inside a cerebral giant aneurysm. 17th international symposium on applications of laser techniques to fluid mechanics, July 7–10 2014, Lisbon, Portugal; 2014.
40. Molyneux AJ, Kerr RS, Yu L-M, Clarke M, Sneade M, Yarnold JA, et al. International subarachnoid aneurysm trial (ISAT) of neurosurgical clipping versus endovascular coiling in 2143 patients with ruptured intracranial aneurysms: a randomised comparison of effects on survival, dependency, seizures, rebleeding, subgroups, and aneurysm occlusion. Lancet. 2005;366:8.

Surgery of Posterior Fossa AVM

21

Ferzat Hijazy, Mardjono Tjahjadi, Aruma O'shahinan, Hanna Lehto, Hugo Andrade, Behnam Rezai Jahromi, Johan Marjamaa, Aki Laakso, Martin Lehecka, and Juha Hernesniemi

21.1 Signs and Symptoms

Prior to the routine use of vertebral angiography, posterior fossa AVMs were usually found unexpectedly during the evacuation of posterior fossa hematomas [1]. In 1932 (May 5th), Olivecrona had reported their first successful radical removal of a left cerebellar AVM in a 37-year-old male who was misdiagnosed of having a posterior fossa tumor. After an 8-h-long marathon surgery under local anesthesia and with a blood transfusion of 2000 ml, the AVM was removed. The postoperative course was uneventful and the patient left the hospital 3 months later [2]. As vertebral angiography became more widely used, the preoperative diagnosis of posterior fossa AVMs became possible. Even so, at that time, neurosurgeons thought that it was possible to operate on small-to-moderate-sized AVMs in silent areas of the brain but were reluctant to touch AVMs in nonsilent areas [2], including the more demanding posterior fossa. Neurosurgeons were, however, disappointed that only very few AVMs could be removed entirely without great risk, which led to the development of other, ineffectual techniques, such as vertebral artery or feeder ligation [1].

In 1961, based on a review of literature and his personal experience, Verbiest showed that small cerebellar AVMs could be removed safely. However large posterior fossa AVMs, even if located outside the brainstem, could be extremely dangerous to operate on, while brainstem AVMs were considered inoperable lesions by their nature [3]. Since that report, the frequency of successful surgical removal of the posterior fossa AVMs has increased with the development of new microsurgical and radiological techniques, modern neuroanesthesia, and refined intensive care principles. Later, Drake with his big series reported that removal of the posterior fossa AVMs even in the more sensitive areas of the hindbrain could also be accomplished with excellent outcomes.

Over the last 30 years, around 1000 patients with AVMs have been treated in two centers in Finland (Helsinki and Kuopio); one tenth of them were posterior fossa AVMs. The accumulated experience in the treatment of these patients is documented in this chapter, as well as the philosophical and practical basis for our current management of these relatively uncommon lesions.

All types of AVMs contribute about 2% of all hemorrhagic strokes. When AVM rupture occurs, it usually affects young adults in third or fourth decade of their life, more often males than

F. Hijazy · M. Tjahjadi · A. O'shahinan · H. Lehto
H. Andrade · B. R. Jahromi · J. Marjamaa · A. Laakso
M. Lehecka · J. Hernesniemi (✉)
Department of Neurosurgery, Helsinki University Central Hospital, Helsinki, Finland
e-mail: Hanna.lehto@hus.fi; Johan.marjamaa@hus.fi; aki.laakso@hus.fi; martin.lehecka@hus.fi; juha.hernesniemi@hus.fi

J. July, E. J. Wahjoepramono (eds.), *Neurovascular Surgery*,
https://doi.org/10.1007/978-981-10-8950-3_21

females. Based on the available data, the estimated rate is about 1:100,000 person-years which is about 1/10 of that of cerebral aneurysms. Posterior fossa AVMs are even more uncommon, and it can be roughly concluded that 1/10 of cerebral AVMs are located in the posterior fossa [1].

21.1.1 Location

The posterior cranial fossa is the largest and deepest of the three cranial fossae, which extends from the tentorial incisura superiorly to the foramen magnum inferiorly. The major contents of it are the cerebellum and the brainstem which consist of the midbrain, the pons, and the medulla oblongata. Posterior fossa AVMs can be generally classified into brainstem (25%), cerebellar vermian (15%), superficial cerebellar hemispheric (40%), and deep cerebellar hemispheric (20%) lesions based on the dominant location of the nidus.

Of the 631 AVM patients admitted to Helsinki University Central Hospital between 1942 and 2005, a total of 64 patients were diagnosed with infratentorial AVMs (Table 21.1).

21.1.2 Signs and Symptoms

In many studies, including ours, hemorrhage is the main clinical presentation of the posterior fossa AVMs accounting for 72–92% of the patients [1, 2, 4–7]. The type of hemorrhage depends on the location of the AVM, e.g., cerebellar AVM cases often come with intraparenchymal hemorrhage, cerebellopontine angle (CPA) AVMs are highly related to subarachnoid hemorrhage, and brainstem AVMs are more likely to cause subarachnoid and intraventricular hemorrhage (Figs. 21.1 and 21.2a). We have earlier reported that the annual rupture rate of posterior fossa AVMs within 5 years after admission is almost three times higher than in their supratentorial counterparts (11.6% vs. 4.3%) [8].

Table 21.1 The locations of the posterior fossa AVMs [4]

	Females *n* (%), 28 (44)	Males *n* (%), 36 (56)	Total *n* (%), 64 (100)
Pontomesencephalic	3 (10.7)	12 (33.3)	15 (23.4)
Medulla oblongata	1 (3.6)	0 (0)	1 (1.6)
Cerebellar vermis	5 (17.8)	4 (11.1)	9 (14)
Superficial cerebellar hemispheric	11 (39.2)	16 (44.4)	27 (42.2)
Deep cerebellar hemispheric	8 (28.6)	4 (11.1)	12 (18.8)

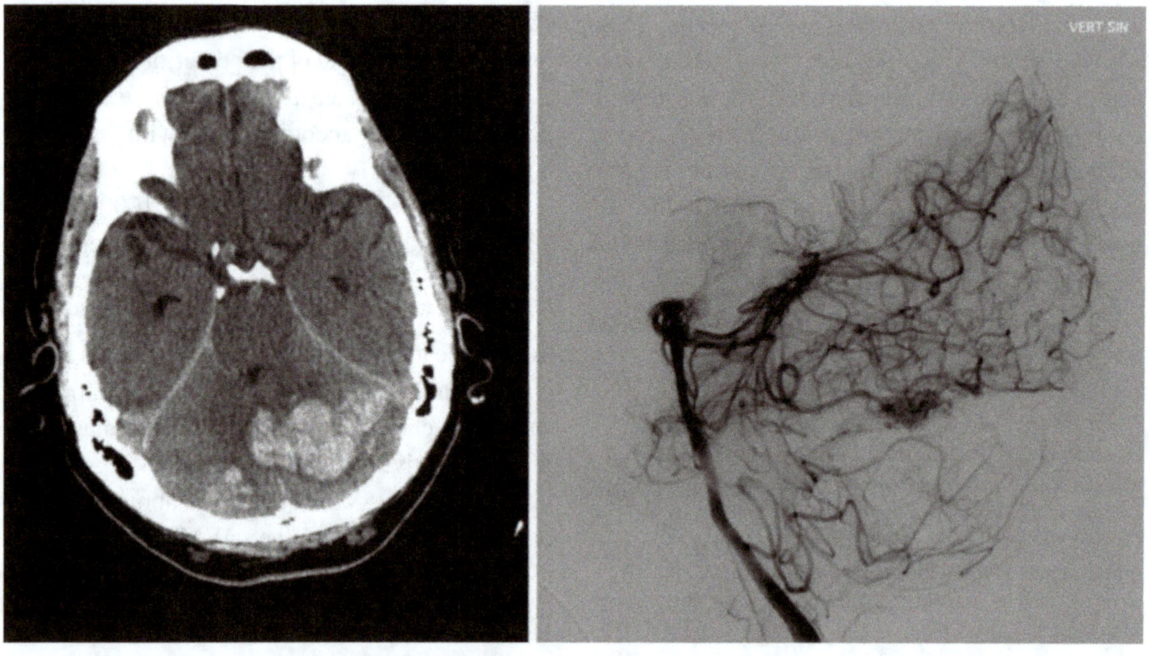

Fig. 21.1 Axial CT scan shows ICH due to AVM rupture, and posterior circulation DSA (lateral view) shows the location of the AVM

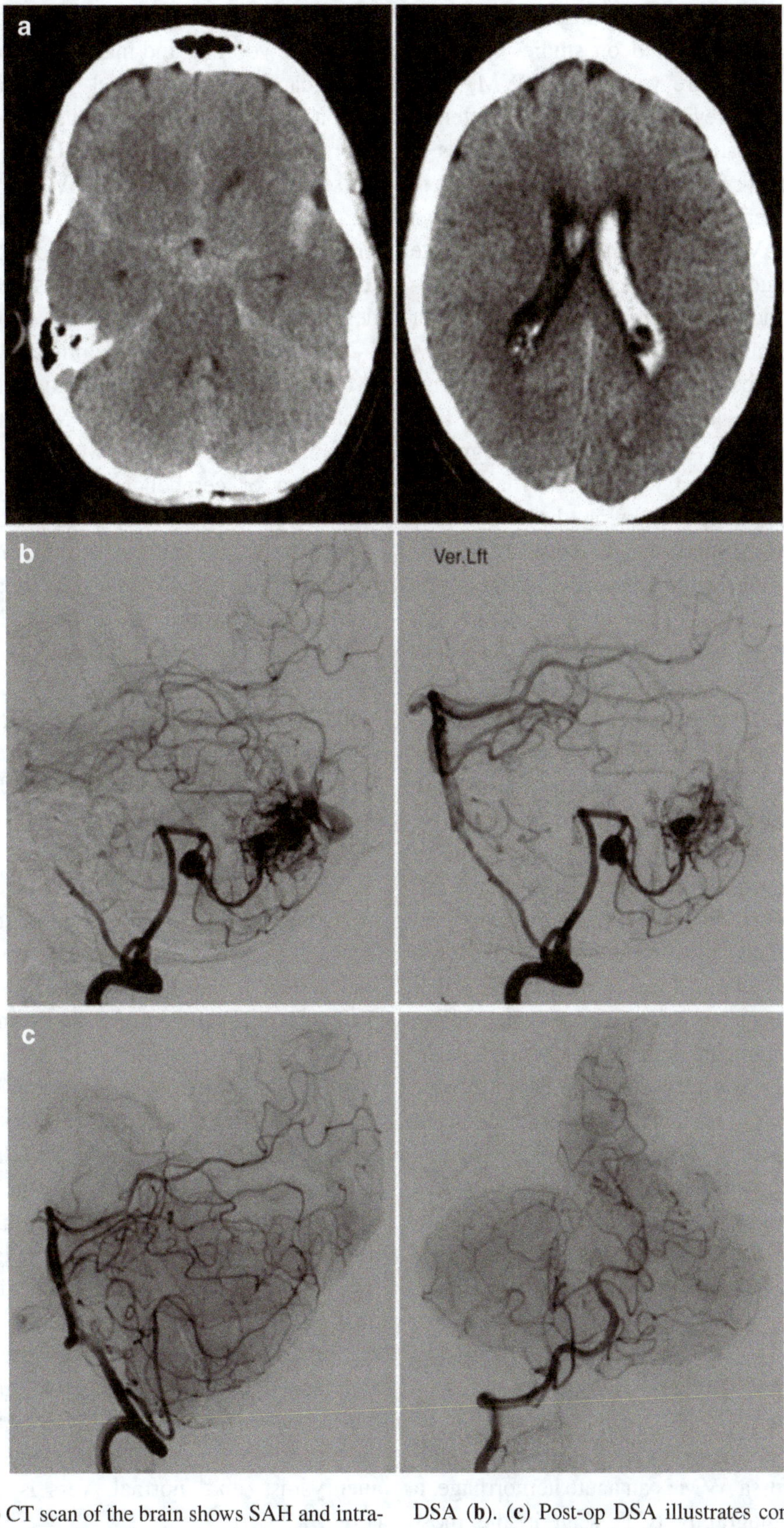

Fig. 21.2 (a) CT scan of the brain shows SAH and intraventricular bleeding due to posterior fossa AVM with associated aneurysm confirmed by left vertebral artery DSA (b). (c) Post-op DSA illustrates complete surgical removal of the AVM and clipping of the associated aneurysms

The risk factors for hemorrhagic presentation of AVMs in general based on studies from the Finnish population are young age, AVM, deep venous drainage, previous rupture, and infratentorial and deep location. Small AVM size tends to have a higher risk for hemorrhagic presentation in almost every series, while large AVM size is also a factor for AVM rupture in most multivariate analyses (including ours) [8, 9]. Some multivariate analyses didn't find large size as a risk factor for AVM rupture, but importantly, small AVM size has never been found as a prospective risk factor for rupture in a multivariate analysis. That is because the small AVMs will not be diagnosed unless they are ruptured, whereas many large ones become symptomatic even before the hemorrhage [10, 11]. AVM-associated aneurysms are found as risk factor for hemorrhage in many meta-analysis studies [10–12]. This risk is highest for the first few years after diagnosis, then it declines, but overall it remains significant for decades [13].

Other clinical presentations are relatively uncommon and depend on the location of the AVM. Cerebellar AVMs are more likely to cause headache, hydrocephalus, and gait disturbances. CPA AVMs may give symptoms of cranial nerve compression such as trigeminal neuralgia or hemifacial spasm. Brainstem AVMs can cause significant neurologic deficits even in the absence of hemorrhage probably due to local mass effect, vascular steal phenomenon, or venous congestion. Overall, progressive neurologic deficits, cranial nerve palsy, headache, and ataxia are possible symptoms of posterior fossa AVMs [1, 7]. In recent years the incidental finding of posterior fossa AVMs has also become more common with the increasing use of modern imaging techniques, making incidental AVMs to account for to 10% in recent studies, compared to that of less than 2% in early studies [14].

21.2 Investigation

Since the most common clinical presenting sign of posterior fossa AVM is an acute hemorrhage, a computed tomography (CT) scan is the most commonly used initial imaging modality. Location, volume, and mass effect of the hemorrhage can be detected quickly with a CT scan as well as signs of hydrocephalus. Any evidence of a previous bleeding or calcification raises the possibility/probability of an AVM as the origin of the hemorrhage (Fig. 21.1). Contrast injection may show feeding arteries and draining veins as linear, vermiform, tubular, or serpentine high-density areas.

Magnetic resonance imaging and angiography (MRI and MRA) provide exquisite detail of the anatomic relations of the AVM. This is particularly useful when the AVM lies in or near the brainstem or cerebellar peduncle, in order to determine the operability or to plan the surgical approach. MRI is superior to other investigations in defining the nidus size and its location in relation to the surrounding structures. Nidus of the AVM is seen as an area of signal void and may have a honeycombed pattern (Fig. 21.3). Tubular signal void structures converging on the nidus represent the feeding arteries and draining veins. Bony artifacts are avoided with MRI, allowing therefore better identification of superficial supply to, or superficial drainage from, the AVM. Gliosis and infarction surrounding the nidus are shown with the hyperintensity area in T2 and FLAIR on MRI. MRI is however an impractical imaging technique for critically ill patients, for example, those harboring a cerebellar clot.

Digital subtraction angiography (DSA) imaging is essential for all patients with AVMs in order to exactly delineate the vascular structures comprising the AVM and for the subsequent management. With DSA the feeding arteries and draining veins can be visualized (Fig. 21.4), but this will necessitate selective injections of contrast material into both the external and internal carotid arteries as well as both vertebral arteries and, occasionally, super-selective injections into the larger feeding arteries. DSA is also vital in the detection of anatomic variants, associated aneurysms, and normal vessels of passage (Fig. 21.2a, b).

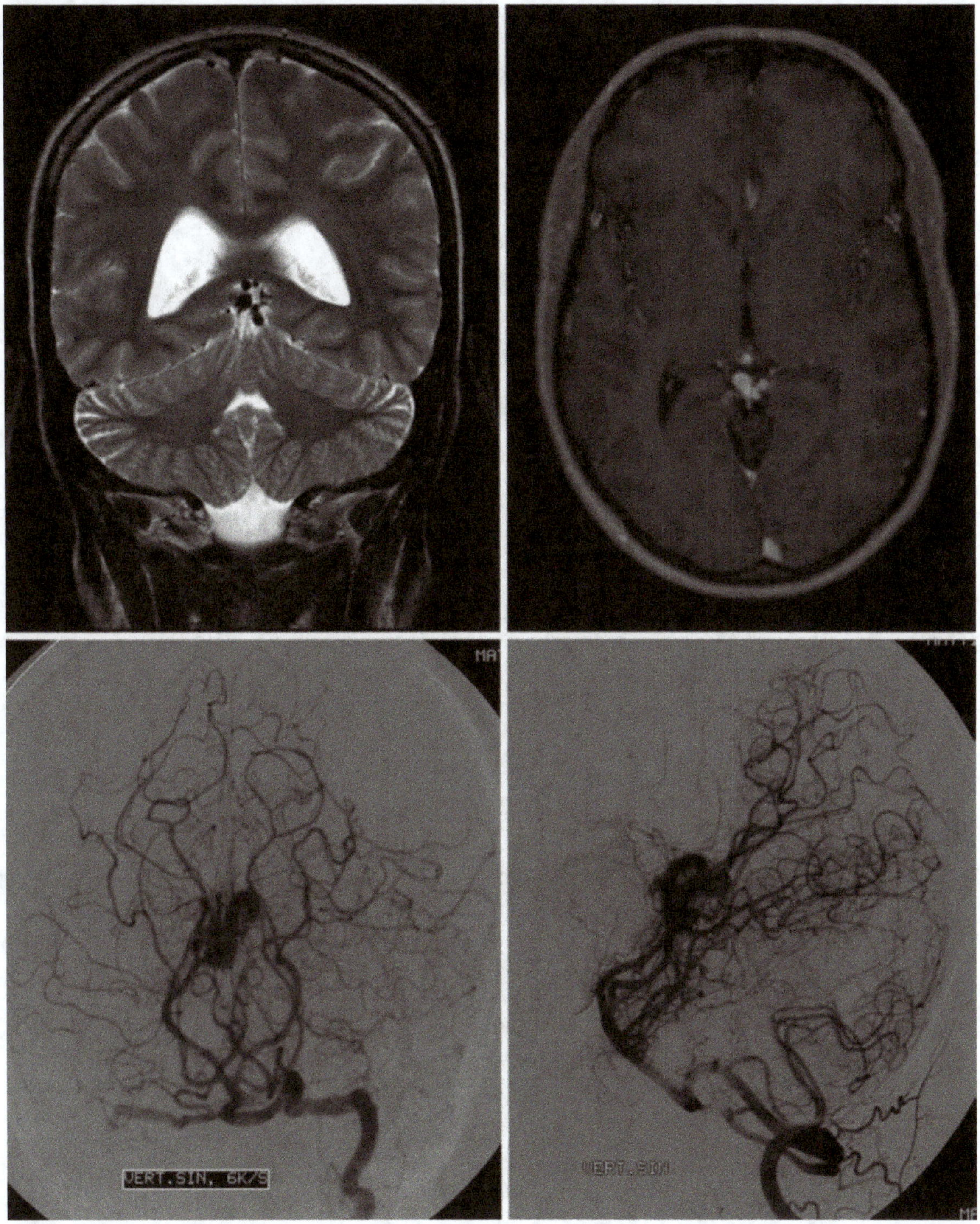

Fig. 21.3 MRI and MRA determine the precise location of the AVM in quadrigeminal cistern after DSA of posterior circulation

21.2.1 Approach

Posterior fossa AVMs are very prone to rupture, and treatment should be considered in every case, except perhaps for the elderly patients with incidental lesions. In AVM treatment, the aim is to eradicate the malformation completely without disrupting normal blood flow. Incomplete treatment provides no significant protection from further hemorrhage.

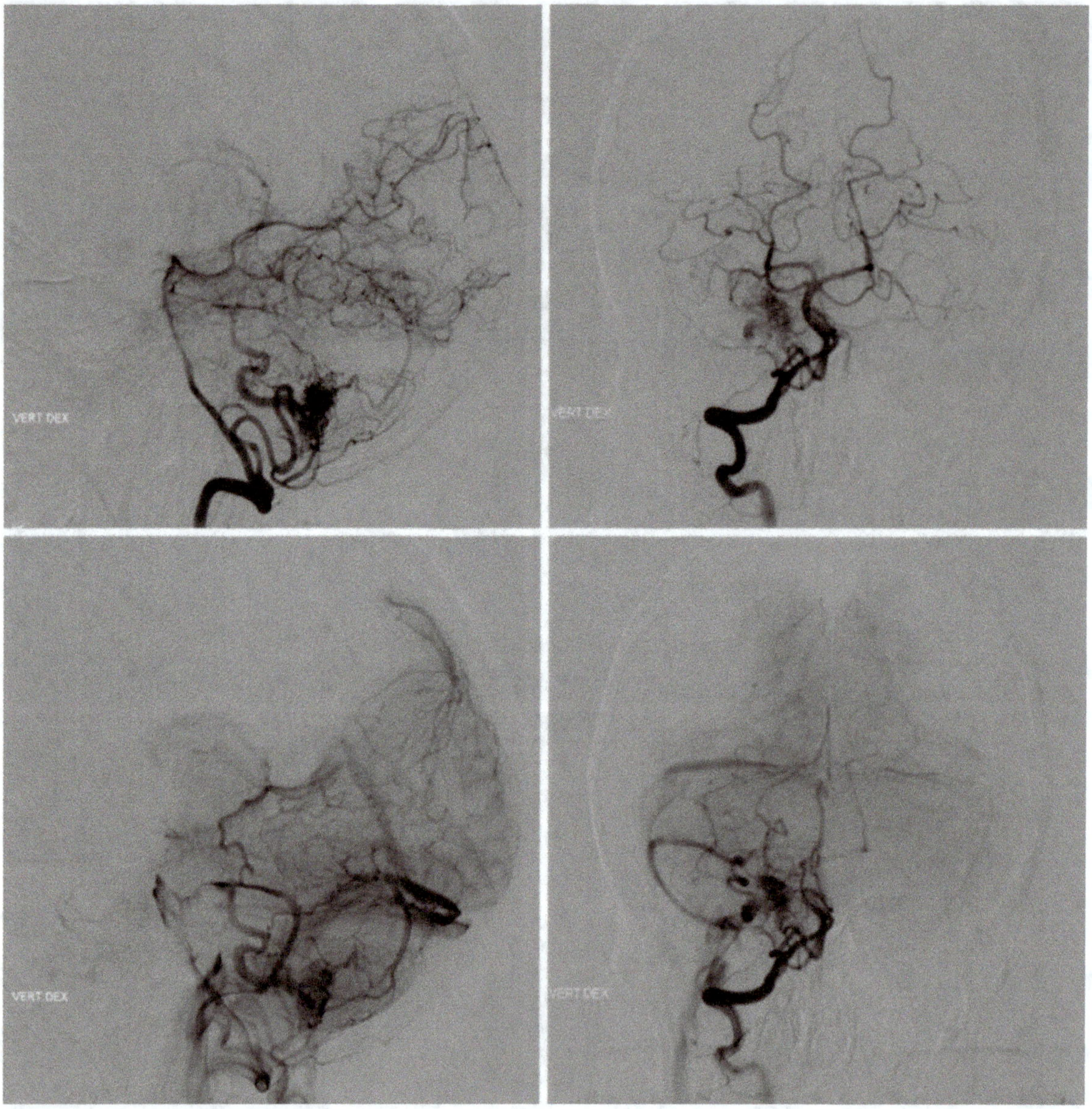

Fig. 21.4 Right vertebral artery angiogram (DSA) demonstrates suboccipital AVM, feeders from PICA, AICA, and SCA

The decision of whether to treat these lesions and the choice of the best treatment modality is difficult. A multidisciplinary team of neurosurgeons, neuroradiologists, and radiotherapists is needed when selecting the best management strategy for each individual patient.

In that process one must take many factors into consideration:

1. The presenting symptom of the lesion.
2. The age and any other comorbid condition of the patient.
3. The anatomical properties of the AVM (location [eloquent, non-eloquent area], size, feeding arteries and its type [terminal, en-passage, deep feeders], and the venous drainage).
4. AVM's relationship to the adjacent brain structures.
5. Presence of a hematoma or not.
6. The associated aneurysm with AVM and which type (intranidal, flow related).
7. Experience of the neurosurgeon.

After the evaluation of all of these factors, the most suitable modality of treatment is chosen as single or combined therapy which directs to prevent future hemorrhage and resolve the related symptoms (Fig. 21.2a–c).

21.3 Modalities of Treatment

21.3.1 Endovascular Techniques

During the last two decades, endovascular techniques have become a therapeutic option in the management of the AVMs. Preoperative embolization aims to devascularize a large AVM with particulate material, mostly by using rapidly (butyl cyanoacrylate, Histoacryl) or more recently by using a slowly setting glue (ethylene vinyl alcohol copolymer, Onyx). Complete obliteration of an AVM by a rapid embolization alone is an uncommon situation and accounts for only about 10% of all our cases, but with a slow technique of Onyx injection, it can be obtained in up to 50% of the selected cases [15].

Until now, however, none of the embolic agents, which have been used to obliterate these lesions, provide total protection against recanalization, regrowing, and rebleeding. Therefore, we use embolization as combined therapy preoperatively to diminish intraoperative bleeding, making the surgery resemble more that of extrinsic tumor removal. Endovascular techniques can also be used to obliterate the feeders that arise from the deep which are usually difficult to reach or controlled with microsurgical techniques, but such vessel may also difficult to reach by microcatheters.

Many complications may follow the embolization procedures, like occlusion of the main draining vein with risk of AVM rupture during or after the procedure, occlusion of arteries in passage, or occlusion of major cerebral arteries. In some locations in the posterior fossa, preoperative embolization may form a hard mass which later can be difficult to dissect from the cranial nerve roots or brainstem. Also, if the preoperative embolization is performed poorly, the result might be of more harm during the surgery rather than benefit; the surgery could become even more difficult especially if they embolized more draining instead of the feeder.

Recently, we started to perform both the embolization and the microsurgical removal at the same day to avoid hemorrhage resulting from the hemodynamic changes inside the nidus, caused by partial embolization of the AVM.

21.3.2 Radiotherapy

Irradiation activates the swelling and degeneration of endothelial cells and perivascular tissue, which promote thrombosis and proliferative fibroblastic repair [1]. These changes in the abnormal vessel walls lead to occlusion of the shunt and finally obliteration of the AVM. The success of this technique depends on the delivery of ionizing radiation in a precise and focused manner to the malformation and avoiding exposure of the surrounding brain. Traditionally, the indication of radiosurgery has been a deep location or a location in eloquent brain that is associated with high surgical morbidity and mortality; such locations include the basal ganglia and brainstem.

The obliteration of AV shunt by radiosurgery takes between 1 and 3 years with a risk of recurrent hemorrhage during this period; actually the rate of recurrent bleeding is 2.98%/year/patient [16], and it seems that the occurrence is the same as if the lesion had been left untreated.

21.3.3 Microsurgery

Microsurgery is considered an ideal treatment for ruptured AVMs. It is, however, controversial in unruptured AVMs, even if radical eradication allows a complete cure of the lesion. ARUBA study found that conservative treatment of unruptured AVMs is superior to the interventional ones (microsurgery, endovascular, and radiosurgery) [17]. The study has nevertheless been criticized because of the short follow-up time, the low number of patients that does not allow subgrouping of the patients according to location or size of AVM, and most patients in the interventional arm being treated by radiosurgical methods.

Laakso et al. studied retrospectively 623 AVM patients [4]. The total follow-up is 10,165 person-years, and this study provides a significant long-term follow-up. In their study, they compare the survival of AVM patients to the general population. Their results show that AVMs are associated with significant and long-lasting excess mortality that is considerably lower in actively treated patients. Even with these results, however, the decision-making regarding incidentally found unruptured AVMs is difficul [4, 5, 13, 18].

The decision of whether to operate on AVMs is based on many factors mentioned before. Size and location are the most important factors in the decision-making; major involvement of the brainstem may increase the risk above acceptable. We found superficial and vermian cerebellar AVMs generally favorable for microsurgical treatment. In ruptured AVMs, the hematoma cavity surrounding the nidus facilitates removal of even deep-seated lesions [5, 19].

Drake et al. in their series had no morbidity or mortality in small AVMs (<2.5 cm), and just over 15% morbidity and mortality in large AVMs (>5 cm) [1].

21.4 Steps of the Surgery

Posterior fossa AVMs are classified into (1) cerebellar hemispheric AVMs (tentorial, suboccipital, and petrosal); (2) vermian AVMs (suboccipital and tentorial); (3) tonsillar AVMs; and (4) brainstem AVMs (midbrain, pontine, and medulla oblongata) [1, 14].

In Helsinki we use four approaches to resect most posterior fossa AVMs: (1) supracerebellar approach for cerebellar tentorial, vermian tentorial, and posterior midbrain AVMs; (2) suboccipital approach for cerebellar suboccipital and vermian suboccipital AVMs; (3) suboccipital telovelar approach for tonsillar AVMs; and (4) retrosigmoid approach for cerebellar petrosal and some brainstem AVMs.

21.4.1 Supracerebellar Approach [20]

Unless contraindicated, e.g., due to old age and cardiac disease, we use the sitting position for the supracerebellar approach. The advantages of this approach are providing better drainage of CSF and possible less bleeding during surgery, provide a relax vein, and being able to observe the superior anatomical view of the AVM and identify the feeder. But we need to be careful with the risk of air embolism, cervical myelopathy, and hypotension.

Instead of the classical midline supracerebellar approach, we prefer paramedian approach. Its advantages are fewer veins in the surgical trajectory, less steep tentorium, and reduced risk of air embolism due to avoidance of exposure to the confluence of sinuses. The disadvantage is the difficulty to identify the best trajectory toward the center of the quadrigeminal cistern.

21.4.1.1 Positioning

The sitting position we use in Helsinki is similar with praying position. We bent the upper torso and head of the patient forward about 30° and downward. By doing that, we expect the tentorium would be almost horizontal. This position will provide a good viewing angle from the most cranial portions of the posterior fossa to the lowest part. Two fingers have to fit between the chin and sternum; it will provide enough room to prevent compression of the airways and jugular veins.

21.4.1.2 Incision and Craniotomy

We make a linear incision 2–3 cm lateral from the midline. The paramedian incision will start about 2 cm cranial to the occipital protuberance and extends until the craniocervical junction. The muscle can be easily split until the occipital bone, along the incision line, and can be held with self-retaining retractor. To spread the wound, we place a curved retractor both from cranial and caudal directions. We detach the muscle insertions with diathermia and expose the occipital bone. Bony exposure is usually enough at 3–4 cm below the transverse sinus.

We place one burr hole 3 cm lateral from the midline, slightly superior to the transverse sinus. We detach the dura from the transverse sinus, gently with blunt and curve dissector. Then we perform craniotomy with 3–4 cm bone flap. The bone flap should be above the transfer sinus to allow retraction of transfer sinus cranially. The bone opening should leave 1 cm edge of bone to the midline.

21.4.1.3 Dural Opening

Sometimes the draining vein or the AVM itself is firmly adherent to the dura. Therefore, we carefully inspect the dura under the microscope to avoid any injury to the draining vein. To avoid injury to the veins or transverse sinus, the dura is opened under microscope. We open the dura in a V-shaped form and the base at the sinus. Many veins at supracerebellar area usually located in the midline such as superior cerebellar vein and could be avoided with this approach. Once the thick arachnoid and few of the bridging veins between tentorium and cerebellum were coagulated and cut, the cerebellum will follow the gravity, allowing a good surgical view without any brain retraction.

21.4.2 Retrosigmoid Approach [20]

This approach is described in detail elsewhere in this book. We describe only our modification of this technique.

21.4.2.1 Positioning

We place the patient in lateral position (park bench), with the head elevated about 20 cm above the heart level. We rotate the upper body slightly (5–10°) backwards, in order that the shoulder is retracted with tape more easily caudally and posteriorly. The head (1) is slightly flexed forward, (2) may be tilted laterally, and (3), if necessary, may be rotated slightly toward the floor.

To gain slack brain, we use spinal drainage with 50–100 ml CSF removed.

21.4.2.2 Skin Incision and Craniotomy

We place a linear incision 2 cm behind the mastoid process. The length of incision varies depending on distance of the AVM from the foramen magnum. Of importance is to have the skin incision long enough to obtain an adequate bony exposure. We place a large-sized curved retractor at the cranial side of incision. We continue to split the subcutaneous fat and muscles with monopolar until we found the yellowish fat at the level of the foramen magnum. This should be a sign for warning of extracranial vertebral artery.

We made one burr hole just at posterior border of the incision and then continue with the craniotomy. A bone flap of 2–3 cm is usually sufficient. If necessary, the bony opening can be extended by drilling mastoid part of the temporal bone. If the mastoid air cells are exposed, they really need to be meticulously closed to prevent the postoperative CSF leak.

21.4.2.3 Dural Opening

The duramater is opened in a curvilinear shape, and the base at the mastoid. The dura edges are tackled with sutures. When the dura cut near the transverse sigmoid junction, the dura will be cut in a three-leaf fashion. One is directed exactly to the junction for better exposure.

The brain should be slack due to the spinal drainage, and once the dura is opened completely, we may close the drain temporarily. If the brain is still tight, opening the cerebellomedullary cistern (cisterna magna) helps to slack the brain. In this approach, the petrosal vein is often the prominent vein seen when approaching the tentorium or the upper cranial nerves. Although some papers mention that we may sacrifice this vein, many surgeons have observed complications after its occlusion. The best suggestion is to preserve it.

21.4.3 Suboccipital Craniotomy [20]

21.4.3.1 Positioning

We usually use the sitting position described previously in this chapter.

21.4.3.2 Incision and Craniotomy

We make the incision on the midline. The incision starts from the external occipital protuberance and extends till the C1–C2 level. We split the muscles at the midline with monopolar all the way to the occipital bone. If we split it exactly at the midline, there will be less vascular tissue. We place one large self-retaining retractor on each end, cranial and caudal. When dissecting the muscles, care is needed to avoid injury to the vertebral artery, which is located 1–2 cm from the midline.

We place one burr hole 1 cm paramedian from the midline, below the transverse sinus. We make two cuts with the craniotomy toward the foramen magnum. At the cranial aspect, the bone flap is secured with strong and large rongeur. If needed, we use a high-speed coarse diamond drill or a small rongeur to extend the lateral exposure of the foramen magnum.

21.4.3.3 Dural Opening

We open the dura under a microscope in a reverse V-shaped form, and the base at the foramen magnum. We start dura cutting below the occipital sinus, and the dural leaf is everted caudally and sutured tightly to the muscles. At this point, usually the arachnoid membrane that covers cisterna magna is usually intact. The arachnoid is opened and attached it to dural leaf using hemoclips. Then under high magnification, we gently push apart the cerebellar tonsils, and we start to enter the fourth ventricle. By changing the table and microscope angle, we may even obtain visualization of superior part of fourth ventricle and aqueduct.

21.4.3.4 Dissection

Mostly microsurgical removal of AVMs is a great challenge. In posterior fossa AVMs, the lesion is located deep in a small compartment close to many critical structures, which makes posterior fossa AVM surgery even more difficult. Therefore, only experienced neurovascular team should operate on these lesions (Table 21.2).

After opening the dura, we inspect the AVM under less magnification to estimate the nidus and their relationships to the adjacent neurovascular structures. We discern also the superficial feeders, the pattern of draining veins, and the plane of cleavage. During this initial inspection of the AVM, we use indocyanine green (ICG) angiography to distinguish arterial feeders from arterialized draining veins. ICG provides great help in this purpose.

We perform all the AVM dissection using maximize magnification. The cleavage plane between the nidus and the neural tissue is distinguished as a yellow gliotic tissue formed by previous hemorrhage(s). The feeders enter the AVM through this plane, and they should be identified, coagulated, and cut at this point. If no clear plane surrounds the AVM, especially in critical areas, dissection must be considered on the AVM itself depending on the axiom that no normal neural tissue between the AVM aggregation.

Besides carefully studying of 3D reconstruction images preoperatively, the large superficial feeding arteries are identified intraoperatively with ICG. We often place temporary clips only on the feeders that terminate in the AVM and avoid the main trunk of en-passage arteries, which also have branches that supply the normal cerebellum and/or

Table 21.2 Characteristics of 64 patients with infratentorial arteriovenous malformation, stratified by result of treatment [4]

	Total occlusion n = 36 (%)	Partial occlusion n = 12 (%)	Conservative n = 16 (%)
Pontomesencephalic	4 (11.1)	3 (25)	7 (43.7)
Medulla oblongata	0 (0)	1 (8.3)	0 (0)
Cerebellar vermis	6 (16.7)	2 (16.7)	1 (6.3)
Superficial cerebellar hemispheric	17 (47.2)	4 (33.3)	6 (37.5)
Deep cerebellar hemispheric	8 (22.2)	2 (16.7)	2 (12.5)
Multiple	1(2.8)	0 (0)	0 (0)

brainstem. Unintended occlusion of these branches may cause devastating brainstem infarction.

The small feeders should be coagulated directly in the cleavage plane. The tiny and fragile feeders, or dilated capillaries around the AVM, remain the most difficult part of the procedure, particularly when these vessels are close to the ventricle. Because of their fragile nature and little tissue to act on, bleeding from these tiny vessels is difficult to control. We use continuous coagulation with nonsticking bipolar forceps, which we quickly interchange when they become soiled. Bipolar is also used to shrink the AVM and to clarify the cleavage plane.

After disconnecting all the feeders, the AVM becomes border-free, bloodless, smaller, and non-tense, and the color of the draining vein(s) changes from red into blue. At this point, the draining vein can be coagulated and divided safely. If the venous drainage is obstructed during the procedure prior to this point, the AVM may become tense and prone to massive uncontrolled bleeding, and also swelling of the cerebellum can occur. If a secondary draining vein impedes the resection, the trick is to occlude this vein by a temporary clip. If no swelling of the AVM or cerebellum is observed, dividing the vein is safe.

Once the total AVM removal is achieved, the cavity should be carefully inspected for any remnants. Our technique is to touch all walls with the cotton and bipolar tip gently. A bleeding may indicate an AVM remnant, and another resection plane should be performed in that location. Hemostasis of the resection cavity must be meticulous. We use hemostatic materials (Tachosil ®, Surgicel ®, fibrin glue) to seal the resection cavity.

The dura should be closed in watertight and few stitches are used to lift it up to the bone edges. We put back the bone flap and secure it before closing the wound in layers.

21.5 Expert Opinion and Suggestions to Avoid Complications

- You cannot “try” AVM surgery – the surgeon always need to be aware that once the AVM surgery started, it has to be carried till it finish, and the nidus should be removed completely (Figs. 21.4 and 21.5).
- Before starting the operation, preoperative study on the images is essential to have clear understanding of anatomy of the main feeders and the relationship between the AVM and the adjacent structures.
- Initiating the dissection around the AVM in the correct plane facilitates the removal of even complex AVM with minor bleeding.
- The whole AVM should be removed as one piece; piecemeal removal causes a massive bleeding which is difficult to control.
- Hemostasis of the deepest part of the AVM with thin-walled feeders is the most difficult part of the surgery. It requires a lot of patience, time, and blunt-tipped bipolar coagulation.
- Persistent bleeding from the resection bed usually indicates the presence of nidus remnant, and then another specific detection is needed.
- To be more familiar with AVM surgery, it is good to know that the small feeders surrounding gliomas are similar to those of AVMs; this helps you to sharpen your skills in AVM surgery.
- The draining veins have to be preserved until the end of the resection.
- Simple ligation of feeding vessels of the AVM is ineffectual. The fistulous connections between the abnormal arteries and veins in the nidus will rapidly change and recruit any vessel and make it even more prominent prior to ligation.

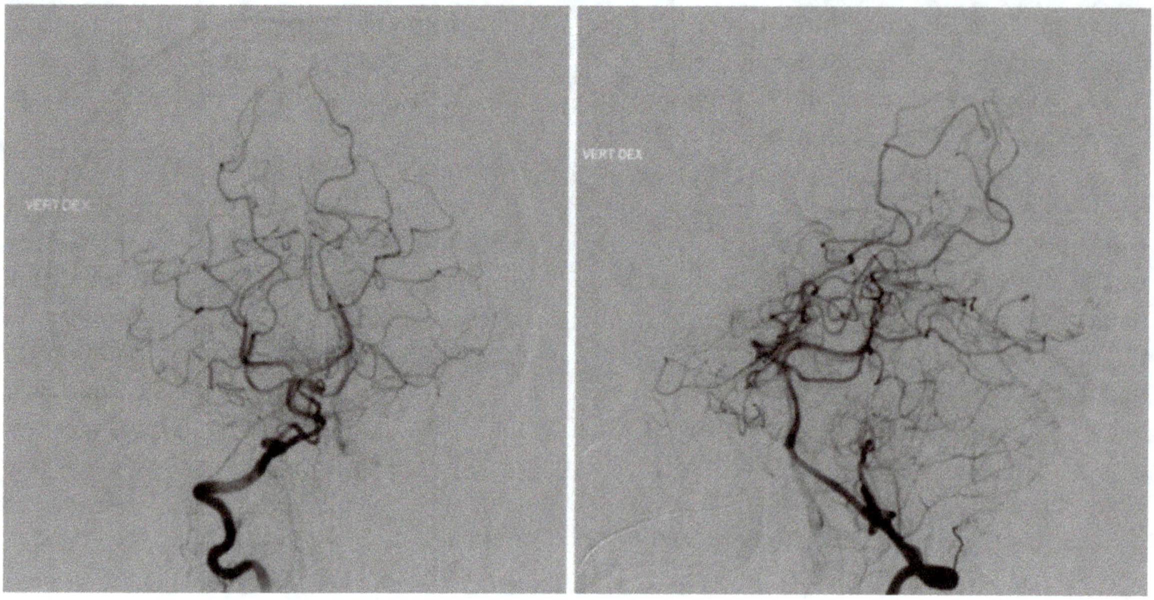

Fig. 21.5 Post-op vertebral artery angiogram demonstrates complete surgical removal of the AVM

21.6 Postoperative Care and Follow-Up

At the end of the procedure, immediate CT and CT angiography are performed directly before awaking the patient to check any postoperative hematoma and to find out any remnant in the AVM resection bed; then the patient is transferred to the neurosurgical ICU, where ECG, arterial blood pressure, central venous pressure, and other vital signs are recorded. Patients with small AVMs are woken up slowly over the period of several hours; those with large or complex AVMs are kept sedated and under moderate hypotension (mean arterial pressure 20% below the patient's normal level) by restricting fluid intake and hypotensive medications for several days. Careful repeat neurosurgical assessments are achieved.

Postoperative DSA is used to check if the AVM is completely eradicated.

Conclusion

Posterior fossa AVMs are very prone to rupture, and their treatment should be considered in almost every case. Microsurgical removal of posterior fossa AVMs is a big challenge in neurosurgical practice. Therefore, only experienced neurovascular team should operate on these lesions. The decision of whether to treat these lesions and choosing the best treatment modality is complex. A multidisciplinary team of neurosurgeons, neuroradiologists, and radiotherapists is important in the selection of the best management in each individual patient.

References

1. Peerless SJ, Hernesniemi J, Drake CG, Arteriovenous malformations of the posterior fossa. In: Wilkins RH, Rengachary SS, editors. Neurosurgery. New York: McGraw-Hill; 1996 p. 2463–76.
2. Yasargil MG. Microneurosurgery, Volume IIIA: AVM of the brain, history, embryology, pathological considerations, hemodynamics, diagnostic studies, microsurgical anatomy. New York: George Thieme Verlag; 1996. p. 11–2.
3. Verbiest H. Arterio-venous aneurysms of the posterior fossa, analysis of six cases. Acta Neurochir. 1961;9:171–95.
4. Laakso A, et al. Long-term excess mortality in 623 patients with brain arteriovenous malformations. Neurosurgery. 2008;63(2):244–53; discussion 253–5.
5. Kuhmonen J, Piippo A, Väärt K, Karatas A, Ishii K, Winkler P, Niemelä M, Porras M, Hernesniemi J. Early surgery for ruptured cerebral arteriovenous malformations. Acta Neurochir Suppl. 2005;94:111–4.

6. da Costa L, Thines L, Dehdashti AR, Wallace MC, Willinsky RA, Tymianski M, Schwartz ML, ter Brugge KG. Management and clinical outcome of posterior fossa arteriovenous malformations: report on a single centre 15-year experience. J Neurol Neurosurg Psychiatry. 2009;80:376–9.
7. Arnaout OM, Gross BA, Eddleman CS, Bendok BR, Getch CC, Batjer HH. Posterior fossa arteriovenous malformations. Neurosurg Focus. 2009;26(5):E12. 1–6.
8. Hernesniemi JA, Dashti R, Juvela S, Väärt K, Niemelä M. Natural history of brain arteriovenous malformation: a long-term follow-up study of risk of hemorrhage in 238 patients. Neurosurgery. 2008;63:823–31.
9. Laakso A, Dashti R, Seppänen J, Juvela S, Väärt K, Niemelä M, Sankila R, Hernesniemi JA. Long-term excess mortality in 623 patients with brain arteriovenous malformation. Neurosurgery. 2008;63:244–55.
10. Gross BA, Du R. Natural history of cerebral arteriovenous malformations: a meta-analysis. J Neurosurg. 2013 Feb;118(2):437–43.
11. Abecassis IJ, Xu DS, Batjer HH, Bendok BR. Natural history of brain arteriovenous malformations: a systematic review. Neurosurg Focus. 2014;37(3):E7.
12. Stapf C, Mohr JP, Pile-Spellman J, Sciacca RR, Hartmann A, Schumacher HC, Mast H. Concurrent arterial aneurysms in brain arteriovenous malformations with haemorrhagic presentation. J Neurol Neurosurg Psychiatry. 2002;73:294–8.
13. Hernesniemi JA, et al. Natural history of brain arteriovenous malformations: a long-term follow-up study of risk of hemorrhage in 238 patients. Neurosurgery. 2008;63(5):823–9; discussion 829–31.
14. Aki Laakso RD, Juvela S, Niemela¨ M, Hernesniemi J. Natural history of arteriovenous malformations: presentation, risk of hemorrhage and mortality. In: Laakso A, Hernesniemi J, Yonekawa Y, Tsukahara T, editors. Surgical management of cerebrovascular disease. Germany: Springer; 2010. p. 65–9.
15. Natarajan SK, Ghodke B, Britz GW, Born DE, Sekhar LN. Multimodality treatment of brain arteriovenous malformations with microsurgery after embolization with onyx: single-center experience and technical nuances. Neurosurgery. 2008;62:1213–25; discussion 1225–1226.
16. Nataf F, Merienne L, Schlienger M, Lefkopoulos D, Meder JF, Touboul E, Merland JJ, Devaux B, Turak B, Page P, Roux FX. Cerebral arteriovenous malformations treated by radiosurgery: a series of 705 cases. Neurochirurgie. 2001;47(2–3 Pt 2):268–82.
17. Mohr JP. A randomized trial of unruptured brain arteriovenous malformations (ARUBA). Acta Neurochir Suppl. 2008;103:3–4. Review.
18. Laakso A, et al. Risk of hemorrhage in patients with untreated Spetzler-Martin grade IV and V arteriovenous malformations: a long-term follow-up study in 63 patients. Neurosurgery. 2011;68(2):372–7; discussion 378.
19. Hernesniemi J, Keränen T. Microsurgical treatment of arteriovenous malformations of the brain in a defined population. Surg Neurol. 1990 Jun;33(6):384–90.
20. Lehecka M, Laakso A, Hernesniemi J. Common approaches. In: Laakso A, Lehecka M, Hernesniemi J, editors. Helsinki microneurosurgery basics and tricks. Helsinki: Department of Neurosurgery, Helsinki University Central Hospital; 2011. p. 111–93.

22 Endovascular Coiling of Intracranial Aneurysms

Naoya Kuwayama

22.1 Introduction

Since the development of Guglielmi detachable coil (GDC), endovascular technique for coiling has become widely accepted as one of the option treatments of intracranial aneurysms.

The randomized trial of ISAT [1] proved the superiority of the aneurysm coiling than clipping for the patients with subarachnoid hemorrhage. Endovascular aneurysm treatment has been rapidly developing in technique, and its indication has been also rapidly spreading with the development of a variety of adjunctive techniques, including simple coiling, catheter- or microwire-assisted coiling, double-catheter technique, balloon remodeling technique, and stent-assisted technique. In this educational chapter, the standard and most updated coiling techniques will be explained including advantages and drawbacks. The flow diverters will not be mentioned here.

22.1.1 Antiplatelet Therapy

Antiplatelet agents (aspirin and/or clopidogrel) should be given to the patients with unruptured aneurysms, 1 or 2 weeks before the treatment, to prevent thromboembolic complications. When using a simple technique, a single agent (aspirin or clopidogrel) will be enough, while when using the adjunctive techniques, dual antiplatelet therapy (DAPT) will be recommended. If using the stents, DAPT is mandatory and should be kept within several months after the treatment. However, we should be aware of the hemorrhagic complications due to the DAPT medication (Match Study) [2]. In cases with ruptured aneurysms, single agent will be given after procedure or during treatment through the nasogastric tube. When using stents, loading dose of aspirin (300 mg) and clopidogrel (300–600 mg) should be given during or immediately after procedure. Increase of blood aspirin level is rapid but that of clopidogrel is slow, taking several hours even if the loading dose is given.

"VerifyNow (Accumetrics)" is an easy, instant, and portable instrument to assess the platelet aggregation activity of the patient immediately before treatment. The degree of suppression of platelet activity with either aspirin (ARU) or clopidogrel (PRU) can be monitored.

22.1.2 Anesthesia

Usually general anesthesia is favorable and selected to get immobilization of the patient particularly in case of ruptured aneurysms. If a patient would bleed in the procedure, vital sign

N. Kuwayama
Division of Neuroendovascular Therapy, Department of Neurosurgery, University of Toyama, Toyama, Japan
e-mail: kuwayama@med.u-toyama.ac.jp

J. July, E. J. Wahjoepramono (eds.), *Neurovascular Surgery*,
https://doi.org/10.1007/978-981-10-8950-3_22

could be controlled much better under intubated condition. Local anesthesia could be selected if the patient could well understand and stay still, but not recommended.

22.1.3 Heparin

Usually femoral arteries are selected for the access routes. After puncture of the artery, heparin should be given to maintain the ACT (activating clotting time) at 1.5–2 times of pretreatment level. We usually give 3000–5000 units in bolus intravenously at first and then 1000 units every 1 h.

22.1.4 Procedures of Coiling

Though the simple technique should be the best, we have to utilize many kinds of adjunctive techniques to protect the parent artery from coil herniation out of the aneurysm dome. The practical techniques with microguidewires, microcatheters, balloons, and stents will be explained.

22.2 Simple Coiling, Basic Techniques, and Follow-Up

A 6Fr guiding catheter is usually selected to prepare for the second microcatheter usage. The first microcatheter is used for coiling and the second microcatheter (balloon catheter) is used for the adjuctive techniques. A microcatheter should be inserted into the aneurysm dome using a microguidewire. The detachable platinum coils are conceptionally divided into three types: framing, filling, and finishing coils. The decision to choose the size of framing coil should be same with or 0.5–1 mm smaller than the aneurysm diameter. When the aneurysm is spherical shaped, the size of framing coil should be the medium diameter between the long and short axes. The filling coils, shorter and smaller, come next and pack inside the framing coil. Then a few finishing coils follow and finalize the treatment. The finishing coil should be much softer and shorter. Final stage, the microguidewiere should be proceeded into the tip of the microcatheter and pulled back together securing the inside coils not coming with the catheter. The optimum packing rate will be 20–25% or more, and it is reported that the higher the packing rate, the less the recurrence rate [3].

The follow-up should be done under the monitor of plain craniogram and MRI time of flight (TOF) sequence. Morphological changes of the coil in the craniogram and/or inside flow into the aneurysm dome in MRI-TOF images will indicate the recurrence of the aneurysms. Then the angiogram should be done to evaluate the necessity of retreatment.

22.3 Adjunctive Techniques

A 6 or 7 Fr guiding catheter is usually selected to go with two or three catheters in combination. Sometimes a balloon-guiding catheter (7 or 8 Fr) is used to stabilize the intracranial remodeling balloon catheter or to control intraoperative bleeding. Here, five kinds of adjunctive techniques will be shown.

22.3.1 # Wire Protection Method (Fig. 22.1)

This is suitable to a small aneurysm arising from a small parent artery. Place a microguidewire passing across the aneurysm neck in the parent artery. It is sometimes useful to prevent the coil from protruding out of the aneurysm neck.

Figure 22.1 shows the anterior communicating artery (AcomA) aneurysm. The microguidewire is coming through the left internal carotid artery (ICA) and going to the distal right A2 segment through the AcomA, while the microcatheter is coming from the right ICA and inserted into the aneurysm dome. The coils do not come out of the dome with the protection of the microguidewire across the aneurysm neck.

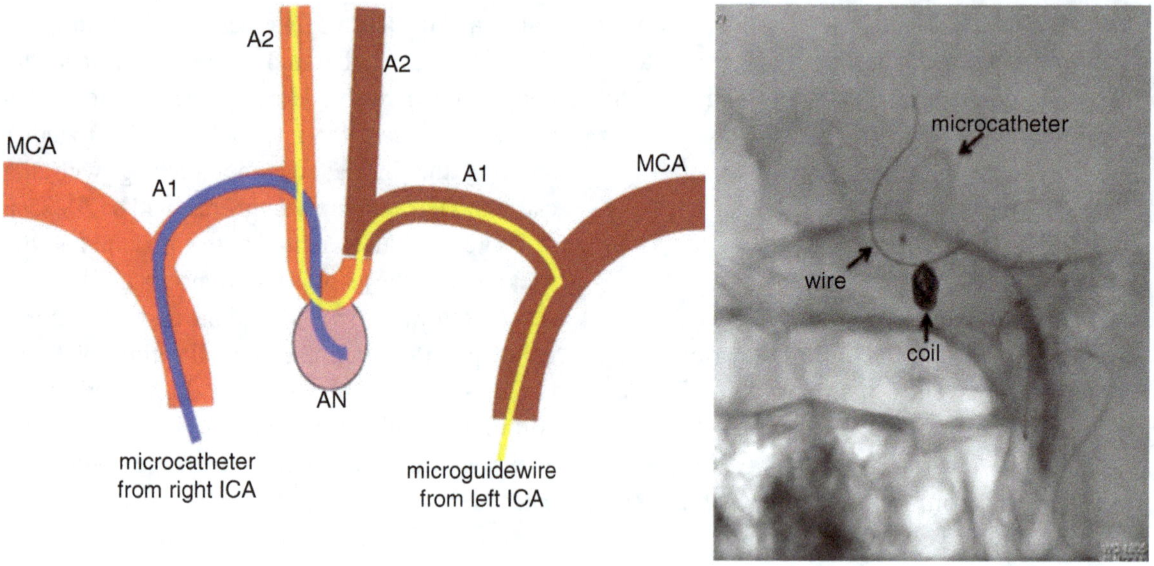

Fig. 22.1 The wire-assisted technique for an aneurysm of the anterior communicating artery

22.3.2 # Catheter Protection Method (Fig. 22.2)

This is a modified method of the wire protection procedure. Place a microcatheter passing across the aneurysm neck in the parent artery. This is available in the small vessel like anterior cerebral arteries and in the posterior circulation.

Figure 22.2 demonstrates the aneurysm of the left VA-PICA. The microcatheter is coming from the contralateral right vertebral artery and going to the left PICA into its distal segment, while the second microcatheter is coming from the left vertebral artery and going into the aneurysm dome.

22.3.3 # Double-Catheter Method (Fig. 22.3)

In case with wide-neck aneurysms, coils are easily herniated from the dome. Sometimes a loop of a detached framing coil may come out of the dome, being pushed by filling coils. In these cases, the double-catheter technique is often useful. First, send the two microcatheters into the aneurysm dome. Then start coiling. When the first coil makes a good frame in the dome, keep the coil undetached and push and hold the catheter slightly pressing the framing coil to the dome side. Then start filling inside the frame with the second catheter. Usually after detaching two or three filling coils inside the dome, the framing coil will be stabilized well and not be herniated to the parent artery. Then the framing coil can be detached. Afterward, both the first and the second catheters can be used for the coil insertion depending on the situation.

Figure 22.3 shows the recurred aneurysm at the right posterior communicating artery (PcomA) after clipping. The previous multiple clips caused the tight stenosis of the ICA proximal to the aneurysm, allowing just one microcatheter to pass through the stenosis. While placing a microcatheter from the right ICA, the second microcatheter was coming from the contralateral left ICA through the AcomA, going down to the right ICA, and finally placed in the aneurysm dome. Thus, the wide-neck aneurysm was completely packed with the double-catheter technique.

22.3.4 # Balloon Remodeling Method (Fig. 22.4)

First, send the balloon catheter to the distal parent artery and then send the microcatheter into

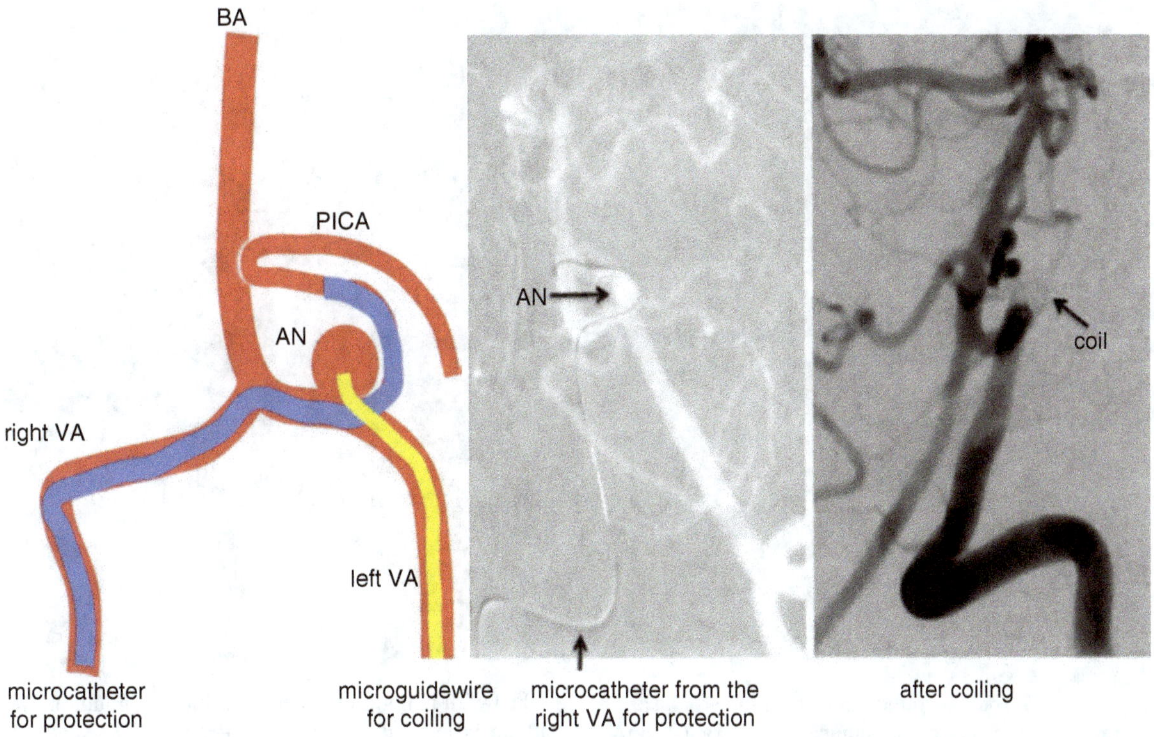

Fig. 22.2 The catheter-assisted technique for an aneurysm of the left vertebral artery (PICA)

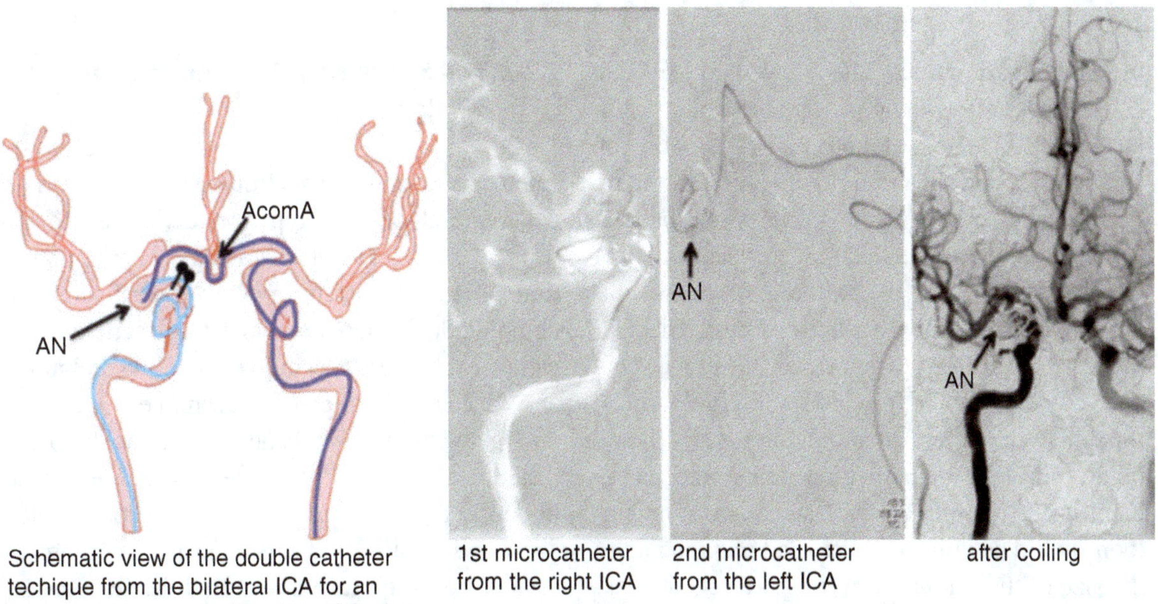

Schematic view of the double catheter techique from the bilateral ICA for an recurrent aneurysm of the right ICA after clipping. The previous clips make the tight ICA stenosis and only one catheter can pass through the ICA. The 2nd catheter is navigated from the left ICA throught AcomA.

Left: 1st microcatheter going from the right ICA to the aneurysm dome. Middle: 2nd microcatheter going from contralateral ICA to the aneurysm through the AcomA. Right: abgiogram after coiling.

Fig. 22.3 The double-catheter technique for a recurrent wide-neck aneurysm of the right ICA after clipping

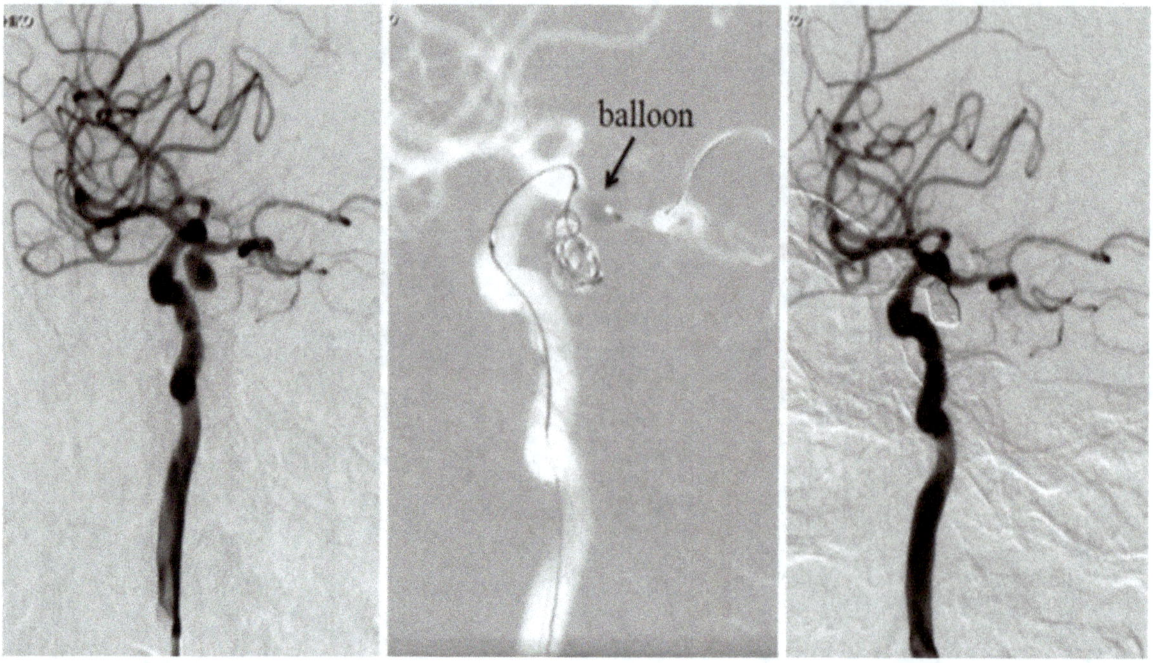

Fig. 22.4 The balloon remodeling technique for an aneurysm of the posterior communicating artery (PcomA). The aneurysm arises from the PcomA. This is the so-called pure Pcom aneurysm (left). The aneurysm is being packed with balloon remodeling technique (middle). The balloon is inflated in the parent PcomA to prevent coil herniation. The aneurysm is completely obliterated with coils keeping the PcomA patent (right)

the aneurysm dome. The movement of one catheter will affect the position of the other catheter by the friction of both catheters. Surgeon should always be aware of the position of the tip of coil catheter, when moving the microballoon catheter, otherwise it may cause perforation of the aneurysm. When the balloon and microcatheter are placed properly, start coiling. The balloon can be inflated, if necessary, to prevent the coil coming out of the dome. Surgeon must remember that the inflated balloon will fix the tip of the coil catheter and prevent its free movement, causing rupture of the aneurysm. The balloon should be inflated under road mapping up to the size of the parent artery, not to cause the vessel rupture.

Figure 22.4 shows the so-called pure PcomA aneurysm (arising from PcomA itself). In the final stage of the procedure, the balloon was inflated in the PcomA preventing the finishing coils from herniating to the parent PcomA.

22.3.5 # Stent-Assisted Technique (Fig. 22.5)

There are several kinds of remodeling stents: open cell type, closed cell type, braided type, etc. To use the stents, DAPT medication before procedure is mandatory to prevent thromboembolic complication. There are two ways to send the coil catheter to the aneurysm: one is jailing technique and the other is trans-cell technique. In case of jailing technique, send the stent catheter to the distal parent artery. Before opening the stent, send the coil catheter into the aneurysm dome. Then open and deploy the stent, and start coiling. In case of trans-cell technique, send the stent catheter to the distal parent artery and then open and deploy the stent. Send the coil catheter to the aneurysm through the cell of the stent, and start coiling. The demerit of the trans-cell method is to have a potential risk of wire or catheter perforation in cases with small aneurysms.

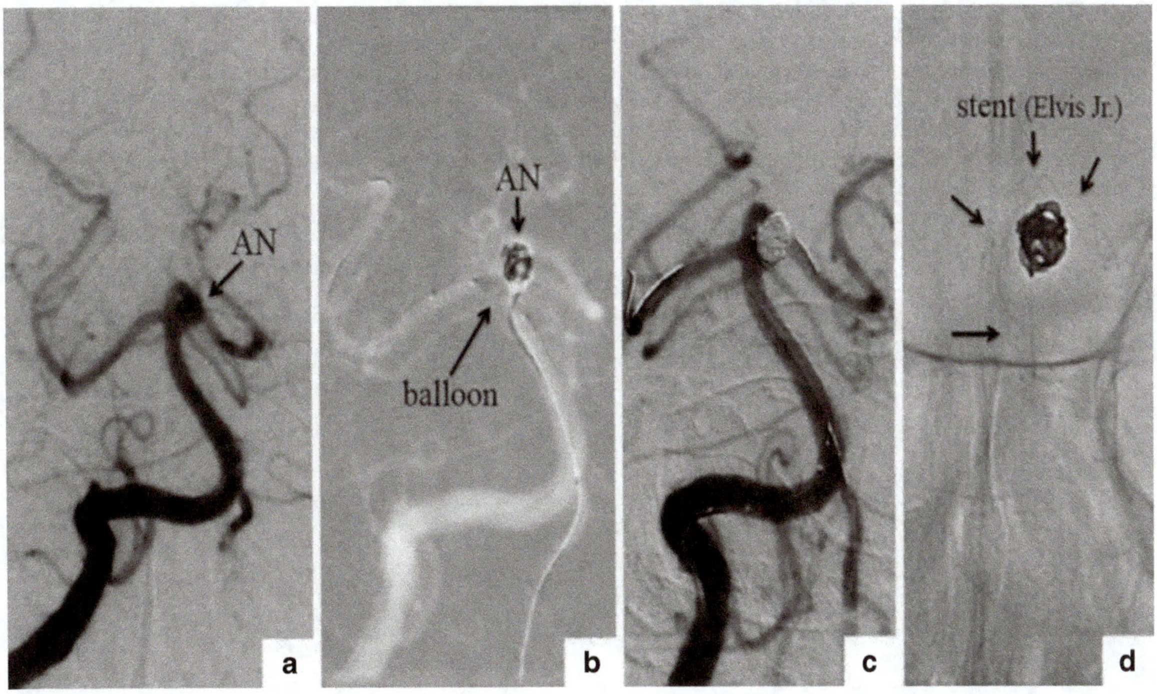

Fig. 22.5 The stent-assisted technique for an aneurysm of the origin of the superior cerebellar artery. (**a**) The aneurysm arises from the origin of the superior cerebellar artery (BA-SCA AN) (**b**) The aneurysm is being packed with balloon-assisted technique at first. The balloon is inflated from the right PCA-P1 segment to the upper basilar artery. (**c**) The aneurysm is completely obliterated with balloon- and stent-assisted technique. (**d**) Note the stent (arrows) is placed from the left PCA-P1 segment to the upper basilar artery

At present, the jailing method seems to be dominantly used. The demerit of the jailing method is to fix the coil catheter preventing the free movement of the tip of the microcatheter. Recently semi-jailing method is frequently used, keeping the stent half open at the neck to secure the free movement of the coil catheter. In other words, the semi-jailing method makes the neck of the aneurysm smaller, allowing free catheter movement and easy and safe coiling. It is reported that stent-assisted coiling has smaller rate of recurrence due to the hemodynamic effect to the aneurysm [4].

Figure 22.5 demonstrates a case with the aneurysm of the superior cerebellar artery treated with balloon- and stent-assisted technique. Coiling started with balloon-assisted technique; then finally the stent (Elvis Jr.) was deployed from the PCA-P1 segment to the basilar artery.

References

1. Molyneux A, Kerr R, Stratton I, Sandercock P, Clarke M, Shrimpton J, Holman R, International Subarachnoid Aneurysm Trial (ISAT) Collaborative Group. International Subarachnoid Aneurysm Trial (ISAT) of neurosurgical clipping versus endovascular coiling in 2143 patients with ruptured intracranial aneurysms: a randomised trial. Lancet. 2002;360(9342):1267–74.
2. Diener HC, Bogousslavsky J, Brass LM, Cimminiello C, Csiba L, Kaste M, et al. MATCH investigators. Aspirin and clopidogrel compared with clopidogrel alone after recent ischaemic stroke or transient ischaemic attack in high-risk patients (MATCH): randomised, double-blind, placebo-controlled trial. Lancet. 2004;364(9431):331–7.
3. Ding YH, Dai D, Lewis DA, et al. Angiographic and histologic analysis of experimental aneurysms embolized with platinum coils, Matrix, and HydroCoil. AJNR Am J Neuroradiol. 2005;26:1757–63.
4. Yang H, Sun Y, Jiang Y, Lv X, Zhao Y, Li Y, Liu A. Comparison of stent-assisted coiling vs coiling alone in 563 intracranial aneurysms: safety and efficacy at a high-volume center. Neurosurgery. 2015;77(2):241–7.

23 Transparent Sheath for Neuroendoscopic Intracerebral Hematoma Surgery

Daisuke Suyama, Jun Hiramoto, Kei Yamashiro, Yasuhiro Yamada, Tsukasa Kawase, and Yoko Kato

23.1 Introduction

Neuroendoscopic procedures for spontaneous cerebral hemorrhage have recently increased. This is a result of the reports published by Nishihara et al. in 2000 [1], describing how to use the neuroendoscopic to evacuate the intracerebral hematoma by using a transparent sheath. Following this, 300 surgical cases of spontaneous intracerebral hemorrhage have been performed with an endoscope in our institution, and in related facilities, between 2000 and 2015. This procedure is commonly performed with only one or two burr holes under local anesthesia. If the transparent sheaths are introduced into hematoma safely, endoscopic procedures will be successful in any location of spontaneous hematomas.

23.2 Preoperative Preparation

Prior to the surgery, if the hematoma is at unusual location, the patient needs an angiography or at least three-dimensional computerized tomographic angiography (3D-CTA) or magnetic resonance angiography (MRA) to rule out the possibility of vascular malformation, such as arteriovenous malformation (AVM), aneurysm, or dural AV fistula.

To decide on surgical approach, 3D-CT was performed with scalp marker. For deep-seated hematoma like thalamic hemorrhage, we used stereotaxic system or navigation system in order to insert transparent sheath.

23.2.1 Surgical Tools

For this surgery, we use endoscope, suction tube, and transparent sheath. There are several different types of transparent sheath depending on the case. Some cases require small diameter of 5 mm, but some require 10 mm. Soft blood clot may need small suction of 2 mm, but hard clot may need bigger one such as 4 mm. Rigid and flexible

D. Suyama (✉)
Department of Neurosurgery, Fuchu Keijinkai Hospital, Tokyo, Japan

Department of Neurosurgery, Fujita Health University, Banbuntane Hotokukai Hospital, Nagoya city, Aichi, Japan
e-mail: daisuke@suyama.org

J. Hiramoto
Department of Neurosurgery, Fuchu Keijinkai Hospital, Tokyo, Japan

K. Yamashiro · Y. Yamada · T. Kawase
Department of Neurosurgery, Fujita Health University, Banbuntane Hotokukai Hospital, Nagoya city, Aichi, Japan
e-mail: kawasemi@hm8.aitai.ne.jp

Y. Kato
Department of Neurosurgery, Fujita Health University, Toyoake, Aichi, Japan
e-mail: kyoko@fujita-hu.ac.jp

J. July, E. J. Wahjoepramono (eds.), *Neurovascular Surgery*,
https://doi.org/10.1007/978-981-10-8950-3_23

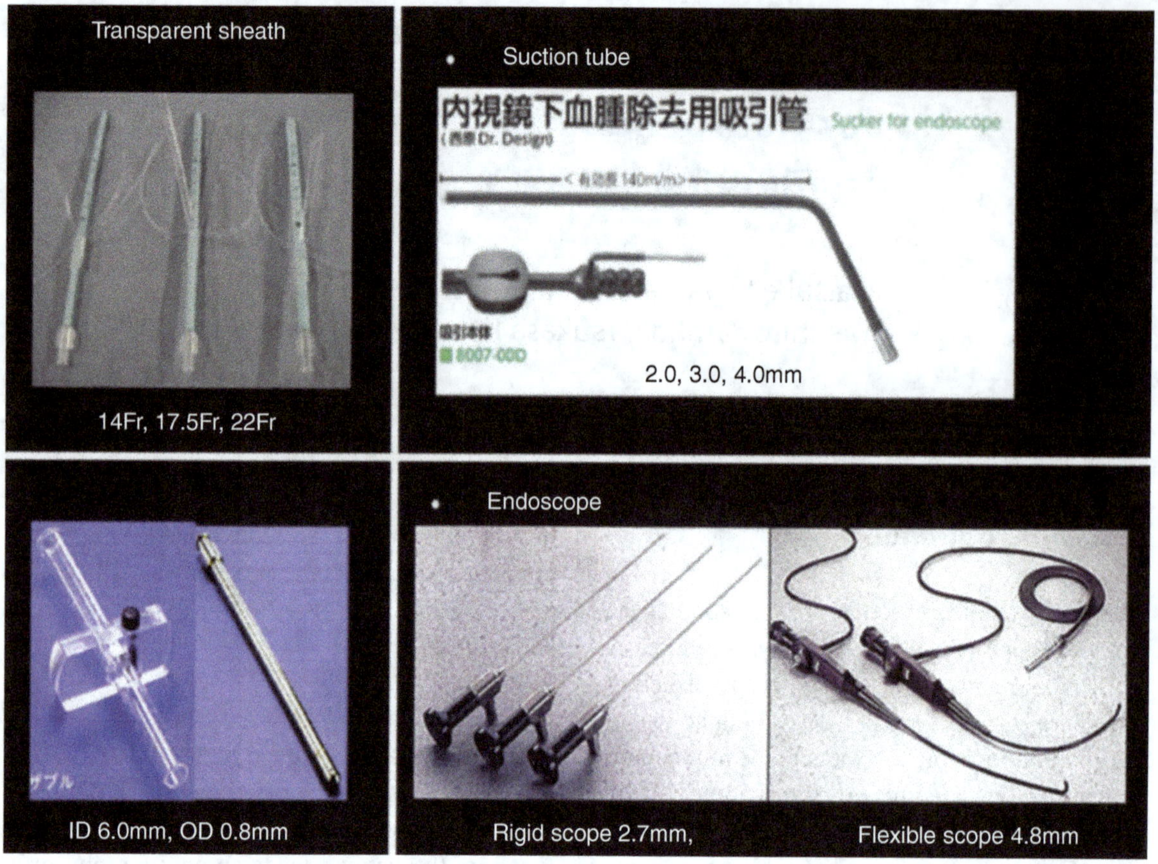

Fig. 23.1 Surgical tools for endoscopic evacuation of intracerebral hematoma

endoscopes are available and their diameter is 2.7 and 4.8 mm (Fig. 23.1).

23.3 Steps of the Surgery

23.3.1 Burr Hole and Hematoma Evacuation

Prior to incision, we need to infiltrate the skin with local anesthesia, and it is very important to infiltrate the periosteum. The periosteum is very sensitive to pain. Linier incision is made and secured with self-retaining retractor. A burr hole is made and should be large enough for the transparent sheath; the sheath is inserted using CT-stereotaxic or navigation guidance until it gets into the hematoma. The transparent sheath (Fig. 23.1) with allows our vison along the tunnel, with the scope and suction tube in it, we will be able to suck out the blood clot. The tube is moveable and has a slippery surface to prevent injury to the brain. If we find the source of bleeding vessel, it could be coagulated with touching the monopolar to the suction tube on the source of bleeding (Fig. 23.2).

23.3.2 Irrigation

When the hematoma is evacuated, we may irrigate the hematoma bed with warm normal saline or ringer solution. Sometimes, when we expand the cavity with the fluid, some residual hematoma is also washed out. The warm fluid usually helps with the local hemostasis, and it's very helpful especially with small oozing blood. Condition with significant bleeding requires bipolar or monopolar. After things are done, the transparent sheath is removed gently and the tract also needs to be washed with warm fluid. No drain is necessary in the hematoma cavity (Fig. 23.3).

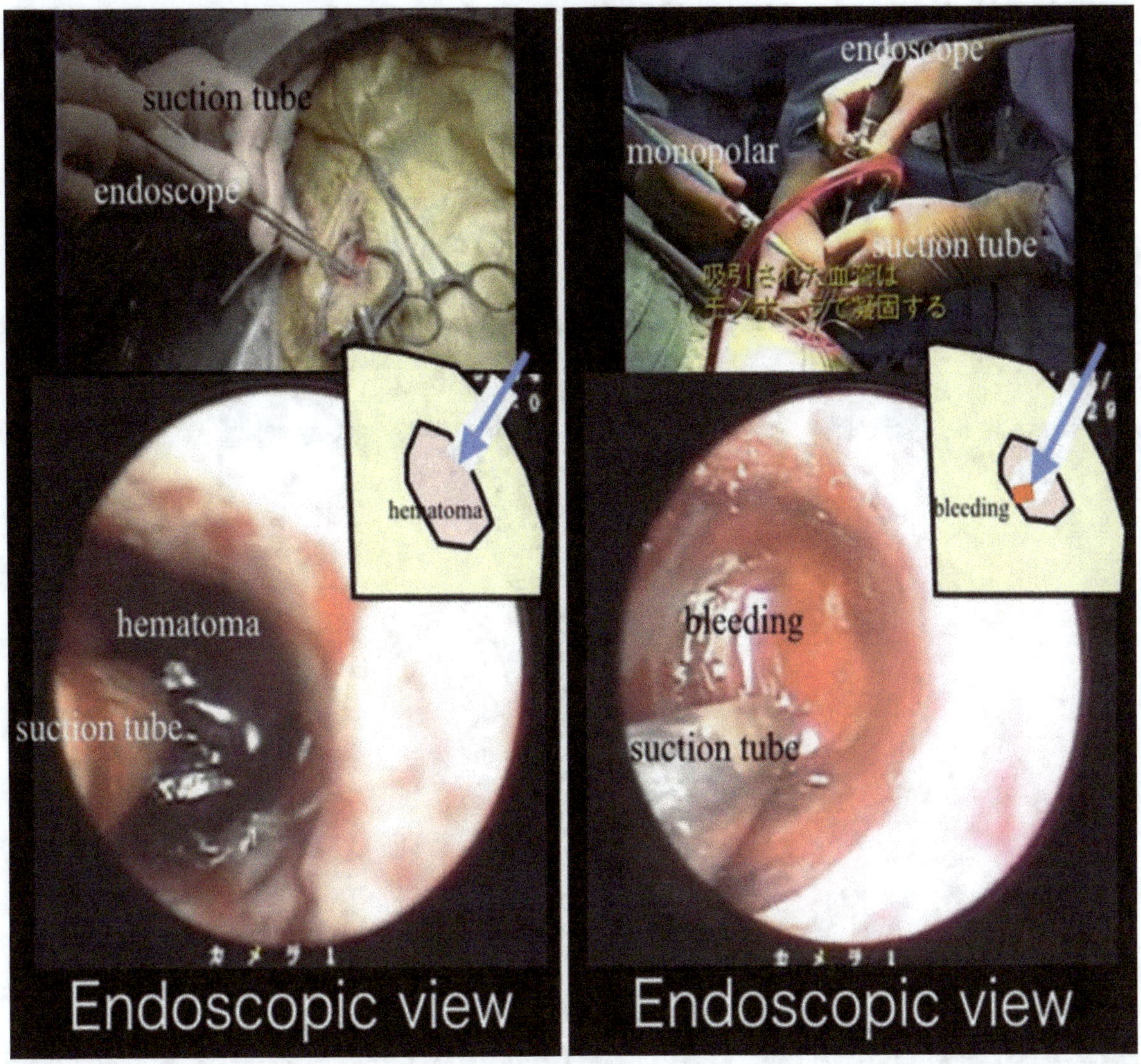

Fig. 23.2 Hematoma evacuation: *left* endoscopic evacuation of the hematoma, *right* endoscopic found and control the source of hemorrhage

23.4 Specific Surgical Technique

The use of endoscope to evacuate the intracerebral hematoma began with endoscopic-assisted stereotaxic aspiration of hematoma, which is popular before 2000 [2, 3]. In contrast to that, recently, the use of endoscope with transparent sheath for evacuation of hematoma is the major role because it provides the direct vision compared to the stereotaxic aspiration surgery. The transparent sheath is movable and provides a clear orientation around the tube. This technique has gain popularity very fast, and it could be done with small incision and with small craniotomy (or burr hole). The entry point for different locations is very important, such as putaminal hematoma, thalamic hematoma, lobar hematoma, and cerebellar hematoma.

23.4.1 Putaminal Hemorrhage

In putaminal hematoma, the burr-hole position should be put at the upper end of the hematoma to the closest vertical trajectory from the cranium. Removing the hematoma and being able to see the brain margin will help the orientation. The hard clot should not be pulled and better to be left

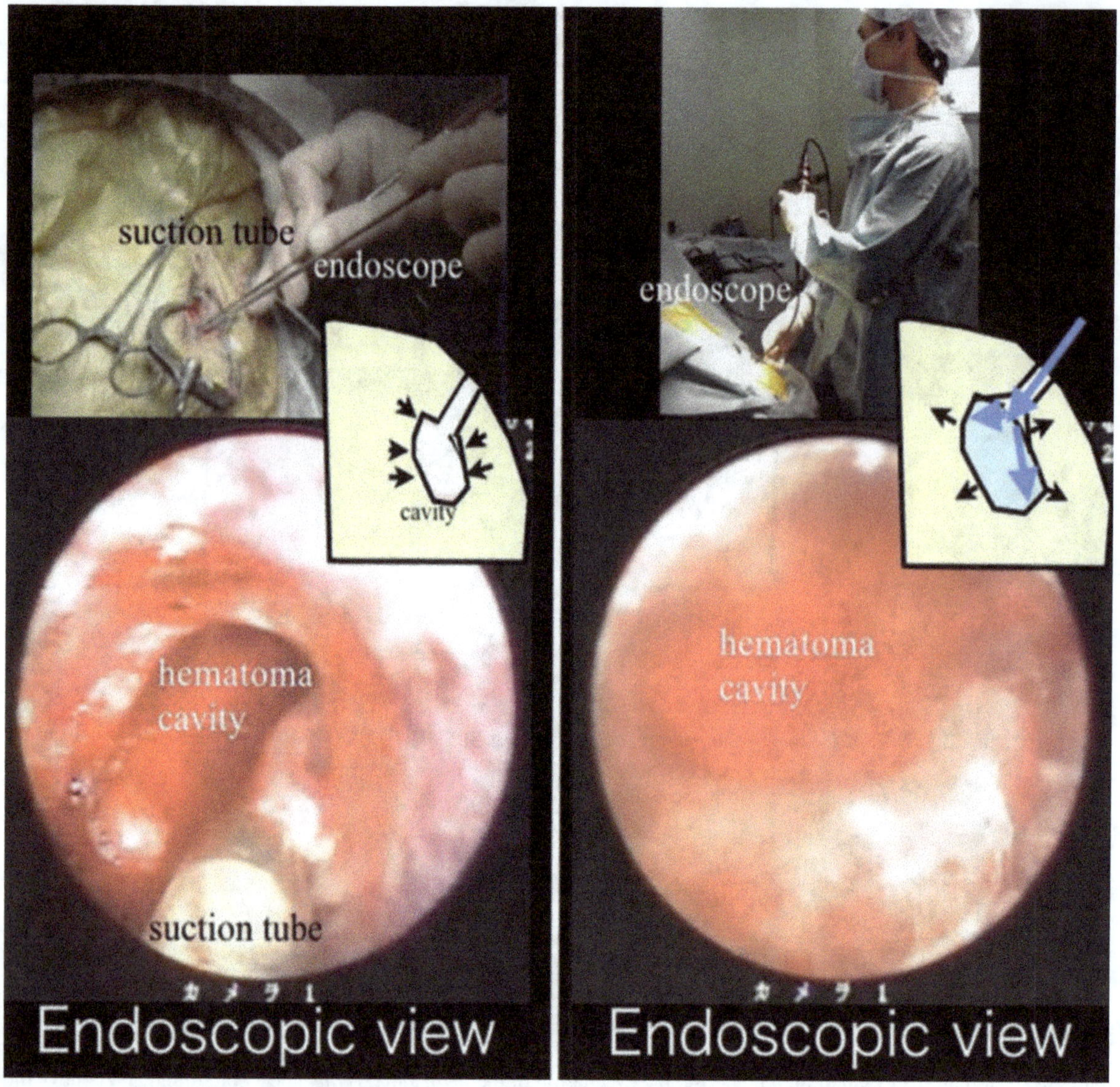

Fig. 23.3 Irrigation of hematoma cavity: *left* rigid scope view, *right* flexible scope view

there. After the hematoma removal, we may irrigate the cavity with warm saline (Fig. 23.4).

23.4.2 Thalamic Hemorrhage

In thalamic hematoma, we have to consider the blood both in the ventricle and in the parenchyma. Also, we need to remember and imagine the location of internal capsule to the blood clot. The surgical approach could be from anterior or posterior transventricular and try to avoid injury to internal capsule, although it's probably already injured by the hemorrhage. But we need to try our best to avoid making more injury to the internal capsule, if there are still some. After evacuating the thalamic hematoma, the blood clot in the ventricle could be aspirated gently. Sometimes we need a flexible scope (Fig. 23.5). But even with rigid scope and lots of irrigation, we may clear the hematoma mostly.

23.4.3 Lobar Hemorrhage

In lobar hemorrhage, the trajectory for lobar hematoma should be planned with navigation or for 3D-CT with scalp marker (Fig. 23.6).

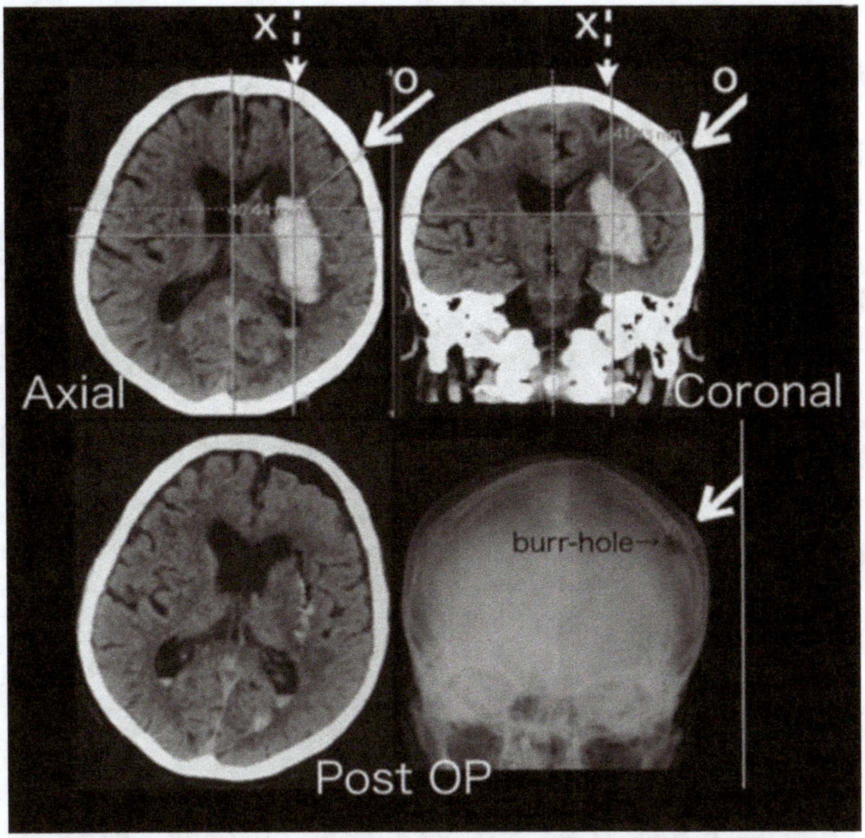

Fig. 23.4 CT scan of putaminal hemorrhage: *O* point of entry, *X* longitudinal axis of the hematoma

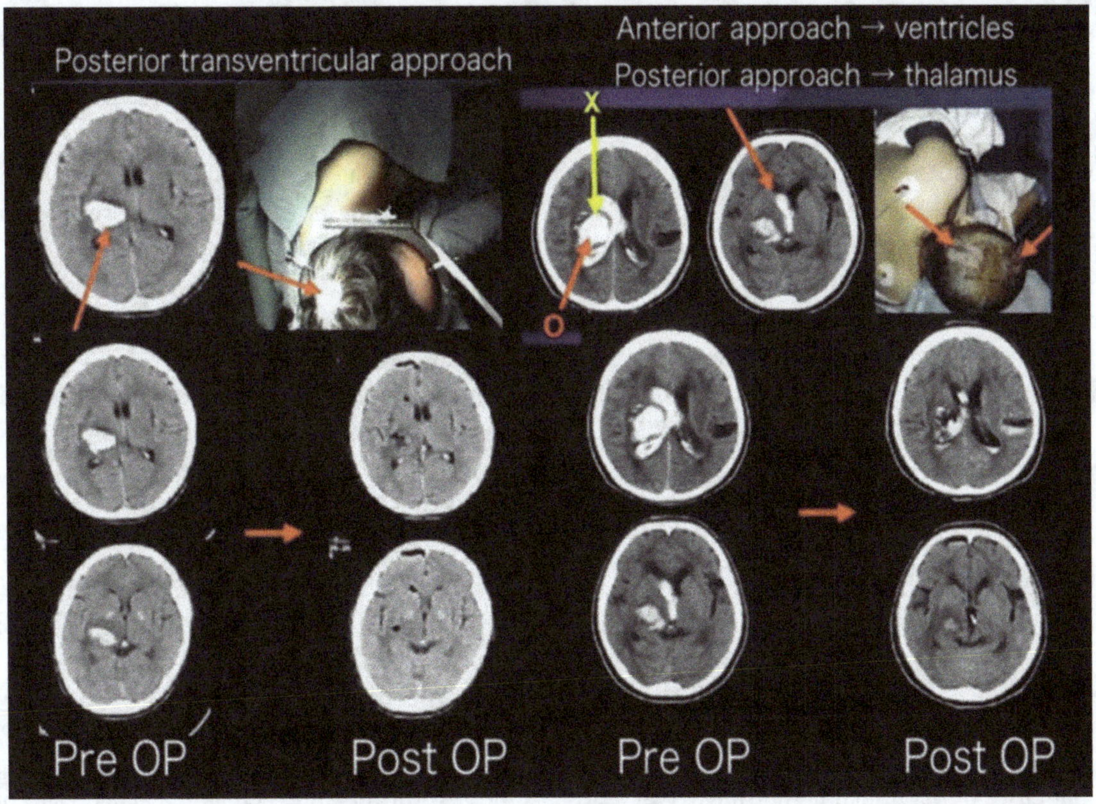

Fig. 23.5 Thalamic hemorrhage: *left*, posterior transventricular removal of the hematoma; *right*, coming from posterior with rigid scope to remove the thalamus hematoma and coming from anterior horn with flexible scope to remove the intraventricular hematoma

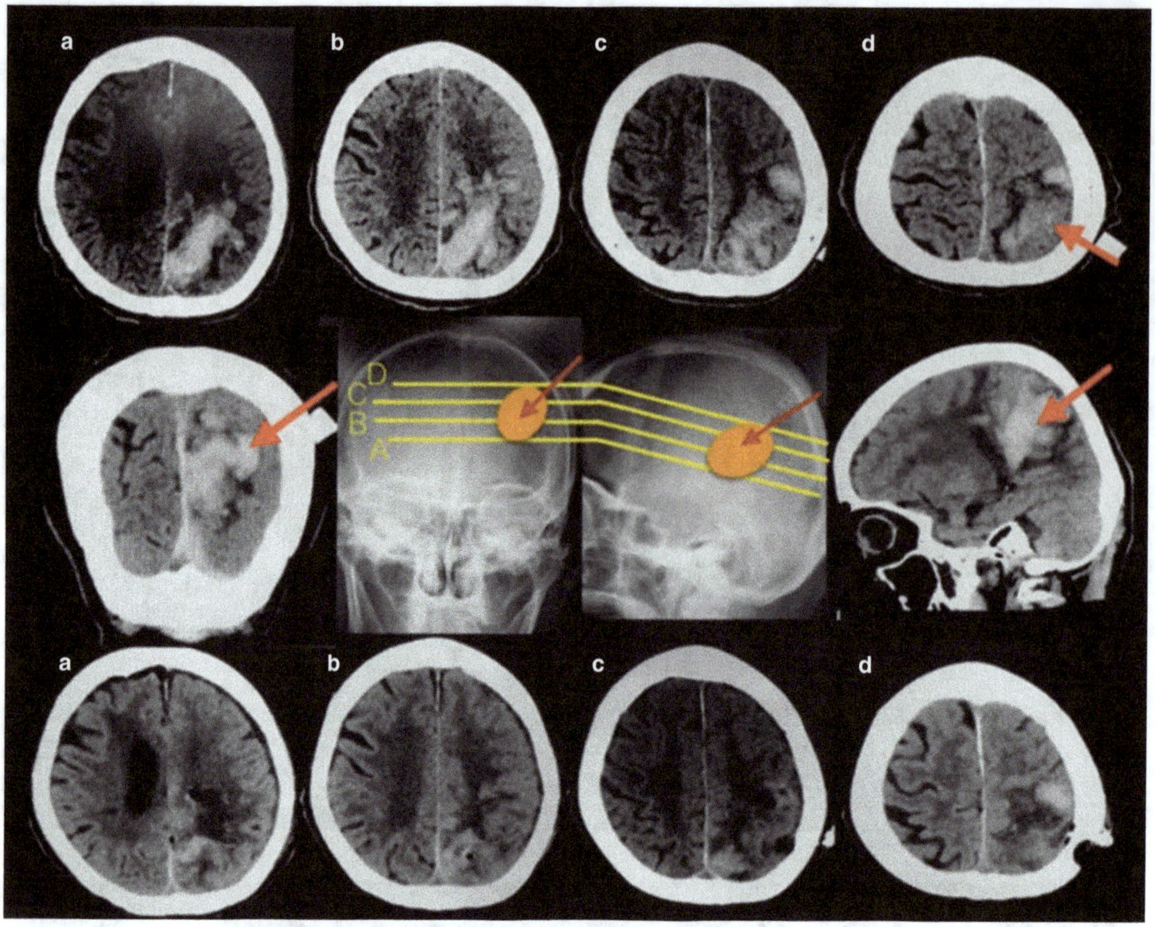

Fig. 23.6 CT scan of lobar hemorrhage, before surgery and after surgery (*lower part*)

23.4.4 Cerebellar Hemorrhage

In cerebellar hemorrhage, burr hole position is very important but it is difficult to decide a proper position only by preoperative scalp surface marker; a midpoint of the line between the inion and the mastoid tip. Burr-hole position should be measured from the foramen magnum on the skull surface during surgery. It is the most reliable marker during surgery, to make a burr hole on the inferior nuchal line in the distance of 3 cm from the foramen magnum (Fig. 23.7).

23.5 Expert Opinion/Suggestion to Avoid Complication

In our cases of putaminal hemorrhage, two cases we switched craniotomy. One case is due to enlargement of the hematoma after surgery, and this probably due to either insufficient hemostasis or rebleeding after surgery. The second case was due to a small AVM that we misdiagnosed at the beginning. It was described by Yasagil in 1987 [4]. The diagnose was proved during craniotomy and the pathology confirmed it. We highly recommend to screen every possible case, especially if the location and the clinical presentation are not typical for hypertensive hemorrhage. If there is a massive bleeding during hematoma evacuation, do not hesitate to switch to craniotomy for hematoma removal. All of such thing should be mentioned in the consent prior to surgery, including the provable micro-AVM [5].

In our cases of thalamic hemorrhage, we have two cases with intraventricular venous; both cases were using an anterior transventricular approach for thalamic hematoma. Therefore, our opinion is considering that a posterior approach is probably better than an anterior approach to

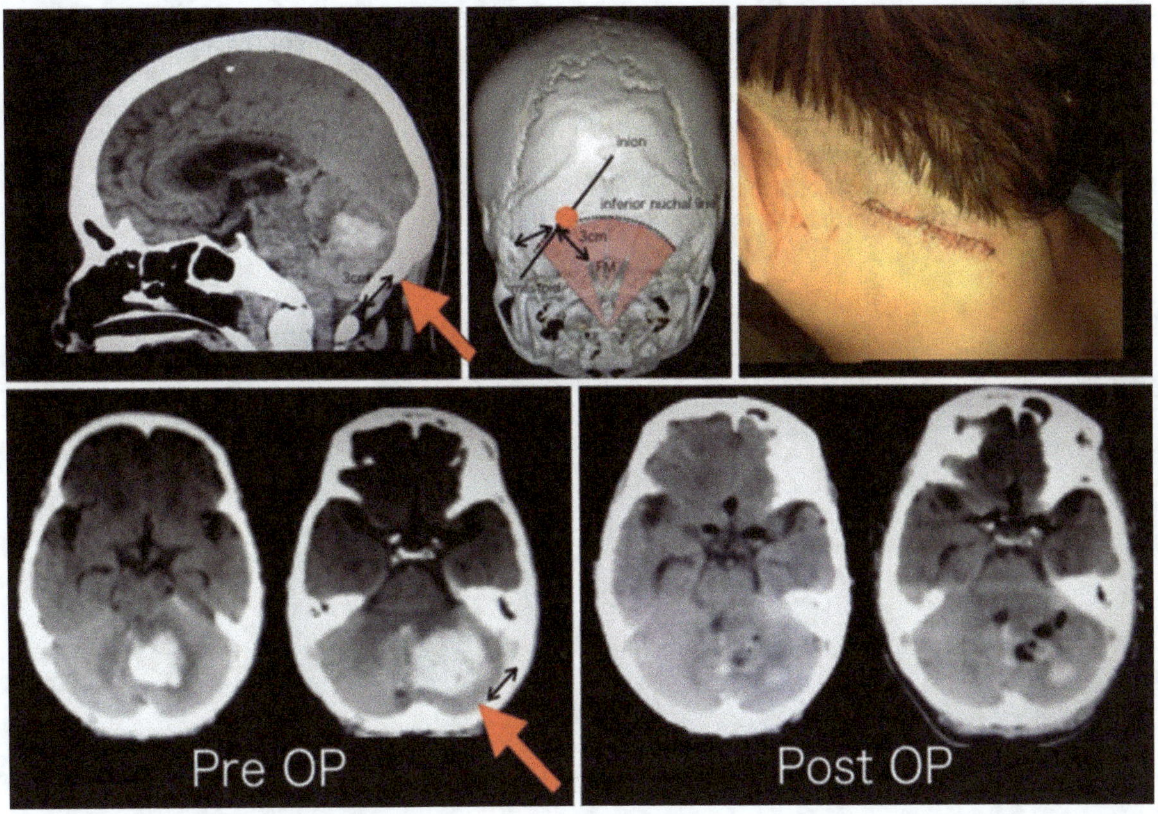

Fig. 23.7 Cerebellar hemorrhage, before and after surgery

remove the thalamic hematoma to avoid injury of intraventricular veins.

Transparent sheath for endoscopic evacuation of intracerebral hematoma will become more and more popular. Once the surgeon becomes familiar and comfortable with this technique, they will less likely go back to the conventional approach with bigger incision and bigger wound. The important points of this surgery is the placement of the burr hole so the track will provide the best direction for hematoma evacuation.

References

1. Nishihara T, Teraoka A, Morita A, et al. A transparent sheath for endoscopic surgery and its application in surgical evacuation of spontaneous intracerebral hematomas. J Neurosurg. 2000;92:1053–5.
2. Auer LM, Holzer P, Ascher PW, et al. Endoscopic neurosurgery. Acta Neurochir. 1988;90:1–14.
3. Kuroda K, Ogawa A. Comparative studies of surgical treatments for intracerebral hemorrhage: mainly on an echo-guide aspiration and a CT-guide aspiration with neuroendoscopy. Jpn J Neurosurg. 1999;8:100–5.
4. Yasargil MG. Microneurosurgery, vol 3B. Stuttgart: Thieme; 1987. p. 18–9.
5. Suyama D, Ito K, Tanii M, et al. A difficult case of endoscopic neurosurgery for intracerebral hemorrhage due to micro-arteriovenous malformation. Surg Cereb Stroke (Jpn). 2003;31:361–4.

Check for updates

24 Surgery of Intracerebral Hemorrhage

Regunath Kandasamy, Zamzuri Idris, and Jafri Malin Abdullah

24.1 Introduction

Spontaneous intracerebral hemorrhage (ICH) due to uncontrolled hypertension is a common clinical entity that affects up to four million people annually [1]. Hemodynamic injury to perforating end arteries (100–400 µm) results in pathological lesions such as lipohyalinosis, fibrinoid necrosis, and Charcot-Bouchard microaneurysm which may predispose to rupture. Common locations where these hemorrhages may occur include the basal ganglia, pons, thalamus, cerebellum, or subcortical white matter (lobar) [2].

Despite numerous multicenter trials, debate still exists on the indication for surgery as well as exact benefits of this treatment modality. Advancement in technology has also provided a number of minimally invasive methods such as endoscopic and stereotactic aspiration for evacuation of clots. The superiority of any one of these methods over the others has still not been completely established.

In the course of training, a young neurosurgeon should be well versed in the basic surgical principles of managing a patient who presents with neurological symptoms due to an intracerebral hemorrhage. Despite the increasing popularity of minimally invasive methods, craniotomy remains a fairly safe and standardized method of clot removal and hemostasis under direct visualization. In cases of hemorrhage with significant perilesional edema, the option of removal of the bone flap may help relieve life-threatening brain shifts and elevation in intracranial pressure.

24.2 Rationale for Surgery

Surgical evacuation of the ICH is aimed at reducing mass effect caused by the clot. This in turn reduces intracranial pressure and prevents life-threatening brain shifts from occurring. The removal of clot also reduces biochemical as well as inflammatory processes that are initiated by toxic blood products.

At present the AHA consensus guidelines suggest that cerebellar hemorrhages >3 cm and supratentorial superficial lobar hemorrhages of >30 cc in volume will benefit from surgical evacuation [3]. Additionally, in our center, we practice the evacuation of superficial (within 1 cm from cortical surface) basal ganglia hemorrhages with significant mass effect in young (age <50 years) viable (GCS > 8) patients suffering from this condition.

Prior to proceeding with clot evacuation, it is imperative to rule out other etiological conditions which may result in intracerebral hemorrhage

R. Kandasamy · Z. Idris · J. M. Abdullah (✉)
Department of Neurosciences, Centre for Neurosciences Services and Research, School of Medical Sciences, Universiti Sains Malaysia Health Campus, Kota Bharu, Kelantan, Malaysia

J. July, E. J. Wahjoepramono (eds.), *Neurovascular Surgery*,
https://doi.org/10.1007/978-981-10-8950-3_24

including aneurysms, vascular malformations, tumor with bleeds, or coagulopathy.

24.3 Signs and Symptoms

Clinical features attributed to an ICH can be divided into general symptoms related to the mass effect of the lesion as well as focal symptoms in relation to the anatomical area of the brain affected. Onset is usually sudden and progression of symptoms typically occurs in minutes to hours. The generalized effects of an ICH are due to dural stretching as well as elevation in intracranial pressure. Initial symptoms include headaches, nausea, vomiting, and blurred vision. Worsening brain shifts can result in deterioration in consciousness, abnormal breathing patterns, as well as motor posturing all related to impending herniation.

Focal symptoms as mentioned depend on the site of the bleeding. Lobar hemorrhages have symptoms related to the affected lobe including seizures, hemiparesis, visual field deficits, aphasia, or impaired higher cortical function. In the basal ganglia, a small clot may not manifest with overt neurological deficits. However, extension of the lesion to the thalamus or internal capsule may often result in hemiparesis or hemisensory loss and visual deficits.

Clots in the brain stem region result in cranial nerve impairment. Depending on which nerve is involved, the location of the bleed can often be predicted. Early onset of deterioration in consciousness with flexor or extensor motor posturing occurs when a brain stem bled disrupts the reticular activating system as well as descending extrapyramidal tracts. Cerebellar hemorrhages on the other hand result in dizziness and vomiting and ataxia. If the clot size is large enough, consciousness may also be impaired due to direct compression of the brain stem.

About a third of patients with ICH will develop secondary intraventricular hemorrhage. In these cases, patients may also develop generalized symptoms due to hydrocephalus causing elevations in intracranial pressure.

A small percentage of patients remain asymptomatic particularly when the hemorrhage volume is small. Often, the only abnormal findings in this group of patients may be a sudden elevation in blood pressure despite being compliant to their regular medications.

24.4 Investigations

On initial assessment, patients suspected with ICH usually undergo a computed tomographic (CT) evaluation of their brain. When reviewing such a scan, it is important to take note of the following points:

1. Site of lesion and extension.
2. Dimension and volume (A × B × C/2).
3. Presence of mass effect, midline shift, as well as hydrocephalus.
4. Atypical features warranting further definitive investigation (*calcifications, perilesional edema incongruent with lesion or in terms of onset of clot development, tortuous vessels, subarachnoid hemorrhage, atypical location*).

If the patient's clinical or radiological features necessitate, further investigations should be performed prior to proceeding with intended surgery. Angiography or CT angiography can be performed to rule out vascular malformation or aneurysm rupture. MRI can be performed if a tumor with bleed is suspected. The surgical strategy and timing for surgery for these conditions may differ from that of a simple ICH, and one runs the risk of uncontrollable intraoperative bleeding or other serious complications if these conditions are not identified and addressed according to their respective treatment protocols.

Alternatively, a CT with contrast maybe performed as a preliminary evaluation. Keep in mind that despite the requirement for complete investigation to rule out the underlying cause for a bleed, it should not occur at the expense of the patient particularly in instances when life-threatening mass effect and herniation are in progress.

MRI with diffusion tensor imaging maybe useful to map out the location of the important motor and sensory fibers in relation to the clot to minimize intraoperative injury. This modality however is often inappropriate for patients with acutely expanding hematomas due to the long duration required to perform this investigation.

Aside from the standard battery of radiological investigations, routine blood investigations such as blood counts, renal profile, coagulation profile, as well blood glucose are essential. It is particularly important that issues such as coagulopathy or thrombocytopenia are duly addressed. Patients with hypertensive ICH usually have a number of coexistent medical problems which may further complicate management. Failure to address these conditions may result in a non-favorable outcome in patients especially those undergoing surgery.

24.5 Preoperative Preparation

Having obtained informed consent from the next of kin, attention should be focused on blood pressure (BP) control, cross-matched blood availability, correction of coagulopathy, and withholding of any drugs which may worsen bleeding (antiplatelet, Coumadin derivatives, etc.). Patients with supratentorial particularly lobar ICH undergoing surgery are usually loaded with an antiepileptic agent due to potential cortical transgression. Antibiotic prophylaxis is also indicated during the time of induction of general anesthesia.

24.6 Steps of Surgery

Preoperative planning of the surgical approach is the key to success in any surgical procedure. It is important to review the preop images carefully in all three surgical planes before deciding on the best approach to use.

Points to consider include exact location and extent of the clot, proximity to eloquent brain regions, and usage of the shortest path with least injury to vital cortical areas. In patients with a lobar hemorrhage in the frontotemporal or basal ganglia region, a frontotemporal craniotomy will usually give adequate access to allow evacuation of the clot. As for parietal or parieto-occipital clots, a more posteriorly placed craniotomy may be more appropriate. Cerebellar hemorrhages can be accessed using a midline or paramedian posterior fossa craniotomy.

To illustrate this point, we will use the clinical case of a typical basal ganglia hemorrhage as shown below.

24.6.1 Case Illustration

A 36-year-old male patient with a history of hypertension presented with sudden-onset weakness over the right side of his body with progressive deterioration in consciousness. He was admitted with GCS (Glasgow Coma Scale) of E2 V3 M5 = 10/15. His BP was recorded as 220/110 on admission. An urgent CT brain was performed as shown below (Fig. 24.1).

The CT scan revealed the presence of a large left-sided basal ganglia hemorrhage causing significant midline shift. The clot had extended to within 1 cm from the surface of the cortex. CT angiography did not reveal any underlying vascular etiology for this bleed. Patient underwent a frontotemporal craniotomy and evacuation of his clots. Following craniotomy and dural opening, one may use one of the three routes to reach the clot. The three routes include either trans-sylvian or via the prefrontal or superior temporal gyri (Fig. 24.2). The choice of the routes would depend on the characteristics of the clot as well clinical condition. The trans-sylvian method is an advantage because only the insular cortex is transgressed during surgery compared to the frontal or temporal cortex where more neurological deficits may occur. Sylvian fissure splitting and dissection can be time consuming in inexperienced hands and difficult in cases where brain swelling is apparent. In this patient given the degree of brain edema, a clot evacuation using the prefrontal cortex was opted for. Due to poor clinical state on admission and intraoperative finding of brain swelling, it was opted to not replace his bone flap after surgery.

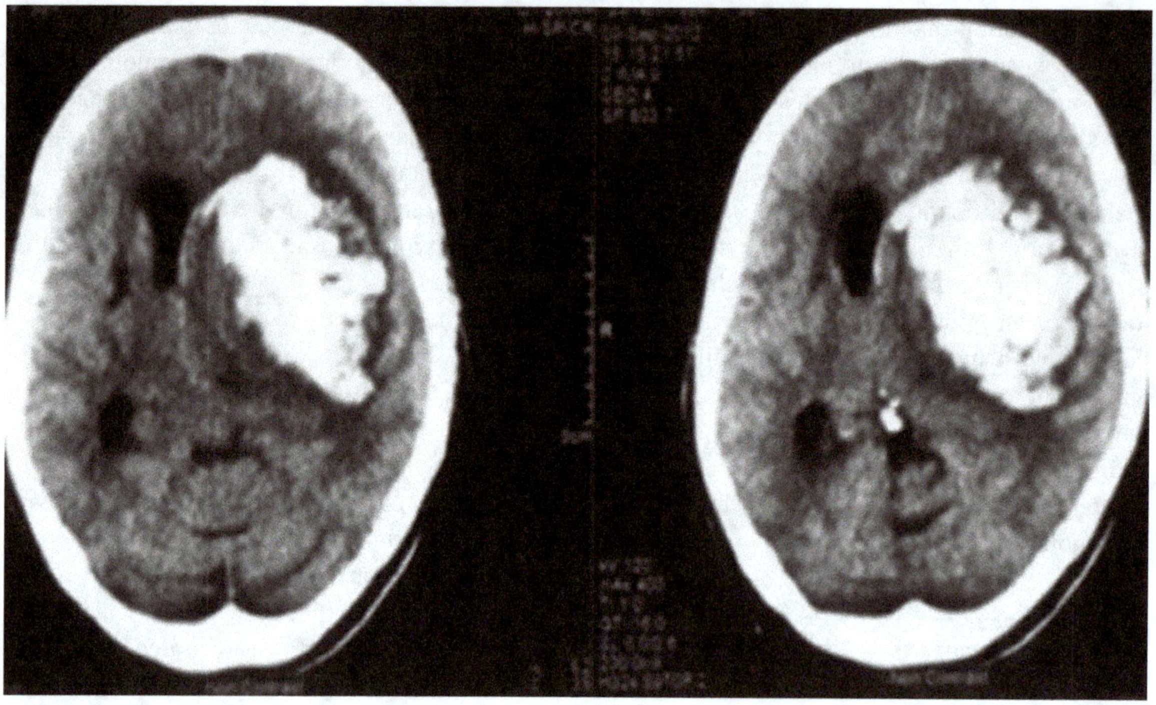

Fig. 24.1 Axial CT brain of the patient

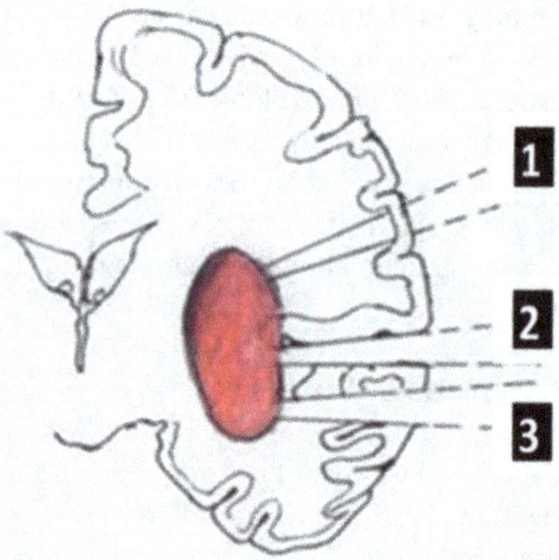

Fig. 24.2 Diagrammatic representation of the surgical corridors that can be utilized for clot evacuation: (1) via the prefrontal cortex, (2) via the Sylvian fissure, and (3) via the superior temporal gyrus

24.6.2 Positioning and Skin Incision

In supratentorial clot evacuation, patients are placed supine with their heads, elevated about 30°, and rotated away from the side of the clot. The patient's head can be fixed in a rigid fixation device (Mayfield clamp) or supported on a horseshoe. Always ensure that the neck is not excessively flexed as this may impair venous outflow from the head (Fig. 24.3).

For clots, predominantly in the frontal region, a hemi-coronal skin incision behind the hairline is usually adequate for exposure. An inverted question mark-shaped incision is however advised when attempting to remove a large ICH. It would allow adequate access to the region of interest without hindrance due to brain swelling.

24.6.3 Flap Elevation and Craniotomy

The skin flap is secured with Raney clips, and the flap raised in two layers to create a mobile fascial flap for later dural closure. The craniotomy is fashioned around three to four entry burr holes and the bone flap is elevated. Once the flap has been elevated, secure hemostasis from dural vessels and perform peripheral tenting (Figs. 24.4 and 24.5).

24.6.4 Dural Opening

The opening of the dura can be performed in a cruciate manner or as a "U"-shaped flap. A size "11" blade or metzenbaum scissors can be used for this. Ensure that the underlying surface of the brain is lined with patties after initial durotomy to avoid possible cortical injury during extension of the dural flap. If the brain is very swollen, an osmotic diuretic may be used or CSF diversion performed if intraventricular hemorrhage or hydrocephalus is present on preoperative imaging.

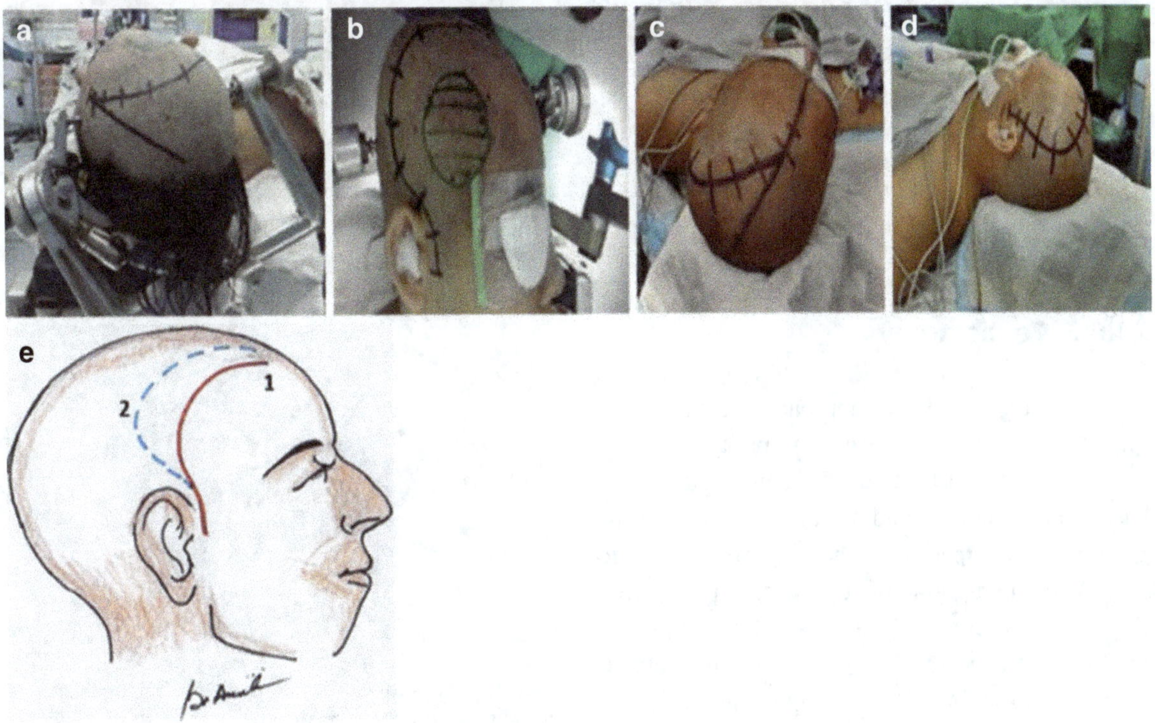

Fig. 24.3 (**a**, **b**) Patient with a frontal lobar hemorrhage with head fixed in a Mayfield device and skin incision fashioned in a question mark shape. (**c**, **d**) Head placement on a horseshoe clamp for a left basal ganglia hemorrhage evacuation. (**e**) Diagrammatic representations of (1) frontotemporal and (2) question mark incisions that can be used for this surgery

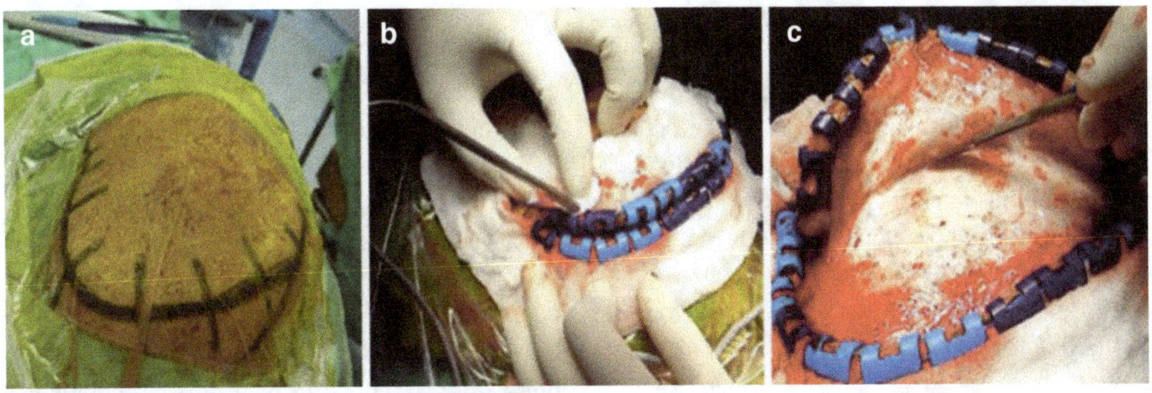

Fig. 24.4 (**a–c**) Skin flap is marked, draped, and subsequently elevated. Skin edges are secured using Raney clips, and elevation of flap is performed as shown

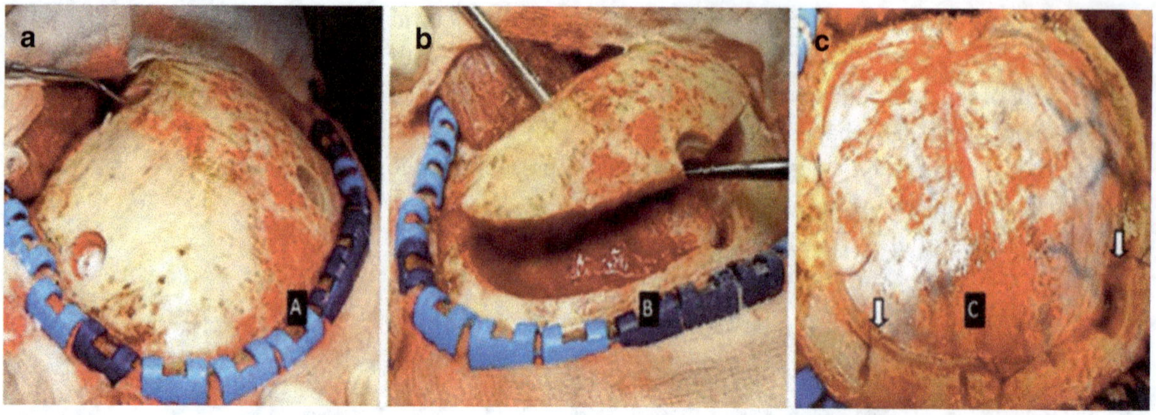

Fig. 24.5 (**a**) Three burr hole are made starting with one over the MacCarty keyhole followed by the temporal region just posterior to the zygomatic root as well over the frontal region anterior to the coronal suture. The dural adhesion to the bone should be released using a blunt dissector prior to cutting the bone flap. (**b**) The flap is elevated while freeing the dural attachment to the bone. (**c**) After elevating the flap, hemostasis is secured by waxing the bone edges and applying tenting sutures peripherally (*white arrow*)

24.6.5 Corticotomy

The decision on how to approach the clot is an important one in view of the morbidity that may result from injury to eloquent brain regions. For basal ganglia clot, we advise an approach via the prefrontal or superior temporal gyrus cortex to minimize disruption of eloquent brain areas (Fig. 24.6). Alternatively, a trans-sylvian approach might be utilized to access a deep-seated clot if brain swelling is not very apparent. Prior to attempted corticotomy, it is wise to use a brain needle to confirm the localization of the clot and subsequently use the tract created by the needle to reach the lesion. This will prevent misadventures due to improper localization that may occur in inexperienced hands. Alternatively, intraoperative ultrasonography may also be used for clot localization. Often, superficial clots may themselves have extended and breached the cortical surface, and in these cases, one should utilize the pre-created path of the clot for evacuation. Once clot location has been confirmed, the operating microscope should be utilized for clot evacuation (Fig. 24.7).

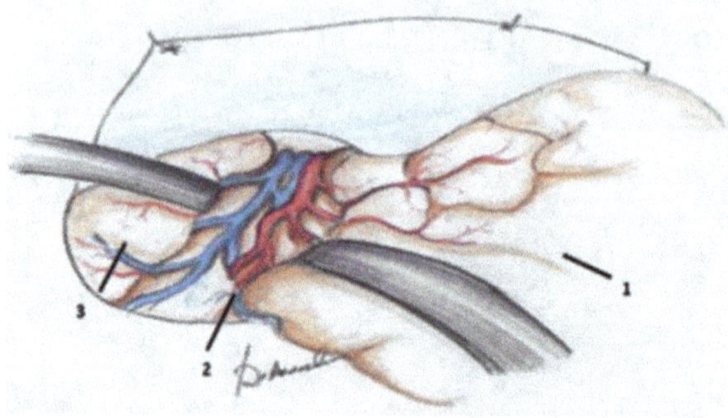

Fig. 24.6 Sites for Corticectomy depending on the surgical approach used: (1) via the prefrontal cortex, (2) via the Sylvian fissure, and (3) via the superior temporal gyrus

24.6.6 Clot Evacuation

Clots can be removed using gentle suction with irrigation. A teardrop suction device at a setting of 100 Kpa is usually very helpful in this setting. It is imperative that clots are removed patiently and slowly in a spiral movement to prevent injury to the surrounding brain. Initially, the liquefied portion of clot can be easily removed. The harder portions may need to be dissected off adjacent the parenchyma prior to successful removal. Dislodged larger clots may be removed using a biopsy of grasping forces. Once the clot has been removed, the raw edges of the brain are usually visible. The aim of this surgery is to remove as much clot as possible to relieve the mass effect. With this in mind, we personally endeavour to remove as much clot that is safely possible due to the fact that aside from direct

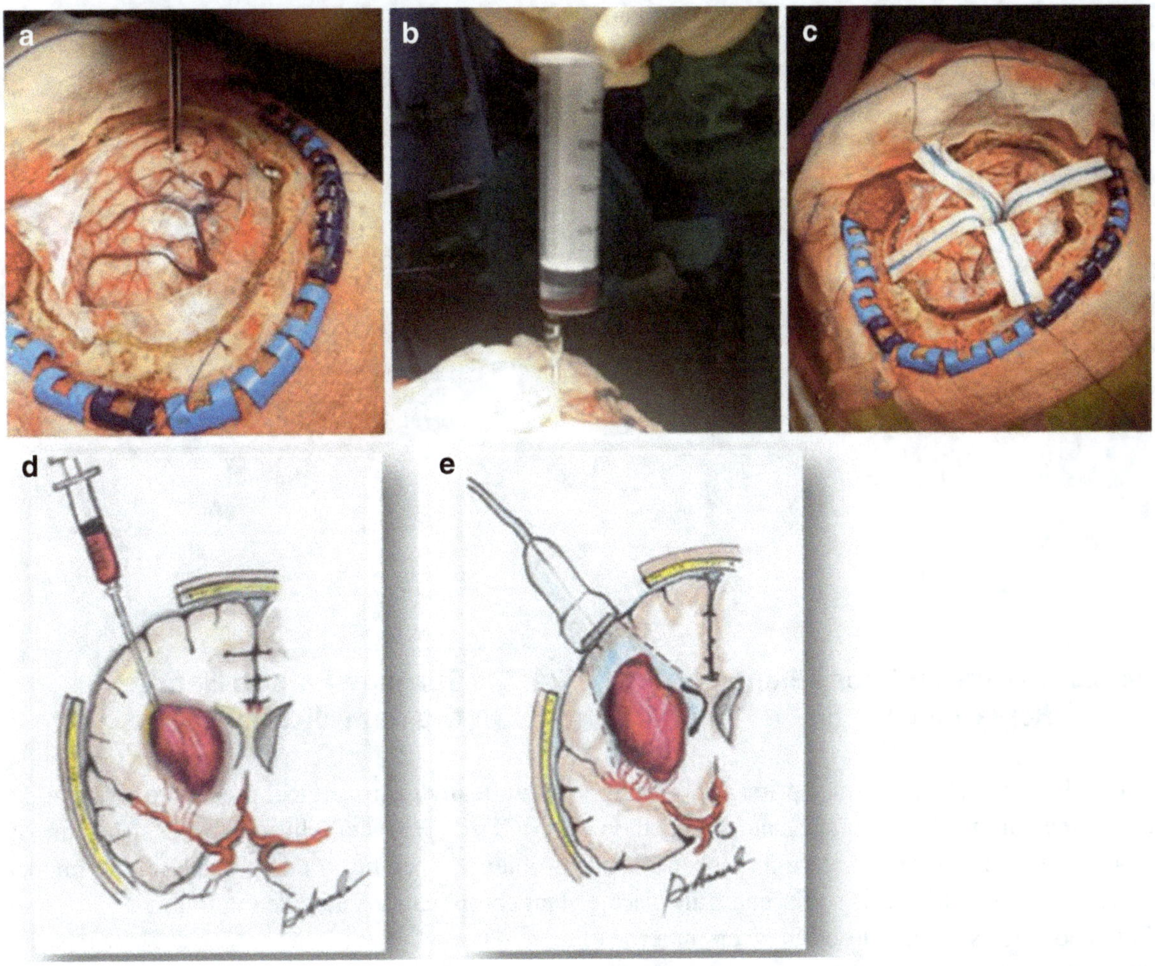

Fig. 24.7 (**a**, **b**) Localization of clots using a brain needle and aspiration. (**c**) Once located, the corticectomy is performed following the trajectory of the needle to the clot. (**d**, **e**) Diagrammatic representation of clot localization using a brain needle or an intraoperative ultrasound probe

mass effect, blood product left in the brain may also be responsible for pro-inflammatory chemical responses that result in persistent brain edema (Fig. 24.8).

24.6.7 Hemostasis

Following clot removal, the authors find that the extent of oozing within the cavity usually significantly reduces. Utilizing cotton pledgets or cotton balls, the cavity can be packed and irrigated with warm saline to stop minimal oozes and to identify overt bleeding vessels. Bleeding sites are best identified and secured by moving from the periphery and walls of the cavity to the base in a systematic manner. It is usually necessary to cauterize the actively bleeding stumps of the end arteries in hypertensive hemorrhages. The cavity is then lined with a mechanical hemostatic agents such as "Surgicel or Fibrillar." Finally, the cavity is again irrigated with warm saline to confirm hemostasis. It is wise to confirm, at this point, the patient's BP reading to ensure that it is not too low. BP can be transiently increased to identify bleeding points; however, this should be performed with great caution, and not excessively lest significant re-hemorrhage occurs.

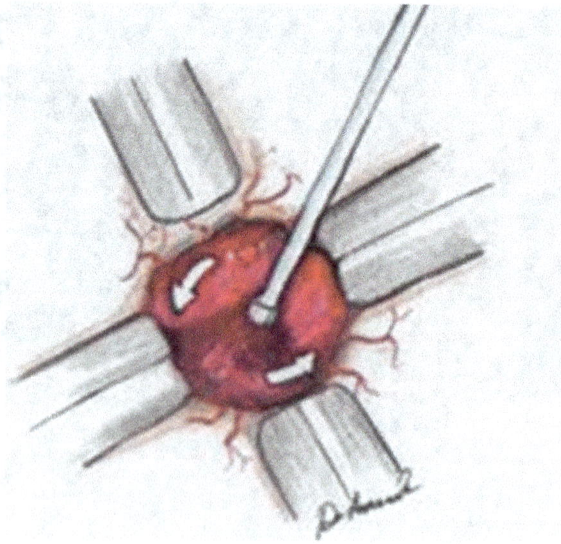

Fig. 24.8 Methods of suctioning and clot aspiration in a spiral manner

24.6.8 Closure and Bone Flap Replacement

Dural closure can be performed primarily or using durofasciaoplasty. A continuous suturing method is advocated to achieve a watertight closure. The bone flap is then replaced and secured in place. Skin and soft tissue are closed in layers in a routine fashion. In cases where brain swelling maybe significant, replacement of the bone flap may not always be advisable. Performing a craniectomy together with clot evacuation has been noted in some series to improve outcome in patients with putaminal hemorrhage in a subset of patients who exhibit brain swelling [4]. Pure decompression alone however without clot evacuation has been found to have limited benefits. In performing a craniectomy, the surgeon should be aware that the size of the bony defect should be large enough to achieve adequate decompression. The middle fossa flow should be removed to ensure that the incisura and brain stem are relieved from pressure. To achieve this, a large skin incision may be required, and it is the reason that we advocate using a question mark incision in cases where brain swelling might be anticipated.

24.7 Surgeon Plan to Handle the Complication

As with any neurosurgical procedure, evacuation of ICH can be complicated by a spectrum of problems. Specific to this procedure, the important complications include the following:

24.7.1 Intraoperative Brain Swelling

Brain swelling maybe encountered at different stages of the surgery. The strategy of management differs slightly in each circumstance. The occurrence of brain swelling at the outset of dural opening can often be predicted based on features such as delayed presentation, poor GCS scores, large clot volume, and significant midline shift. Even in patients with moderate-sized clots on imaging, intraoperative brain swelling is still possible due to clot expansion during the interim period of going to the operation room and induction of anesthesia. One common cause for expansion relates to poorly controlled BP. Thus, it is very important to ensure that the patient's BP is constantly monitored and adequately controlled. If a significant deterioration of the patient's GCS occurs prior to transfer to the OR, a CT scan can be performed to elucidate the extent of expansion or if hydrocephalus has developed (*but not at the expense of timely surgical intervention*). In cases like these, the surgical strategy should also include decompression and/or CSF diversion aside from clot evacuation.

If brain swelling is encountered during or after clot evacuation, firstly ensure that hemodynamic parameters such as BP and PC02 are normal. Additionally, CSF diversion can also be performed if a search of the clot cavity post evacuation reveals no evidence of a new clot formation.

24.7.2 Re-accumulation of Clots

After clot evacuation, rebreeding with recollection may occur immediately or in a delayed manner. If it occurs intraoperatively, it may be heralded by brain swelling, and the surgeon can usually reexplore the clot cavity and evacuate it. In the postoperative period, re-accumulation of clots is often associated with elevations in blood pressure which were not adequately addressed. They may come to attention during routine postoperative CT scanning or due to deterioration in the patient's conscious level after initial recovery. If needed, then a repeat surgery may be required to remove the new clot.

24.7.3 Hydrocephalus

In patients with intraventricular extension of their ICH, hydrocephalus may occur early or late depending on the extent and location of blood in the ventricular system. Patients with hydrocephalus at the outset should get early CSF diversion. Alternatively, the hydrocephalus may manifest as brain swelling intraoperatively or in the postoperative period during patient recovery. A patient who develops a subgaleal CSF collection or leak should be investigated to rule out underlying hydrocephalus. Permanent CSF diversion is usually not necessary for a majority of patients, and these can be managed using temporary diversion methods.

24.7.4 Injury to Parenchyma During Clot Evacuation

It is advised that a microscope be used for clot evacuation to enable clear differentiation between the clot and adjacent brain. Gentle suction and irrigation are to be used during clot evacuation. If any large vessels are seen during surgery, cover them with a thin layer of hemostatic material and patties to avoid inadvertent injury during clot removal.

24.8 Expert Opinion to Avoid Complications

- Review all investigations prior to surgery.
- Plan surgical approach based on CT imaging.
- Anticipate brain swelling and plan early measures to alleviate it.
- Plan skin flap, keeping in mind the need for a larger bone flap in some patients.
- Localize clot using a brain needle.
- Gentle clot evacuation assisted by microscope.
- Check operative field to ensure hemostasis prior to closure.
- Maintain judicious blood pressure control in postoperative period.

Do not forget hydrocephalus as a cause for delayed duration or operative wound CSF leak.

24.9 Postoperative Care and Follow-Up

Following surgery, patients should be monitored in an intensive care setting with hourly assessment of vital signs and neurological status. Careful attention to BP readings is vital to prevent postoperative re-accumulation of clots. If patients have significant brain swelling intraoperatively, postoperative sedation and weaning after repeat CT scanning are advisable.

References

1. Van Asch CJ, Luitse MJ, Rinkel GJ, van der Tweel I, Algra A, Klijn CJ. Incidence, case fatality, and functional outcome of intracerebral haemorrhage over time, according to age, sex, and ethnic origin: a systematic review and meta-analysis. Lancet Neurol. 2010;9:167–76.
2. Siddique SM, Mendelow AD. Surgical treatment of intracerebral haemorrhage. Br Med Bull. 2000;56:444–56.
3. Morgenstern LB, Hemphill JC, Anderson C, et al. Guidelines for the management of spontaneous intracerebral hemorrhage: a guideline for healthcare professionals from the American Heart Association/American Stroke Association. Stroke. 2010;41:2108–29.
4. Hayes SB, Benveniste RJ, Morcos JJ, Aziz-Sultan MA, Elhammady MS. Retrospective comparison of craniotomy and decompressive craniectomy for surgical evacuation of nontraumatic, supratentorial intracerebral hemorrhage. Neurosurg Focus. 2013;34:E3.

25 Intracranial Dural Arteriovenous Fistula: Microneurosurgery Basics and Tricks

Anna Piippo, Mardjono Tjahjadi, and Juha Hernesniemi

25.1 Introduction

Intracranial dural arteriovenous fistulas (DAVFs) are acquired lesions characterized by a region of abnormal arteriovenous fistulous connection within the dura. DAVFs contribute to 10–15% of all AVM intracranially as reported by Newton et al. from 1969 [1]. In common population the probable rates were 0.15–0.29 per 100,000 people per year [2, 3]. Median age of DAVF patients is between 50 and 60 years, but it may present at any age [4, 5].

25.2 Classification

There are several classifications for DAVF, but the most commonly used ones are the simplified Borden classification and the Cognard classification, which is a modification of Djindjian classification [6–8].

25.2.1 Simplified Borden Classification

Lesion type	Definition
I	Drains directly anterograde to major sinus of the vein
II	Drains to sinus of the vein with retrograde drainage back to subarachnoid veins
III	Drains directly to subarachnoid veins (CVD only)

25.2.2 Cognard Classification

Lesion type	Definition
I	Drains to dural venous sinus (DVS) with anterograde flow
IIa	Drains to DVS with retrograde flow
IIb	Drains to DVS with anterograde flow + CVD
IIa + b	Drains to DVS with retrograde flow + CVD
III	Drains directly to subarachnoid veins (CVD only)
IV	Drains directly to subarachnoid veins with ectasia of the draining vein
V	Drains directly into spinal perimedullary veins

A. Piippo · M. Tjahjadi · J. Hernesniemi (✉)
Department of Neurosurgery, Helsinki University Central Hospital, Helsinki, Finland
e-mail: anna.piippo@hus.fi; juha.hernesniemi@hus.fi

J. July, E. J. Wahjoepramono (eds.), *Neurovascular Surgery*,
https://doi.org/10.1007/978-981-10-8950-3_25

25.3 Signs and Symptoms

Clinically, DAVF presentation is determined by their location and pattern of venous outflow. Below are common clinical signs and symptoms in relationship with their location.

DAVFs at transverse-sigmoid sinus	Pulsatile tinnitus
DAVFs at cavernous sinus	Exophthalmos, chemosis, and blindness (Fig. 25.1)
Superior sagittal sinus DAVFs	Hemorrhage, local venous congestion, brain edema, and ischemia
DAVFs with perimedullary draining vein	Myelopathy and progressive tetraplegia

25.4 Investigation

25.4.1 DSA

Digital subtraction angiography (DSA) is still the best way to show DAVF. DSA accurately illustrates the flow dynamic of the fistula and the cerebral circulation of the brain. This information is critical both for the surgical planning and for the evaluation of the treatment (Fig. 25.2).

25.4.2 MRA (Magnetic Resonance Angiography) (Fig. 25.3)

In case of Borden type 1 DAVFs without CVD, MRI is usually normal. It may show vein dilatation, venous occlusion, or, after contrast enhancement, increased vascularity around the involved sinus. Venous congestion may be seen on MRI T2 as a signal changes to hyperintensity that diffusely involves the cortex in DAVFs with CVD, either at the cerebrum or cerebellum. Time-of-flight MRI (TOF MRI) now is widely available and usually the primary screening tool when the DAVF is suspected [9–11]. With time-resolved imaging of contrast kinetics (TRICKS) technique introduced

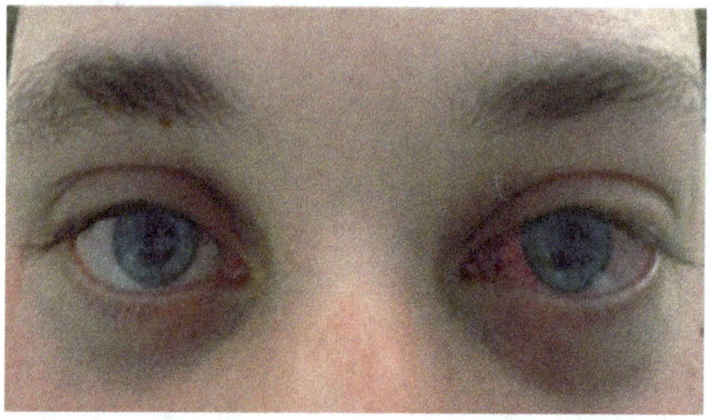

Fig. 25.1 Slight chemosis and exophthalmos of the left eye in a patient with left cavernous sinus DAVF

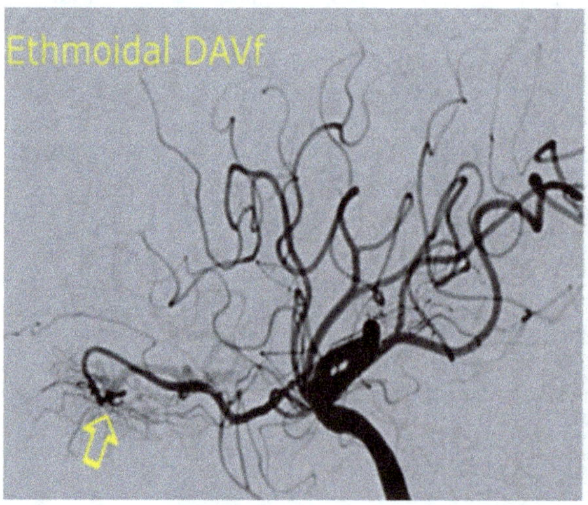

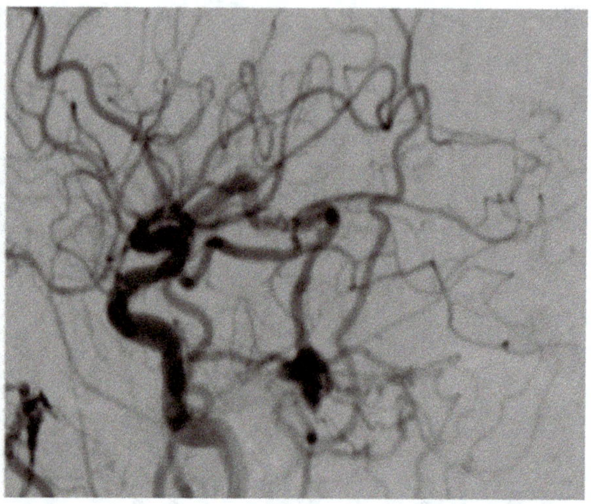

Fig. 25.2 *Left*: The DSA of the ethmoidal DAVF showing the fistula connection Borden type III fed by ophthalmic artery and drained through the cortical veins. *Right*: Tentorial DAVF Borden type III fed by meningohypophyseal branch and drained through the cortical veins

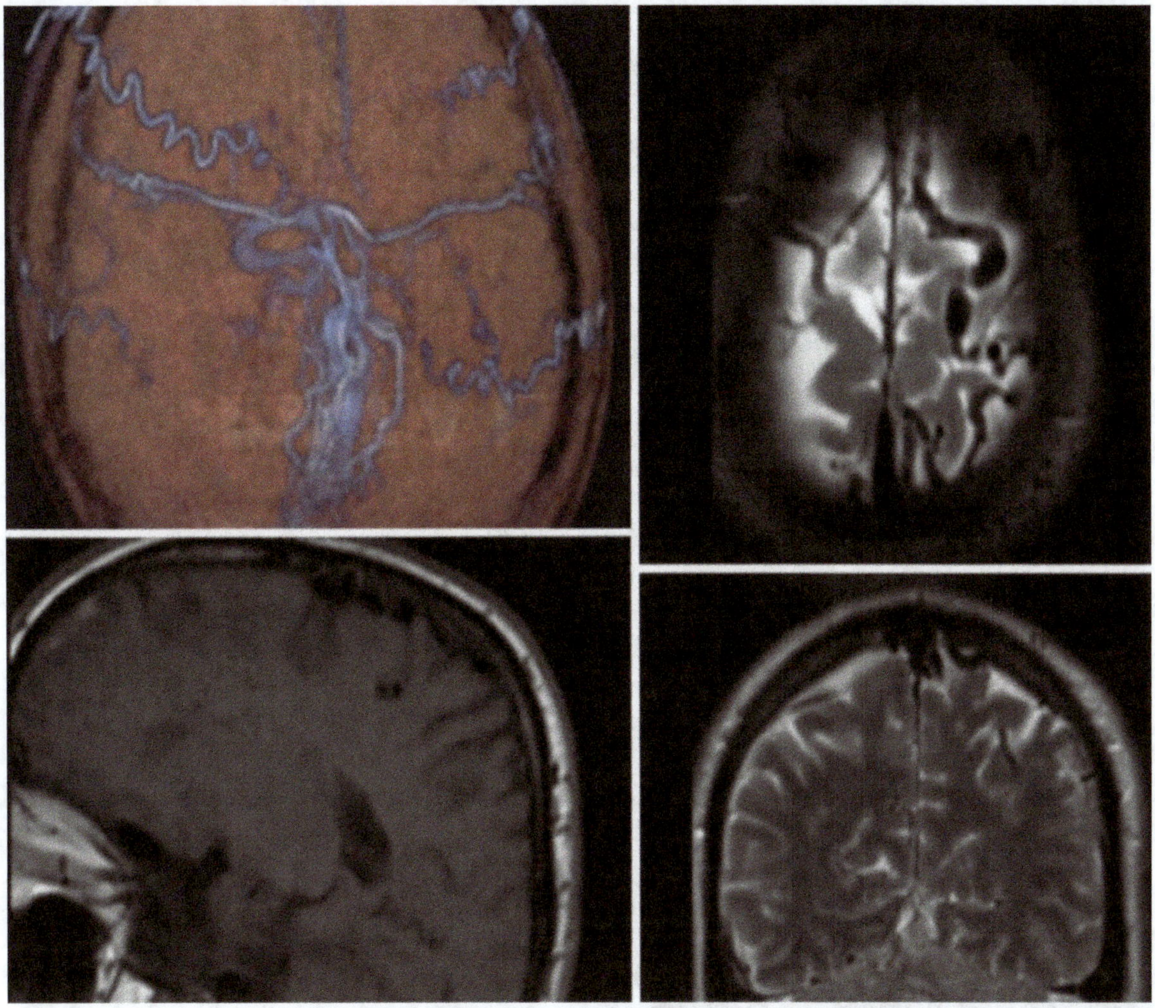

Fig. 25.3 MRA shows a superior sagittal sinus DAVF Borden type II fed by the meningeal arteries and drained through the superior sagittal sinus with retrograde flow to the cortical veins

in 1996 [12], arterial and venous phases of contrast passage through the brain can be separated, showing the flow dynamics of the DAVFs. TRICKS has a better sensitivity over TOF MRA to detect DAVFs and a useful noninvasive imaging method during the treatment and follow-up [13, 14]. TRICKS has less accurate spatial resolution than DSA, and therefore DSA is still needed for studying the detailed anatomy of DAVFs.

25.4.3 CTA (Computed Tomography Angiography)

Computed tomography is the primary method for ruptured DAVFs showing intracerebral hemorrhage (ICH), sometimes subdural hemorrhages (SDH), subarachnoid hemorrhages, or intraventricular hemorrhages (IVH). CT and CTA can show abnormal vessels, venous ectasia, and pouches related to the DAVFs, but the drawback is its lack of temporal solution [15]. Dynamic CTA can show pathologic flow dynamics in intracranial vessels indicating the presence of DAVFs [16].

25.5 Preoperative Preparation

Careful analysis of the angiographic images and angioarchitecture of DAVF when planning the surgery is crucial for achieving complete eradication of the fistula, preserving normal vasculature and avoiding pitfalls of the surgery. Preoperative embolization of the DAVF can reduce the bleeding during operation. Bleeding can also be reduced by sustaining moderate hypotension (systolic blood pressure around 100 mmHg) during the operation.

25.6 Approach and Step of Surgery

25.6.1 Transverse and Sigmoid Sinus DAVFs

It could be approached through lateral suboccipital approach. Patient is set up with park-bench position and the head is higher than the heart level. The head is tilted laterally to the opposite side, and the shoulder is retracted caudally with tape to achieve a correct trajectory of the approach.

25.6.1.1 Steps of Surgery

- A curved incision or the shape of question mark incision is placed about 1 in. behind the mastoid process (Fig. 25.4).

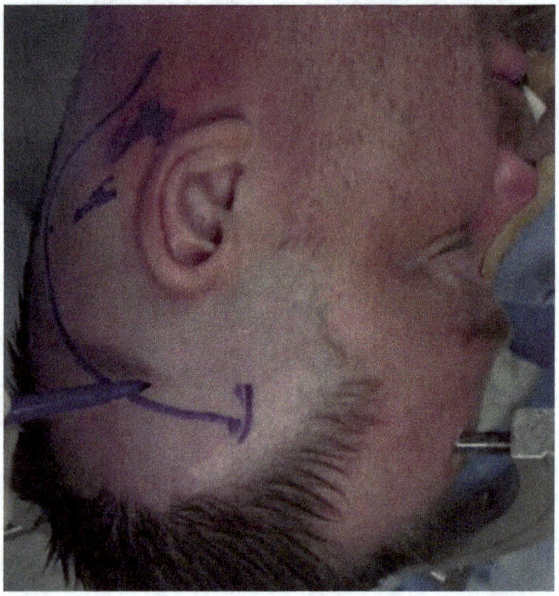

Fig. 25.4 Large question mark skin marking for lateral suboccipital approach to treat the transverse-sigmoid sinus DAVF

- Any bleeding from the skin should be cautiously coagulated to prevent a later excessive bleeding.
- Several burr holes (three to four) are placed, and a large suboccipital bone flap is removed by cutting the medial part with craniotome, and the lateral margin by drilling off the bone.
- Lateral margin of the opening is further drilled away as far as laterally as possible to achieve a good visibility and control around the sigmoid sinus.
- If we get into the mastoid air cells, they have to be meticulously sealed with fat or muscle graft, and then add the fibrin glue to avoid CSF leak.

25.6.1.2 Occlusion of the Fistula

- If the venous sinus is open and it serves as a main venous drainage, the feeding arteries are coagulated and cut.
- In case the sinus is occluded or nonfunctional, or we find a retrograde flow into the veins at the cortex, then it may be removed.
- The medial part of the sinus is ligated first. Then using the lateral part of the sinus is resected, and the remaining part of the proximal sinus is filled using oxidized cellulose (Surgicel®) or another option is using muscle then ligated.
- The vein of Labbé should be preserved to prevent venous infarction.

25.6.2 Middle Fossa and Cavernous Sinus DAVFs

It could be approached through lateral supraorbital (LSO) approach. Position of the patient is supine, and the head is higher than the heart level, rotated 30° to contralateral side and tilted slightly (Fig. 25.5).

25.6.2.1 Steps of Surgery

- One-layer frontotemporal skin and muscle flap is made extending about an inch above the zygomatic arch (Fig. 25.6).

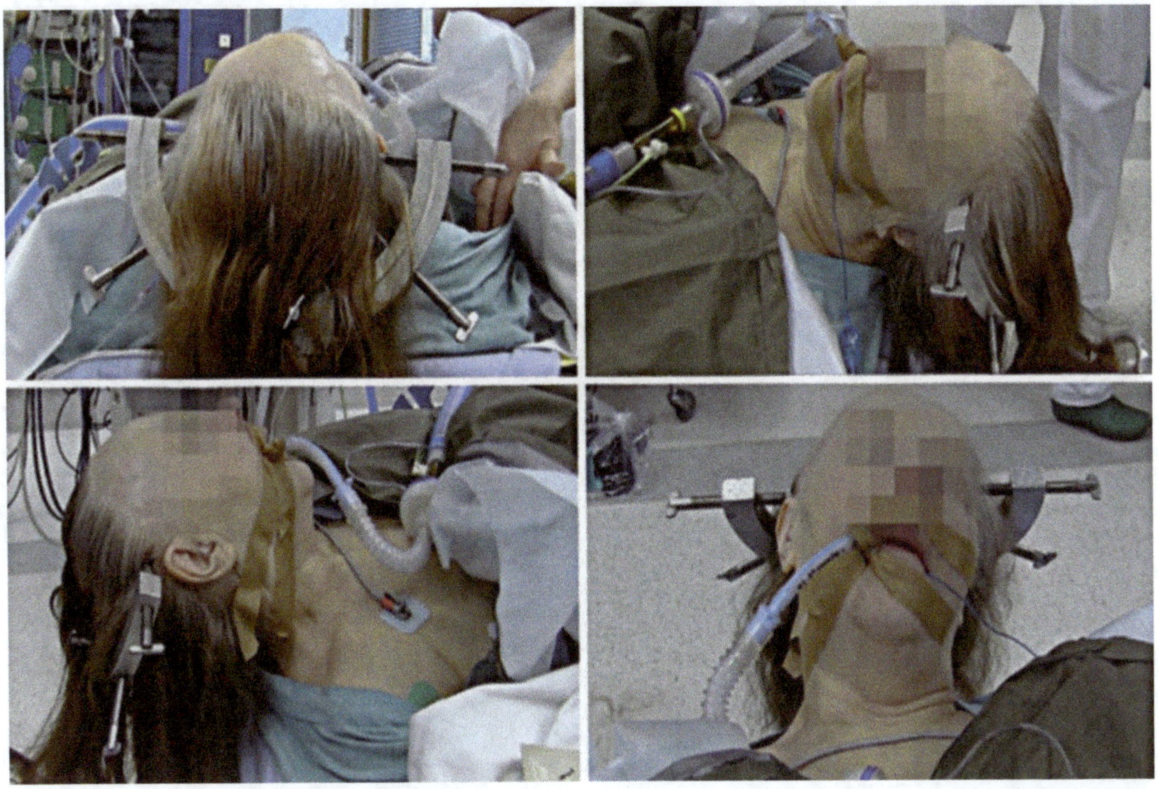

Fig. 25.5 Positioning of the right LSO approach. The LSO approach is usually used to operate on cavernous sinus DAVF and sometimes for the ethmoidal/frontobasal DAVF

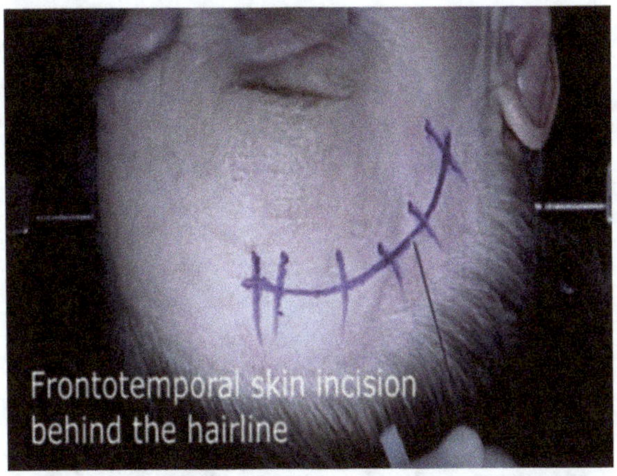

Fig. 25.6 Frontotemporal skin incision for LSO approach is done behind the hairline

- One burr hole is made on the superior insertion of the temporalis muscle and a small bone flap 3 × 5 cm is elevated.
- Sphenoid ridge at its lateral part should be drilled with a diamond high-speed drill.
- The medial part of sphenoid ridge including anterior clinoid process is removed with Sonopet drill.

25.6.2.2 Occlusion of the Fistula (Fig. 25.7)

- After exposing the wall of the cavernous sinus, it is opened with a very small incision.
- From this opening, fibrin glue is injected with blunt needle, and a pack of Surgicel® is applied on top of it.
- Then do another one repetitively at multiple places of cavernous sinus wall, and keep doing the same thing until we occlude all the fistulas.
- While doing the injections, it is important to make sure and keep the carotid artery flow adequately.

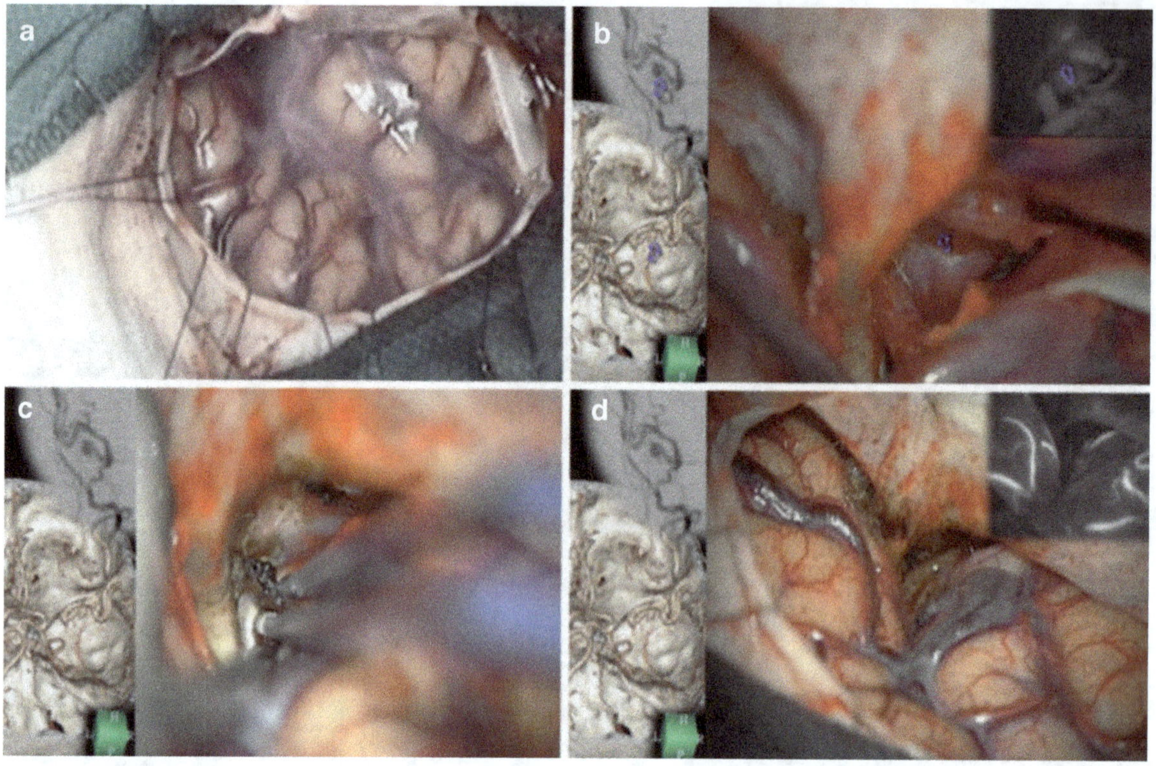

Fig. 25.7 *Steps of surgery*. (**a**) Exposure after the dura opening. (**b**) Confirmation of the draining veins. (**c**) Coagulation of the draining veins and disconnection of the fistula. (**d**) ICG-VA confirmed the disconnection of DAVF

- If the fistula does not involve the cavernous sinus, then identification of the draining veins should be done with the guidance of ICG-VA.
- Coagulation and disconnection of the draining veins should be performed cautiously to avoid the injury of the normal draining veins.
- To verify the occlusion of the fistula and the patency of the carotid artery, intraoperative indocyanine green video angiography (ICG-VA) or conventional angiography is performed.

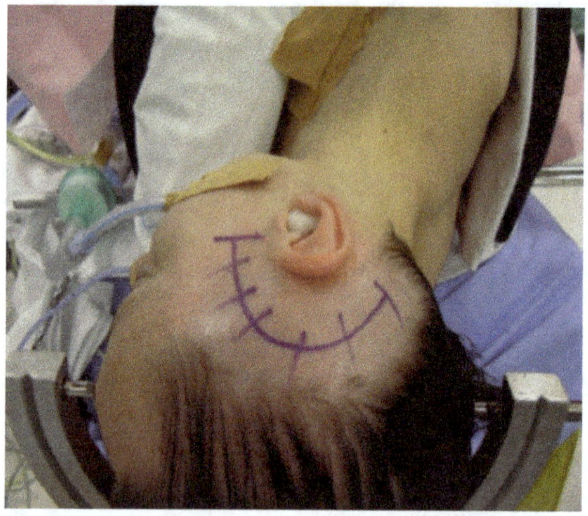

Fig. 25.8 The position and skin incision marking for subtemporal approach

25.6.3 Tentorial DAVFs

It could be approached through subtemporal approach. Position of the patient is following park-bench position.

25.6.3.1 Steps of Surgery

- A small horseshoe-like incision from above the zygomatic arch curving posteriorly just above the ear lobe is placed (Fig. 25.8).
- Two burr holes are placed, one close to the origin of zygomatic arch, where the dura is often tightly attached to the bone, and another at the cranial border, to elevate a small bone flap.
- The temporobasal bone is drilled until the origin of the floor of the middle fossa to widen the bone opening.
- Cut the dura at its base caudally to expose subtemporal space.

- Tentorial edge is then quickly reached and cisterns opened to relax the brain with minimal retraction of the temporal lobe.
- The temporal lobe is elevated gradually starting anteriorly from the temporal pole and moving posteriorly.
- The retraction should be increased gradually. Finally, a rather wide retractor is placed to retain space.

25.6.3.2 Occlusion of the Fistula

- To get a better visualization to the fistulous site, the tentorial edge is cut at posterior to the insertion of trochlear nerve and then lifted upward using small Aesculap® clip.
- The feeding arteries along the dura are coagulated and cut.
- The occlusion of the fistula can be verified by using intraoperative ICG-VA or DSA.

25.6.4 Frontobasal DAVFs

It could be approached through anterior interhemispheric approach. The patient is seated in a semi-sitting position.

25.6.4.1 Steps of Surgery

- A linear incision is placed behind the hairline.
- Make two burr holes at midline over SSS.
- Bone flap is cut with a craniotome extending both sides of the sinus.

25.6.4.2 Occlusion of the Fistula

- Frontobasal DAVFs often have feeding arteries from both sides.
- The falx is coagulated and divided close to crista galli to reach the feeders from the contralateral side.
- Feeding arteries within dura and draining cortical veins are coagulated and cut from both sides of the falx.

25.6.5 Superior Sagittal Sinus DAVFs

It could be approached through midline approach. Position of the patient is semi-sitting or we also may do it with supine position.

25.6.5.1 Steps of Surgery

- A linear incision is placed behind the hairline.
- Making two burr holes at midline over SSS.
- Bone flap is cut with a craniotome extending both sides of the sinus.
- If the frontal sinus opens during approach for frontobasal DAVFs, the endonasal mucosa is stripped of and the sinus is packed with fat and covered with pericranium and fibrin glue.

25.6.5.2 Occlusion of the Fistula (Fig. 25.9)

- Superior sagittal sinus DAVFs also often have feeding arteries from both sides.
- Feeding arteries within dura and draining cortical veins are coagulated and cut from both sides of the SSS.
- Tack-up sutures are used to lift the dura and prevent excessive bleeding and formation of epidural hematoma.
- Preserving SSS is extremely important in the lesions of the posterior part of the SSS because it serves as the major route for venous outflow of the cerebral hemispheres.
- If the DAVF is located in anterior third of SSS, this part of sinus can be resected.
- Dura is left open to prevent recurrence of the fistulous connections.

25.7 Expert Opinion/Suggestion to Avoid Complication

- Microsurgery is the first-line treatment in tentorial or frontobasal DAVFs. Others should primarily be treated by endovascular and/or radiosurgical means. Microsurgery is also recommended if the endovascular and/or radiological effort could not achieve total occlusion, and the patient presents with intolerable symptoms or CVD is still present.
- The most dangerous complications of DAVF treatment, whether it was microsurgical or endovascular, are severe brain swelling and hemorrhagic infarction due to sudden occlusion of the DAVF.
- The best way to avoid these complications is to carefully study the angioarchitecture and flow dynamics of the DAVF before treatment.

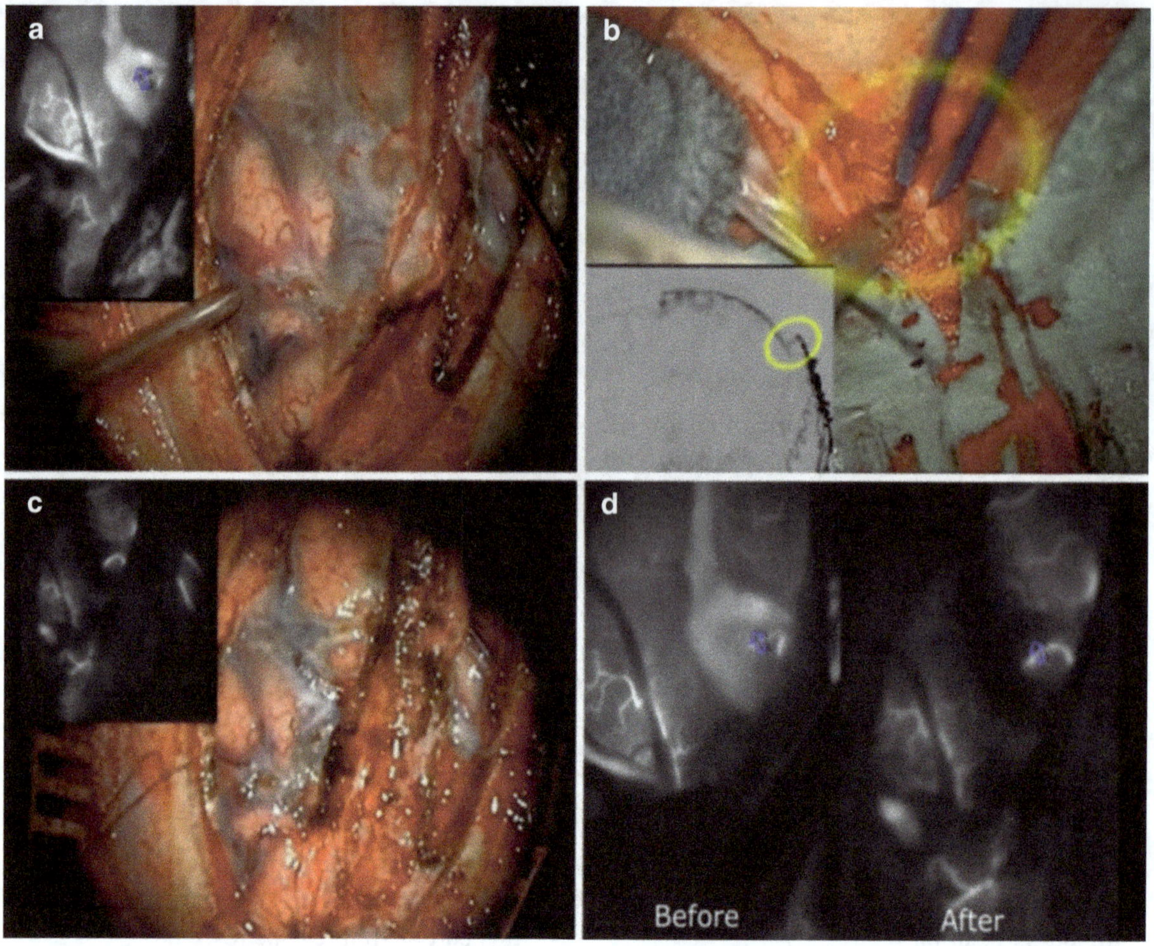

Fig. 25.9 *Steps of surgery*. (**a**) Exposure after the dura opening reveals an early venous filling. (**b**) Coagulation of the feeder arteries from dura mater which was shown from the preoperative DSA. (**c**) Condition after the feeding arteries coagulation. IVG-VA showed no early venous filling anymore. (**d**) Comparison of ICG-VA before and after feeding artery coagulation

- Identification and preservation of the vein of Labbé during the microsurgery of transverse and sigmoid sinus DAVF are crucial.
- Heavy arterial bleeding from the enlarged extracranial feeding arteries with high flow through the bone into the fistula can make the microsurgery a great challenge already from the skin incision.
- To prevent the highly vascularized DAVFs from bleeding extensively, hemostasis should be done carefully in every phase of the surgery using a high-power bipolar coagulation.
- To achieve a good control of all the fistulous connections, large craniotomies with three to four burr holes are used to expose the lesion.
- The bleeding from the bone margins is managed by the heat produced by drilling the bone with a large diamond drill without irrigation ("hot drilling").
- Using operative microscope from the early stages of the surgery is crucial to visualize and control the bleeding.
- In of case heavy bleeding during surgery from the affected sinus, then we may use Surgicel®, fibrin glue, and muscle are packed over the sinus.
- A slight hypotension (systolic pressure 100 mmHg) is recommended during the surgery and 1–2 days after it to prevent postoperative hematomas.

25.8 Verification of Complete Occlusion

25.8.1 Intraoperative Imaging

- Indocyanine green (ICG) angiography is a helpful tool for intraoperative imaging in DAVF cases.
- The fistulous site can be detected during the opening, and the occlusion of the fistula can be verified intraoperatively.

25.8.2 Postoperative Imaging

- The primary method for verification of DAVF occlusion postoperatively is DSA, because all the small feeding arteries may not show in ICG-VA or CTA.
- Later during follow-up, MRA and/or TRICKS is used to verify the occlusion of the fistula.

25.9 Complications of Microsurgery

In our series, the complications were: [4]

- Severe bleeding more than 1000 ml occurred in 10 (8.6%).
- Ischemic complication. Seventeen (15%) patients had postoperative infarction.
- Hemorrhagic complications. Three (2.6%) patients developed intracerebral hemorrhages (ICH) that were observed, and two (1.7%) patients developed epidural hematomas necessitating evacuation.
- Other complications include postoperative septicemia, urinary tract infection, pneumonia, postoperative meningitis despite routine prophylactic antibiotics, wound infection, pulmonary embolism, cardiac infarction, gastrointestinal bleeding, and deep venous thrombosis.

25.9.1 Neuro-fuctioning ourcome

The length of follow-up is up to 15.9 years, with a median of 3.2 years. There are 103 patient's data available for this follow-up. The Glasgow Outcome Scale at 3 months shows 98 (84%) patients had GOS 4–5, 2 (1.7%) were severely disabled, and 3 (2.6%) died.

References

1. Newton TH, Cronqvist S. Involvement of dural arteries in intracranial arteriovenous malformations. Radiology. 1969;93(5):1071–8.
2. Al-Shahi R, et al. Prospective, population-based detection of intracranial vascular malformations in adults: the Scottish Intracranial Vascular Malformation Study (SIVMS). Stroke. 2003;34(5):1163–9.
3. Satomi J, Satoh K. Epidemiology and etiology of dural arteriovenous fistula. Brain Nerve. 2008;60(8):883–6.
4. Piippo A, et al. Characteristics and long-term outcome of 251 patients with dural arteriovenous fistulas in a defined population. J Neurosurg. 2013;118(5):923–34.
5. Piippo A, et al. Early and long-term excess mortality in 227 patients with intracranial dural arteriovenous fistulas. J Neurosurg. 2013;119(1):164–71.
6. Borden JA, Wu JK, Shucart WA. A proposed classification for spinal and cranial dural arteriovenous fistulous malformations and implications for treatment. J Neurosurg. 1995;82(2):166–79.
7. Cognard C, et al. Cerebral dural arteriovenous fistulas: clinical and angiographic correlation with a revised classification of venous drainage. Radiology. 1995;194(3):671–80.
8. Davies MA, et al. The validity of classification for the clinical presentation of intracranial dural arteriovenous fistulas. J Neurosurg. 1996;85(5):830–7.
9. Chen JC, Tsuruda JS, Halbach VV. Suspected dural arteriovenous fistula: results with screening MR angiography in seven patients. Radiology. 1992;183(1):265–71.
10. Kitajima M, et al. Retrograde cortical and deep venous drainage in patients with intracranial dural arteriovenous fistulas: comparison of MR imaging and angiographic findings. AJNR Am J Neuroradiol. 2005;26(6):1532–8.
11. van Vaals JJ, et al. "Keyhole" method for accelerating imaging of contrast agent uptake. J Magn Reson Imaging. 1993;3(4):671–5.
12. Korosec FR, et al. Time-resolved contrast-enhanced 3D MR angiography. Magn Reson Med. 1996;36(3):345–51.

13. Pekkola J, Kangasniemi M. Posterior fossa dural arteriovenous fistulas: diagnosis and follow-up with time-resolved imaging of contrast kinetics (TRICKS) at 1.5T. Acta Radiol. 2011;52(4):442–7.
14. Pollock BE, et al. Magnetic resonance imaging: an accurate method to evaluate arteriovenous malformations after stereotactic radiosurgery. J Neurosurg. 1996;85(6):1044–9.
15. Narvid J, et al. CT angiography as a screening tool for dural arteriovenous fistula in patients with pulsatile tinnitus: feasibility and test characteristics. AJNR Am J Neuroradiol. 2011;32(3):446–53.
16. Pekkola J, Kangasniemi M. Imaging of blood flow in cerebral arteries with dynamic helical computed tomography angiography (DHCTA) using a 64-row CT scanner. Acta Radiol. 2009;50(7):798–805.

Part III

The Miscellaneous Chapter

26 Moyamoya Disease, Basic Concepts of Diagnostics, and Treatment

Dilshod Mamadaliev, Alberto Feletti, Tushit Mewada, Kei Yamashiro, Yasuhiro Yamada, Tsukasa Kawase, and Yoko Kato

26.1 Introduction

Moyamoya disease (MMD) is a rare condition where the supraclinoid part of internal carotid artery is slowly and progressively becoming stenotic, and also it often involves both middle cerebral arteries and anterior cerebral arteries (Fig. 26.1) [1]. The term moyamoya means *a puff of smoke* in Japanese, and it was first reported by Takeuchi and Shimizu in 1957 with Japanese language [2].

Its etiology still remains unknown. The *moyamoya syndrome* (MMS) has similar clinical and angiographic characteristics to MMD but might be associated with Down's syndrome, neurofibromatosis type 1 (NF-1), prior irradiation, and sickle-cell disease.

Although MMD was initially found in Asian patients, it has been increasingly reported in patients of all demographic groups; the exact incidence is not completely known [3].

Japanese studies report an annual incidence between 0.35 and 0.94/100,000 persons per year and annual prevalence between 3.16 and 10.5 per 100,000 persons [4–6]. Female has twice the number compare with male [4, 5].

26.2 Signs and Symptoms

There is a classification that is supported by the Ministry of Health and Welfare of Japan, which classified the moyamoya diseases (MMD) based on its presentation in to four: ischemic, hemorrhagic, epileptic, and "other." In children, it is more common to see the ischemic type, while in the adult it is more common to see they present with hemorrhage. It is reported that

D. Mamadaliev
Department of Neurosurgery, Fujita Health University, Banbuntane Hotokukai Hospital, Nagoya city, Aichi, Japan

Republican Scientific Center of Neurosurgery, Tashkent, Uzbekistan

A. Feletti
Department of Neurosurgery, Fujita Health University, Banbuntane Hotokukai Hospital, Nagoya city, Aichi, Japan

Department of Neurosurgery, NOCSAE Modena Hospital, Modena, Italy

T. Mewada
Department of Neurosurgery, Fujita Health University, Banbuntane Hotokukai Hospital, Nagoya city, Aichi, Japan

G. B. Pant Institute of Post Graduate Medical Education and Research, New Delhi, India

K. Yamashiro · Y. Yamada · T. Kawase
Department of Neurosurgery, Fujita Health University, Banbuntane Hotokukai Hospital, Nagoya city, Aichi, Japan
e-mail: kawasemi@hm8.aitai.ne.jp

Y. Kato (✉)
Department of Neurosurgery, Fujita Health University, Toyoake, Aichi, Japan
e-mail: kyoko@fujita-hu.ac.jp

J. July, E. J. Wahjoepramono (eds.), *Neurovascular Surgery*,
https://doi.org/10.1007/978-981-10-8950-3_26

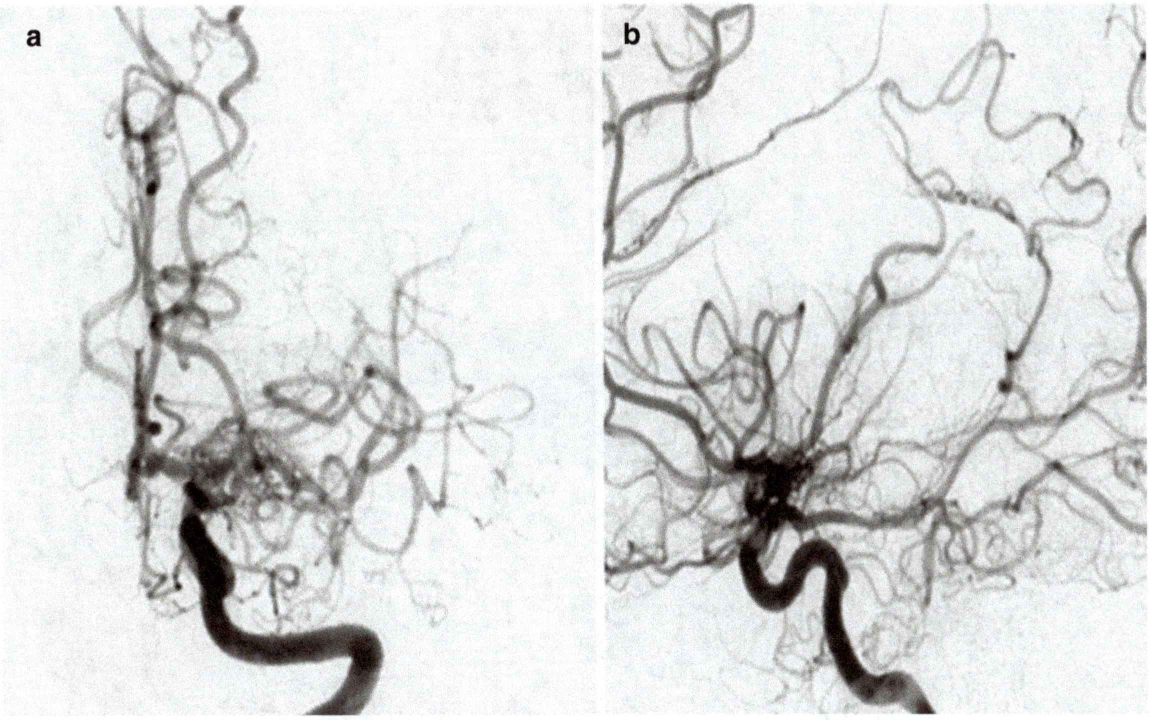

Fig. 26.1 Left ICA anterior-posterior and lateral injections demonstrating supraclinoid internal carotid artery stenosis and M1 occlusion with resultant moyamoya vessels

the hemorrhage presentation of MMD is approximately seven times higher in adult patients (14.6%) if we compare with the pediatric group (2.1%) [7]. Occasionally patients may also present with seizure, headaches, or behavioral changes. Some studies suggest a relation between headaches and hypoperfusion leading to cortical depression and associated migraine symptoms [8]. Others have suggested that dilation of dural and meningeal vessels irritate the pain fibers on the dura, resulting in a migraine-like headache that is refractive to medical therapies [9]. This headache initially persisted in 63% of patients even after cerebral revascularization, although it would often improve over time. Based on angiographic studies, the typical course of disease can be classified into six stages. The first description was written by Suzuki and Takaku (1969). They describe it in six stages. *Stage I*: on the early stage, it is started with the narrowing of carotid bifurcation at the neck and also the ICA bifurcation. *Stage II*: it is also called moyamoya initiation, which is characterized by dilated ACA, MCA, and further narrowing of ICA bifurcation. *Stage III*: this stage is called moyamoya intensification; the ICA bifurcation is much narrower, and ACA and MCA now become narrow as well. *Stage IV*: this stage is called moyamoya minimization; the occlusive changes in ICA and tenuous ACA and MCA happened slowly. *Stage V*: This stage is called moyamoya reduction; the occlusion of ICA, ACA, and MCA becomes very severe. *Stage VI*: this stage is called moyamoya disappearance; the ICA is totally occluded, and the brain tries to get supplied from ECA.

On histopathologic examination, the internal carotid artery wall shows eccentric fibrocellular thickening of the intimal layer, and the smooth muscle cells proliferate too much. The ICA becomes tortuous, and frequently we will find the duplication of internal elastic lamina, and it does not show any inflammatory reaction or any atheromatous forming, resulting in artery stenosis/occlusion [10]. The hypoxia induces supply from other parts to form collateral flow, and the arteries become tortuous and dilated (Fig. 26.2). These "moyamoya" vessels have many fibrin deposits at its wall, but the media layer is thin, the elastic lamina becomes fragmented, and so there

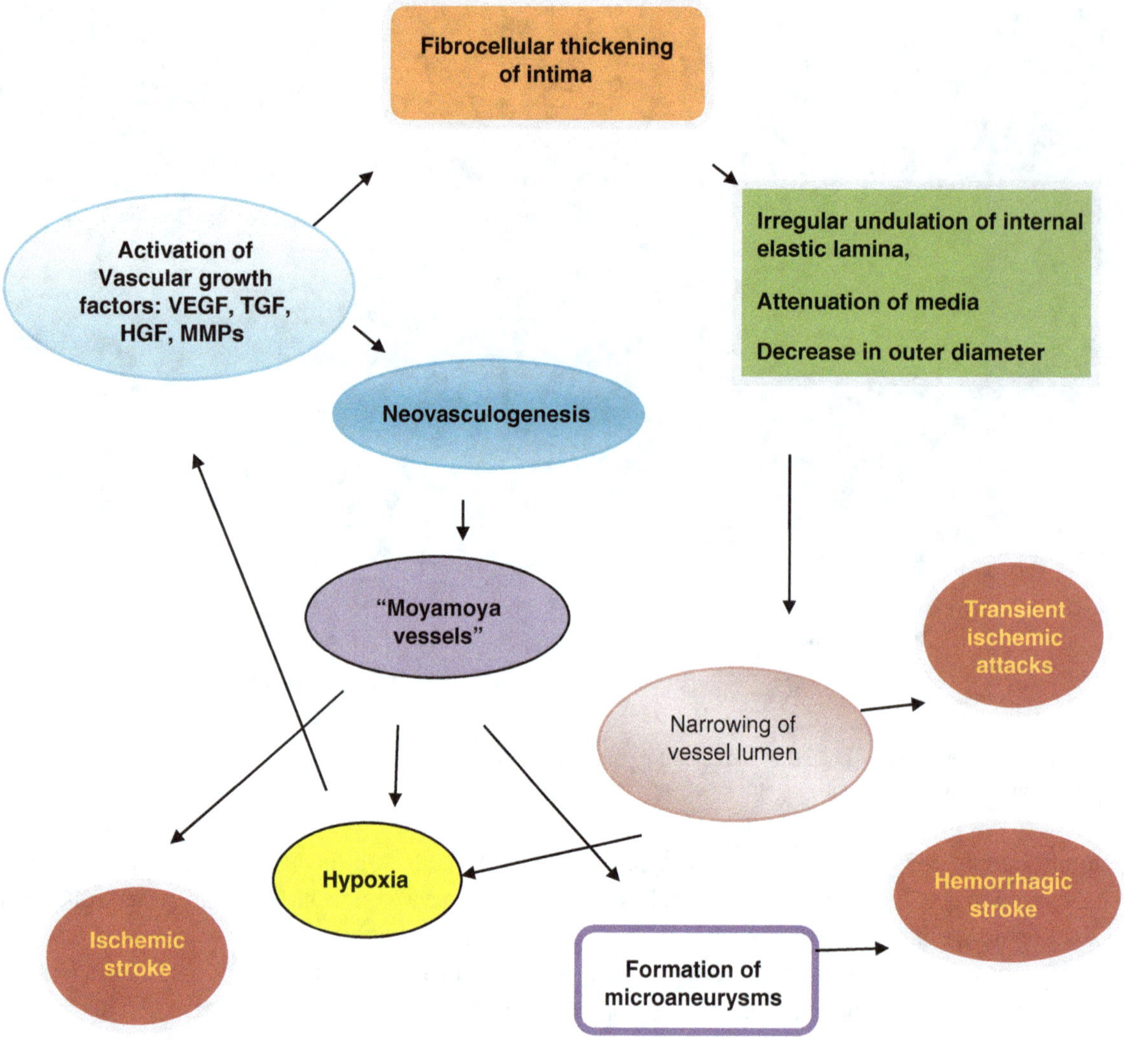

Fig. 26.2 Pathophysiology of moyamoya disease

is a high chance to have microaneurysm formation. It has been reported that the aneurysm formation might be associated with over-expression of several growth factors such as matrix metalloproteinases (MMPs), hypoxia-inducible factor 1 (HIF-1), vascular endothelial growth factor (VEGF), basic fibroblast growth factor (bFGF), transforming growth factor-beta (TGF-beta), and hepatocyte growth factor (HGF) [10]. It is also reported that autosomal dominant inheritance may play a role up to 15% of MMD patients, and some genome are widely studied from the family who carry the inheritance of MMD. The result shows some association with certain chromosomal regions including 3p24.2-p26 [11], 6q25 [12], 8q23 [13], 12p12 [13], and 17q25 [14].

26.3 Natural History and Prognosis

The disease inevitably progresses if left untreated. In a patient whose both side vessels are narrowing, the risk of stroke after 5 years is up to 82% [15]. The National Register of all asymptomatic moyamoya in Japan finds that 3.2% of them will get stroke even if they were treated medically [16]. On the other hand, the stroke or death rate prior, during, and after the surgical revascularization is something between 5.5% [7] and 17% [15] over 5 years, and this results in demonstrating that the surgery may offer a benefit to the patients.

26.4 Investigation

The diagnoses of MMD or MMS should be considered in any patient, especially in a child or young adult who presents with neurologic deficits or symptoms secondary to cerebral ischemia or hemorrhage. Radiologic evaluation may include CT; MRI; cerebral angiography and cerebral perfusion studies, including CT perfusion, xenon-enhanced CT, or PET; MR perfusion; and SPECT or CT imaging without and with acetazolamide challenge. Cerebral angiography, CT angiography, and MR angiography imaging can reveal intracerebral vascular occlusion along with the resulting moyamoya vessels. CT and MRI can reveal hemorrhage or ischemic changes.

26.5 Approach and Steps of Surgery

Currently we still do not have a good randomized study that compares medical treatment versus surgical revascularization for patients with MMD, but in good hand surgeon, they claim that the stroke rate is significantly reduced in surgically treated group. As discussed in the previous section, the natural history of these patients is to progress, and the risk of recurrent stroke is extremely high with medical management only. The main medical treatment option for these patients is antiplatelet therapy. All patients are on aspirin pre- and postoperatively. Full anticoagulation drugs such as warfarin are rarely used.

One of the obvious indications to recommend surgery for moyamoya patients is multiple episodes of TIA (transient ischemic attack), RIND (reversible ischemic neurological deficit), or even stroke. The purpose of the surgery is to prevent the next episode by reestablishing adequate blood supply to the affected cortex. There are two ways to reestablish the blood supply to the brain. Adult and older children may have **direct bypass** surgery to revascularize the brain vessels, and the children under 10 years old may have **indirect bypass surgery** because their vessels are very tiny and tend to fail if we do direct bypass.

26.5.1 Bypass Surgery of the Brain

Bypass surgery of the brain is a revascularization either between extracranial vessel and intracranial vessel or between intracranial vessel and another intracranial vessel by using graft (saphenous vein, radial artery, etc.) The purpose of the bypass is to reestablish another route or reroute blood flow from the narrowed, blocked, or damaged vessel and supply the distal part of the artery. It is very common to just use the natural provided artery such as from the STA (superficial temporal artery) and directly bypass it to the MCA (middle cerebral artery). Just after the bypass, it may show an instant upgrading blood flow to the distal part of the narrowed artery. Certain people may have a very tiny superficial temporal artery, and we might think the size is not big enough to provide long-term support, and then saphenous vein or radial artery may be harvested to make an anastomosis from the extracranial carotid artery to the distal part of the narrowed vessel. The surgeon will look at the angiogram or nowadays the CT angiogram to decide and plan the surgery.

26.5.2 EDAS (Encephaloduroarteriosynangiosis)

EDAS (encephaloduroarteriosynangiosis) surgery is considered as an indirect way of establishing new vascularization in the brain. It is using the superficial temporal artery that was dissected from the surrounding soft tissue and is placed in direct contact with the cortical surface. The artery should not be kinking at its entry point to the cortical surface and at its distal part where it is going back to supply the scalp. Some fine suture should be placed to hold the artery on the cortical surface. The bone flap is repositioned and secured with miniplate and screw, but the entry and exit of the STA have to make sure there is no pressure at all. Over a period, we expect some new vessel forming to supply the brain. It is important to remember that the STA is always kept intact, so it will give branches to the brain.

26.5.3 EMS (Encephalo-Myo-Synangiosis)

EMS (encephalo-myo-synangiosis) surgery is also considered as indirect way of establishing new vascularization by using temporalis muscle as the source of the angiogenesis to the brain. The muscle is gently dissected, and through the opening of the bone at the temporal base, the muscle is laid on top of the cortical surface. It is very important to have a meticulous bleeding control to avoid postoperative blood accumulation, but be careful not to coagulate too much of the temporal muscle because we don't want to make the muscle de-vascularized. Closing the dura with the muscle underneath it is sometimes challenging, but surgeons need to do the closing meticulously. The muscle is a very good source of blood supply to the brain, and they may spread angiogenesis all over the brain.

26.5.4 EDAMS (Encephalo-Duro-Arterio-Myo-Synangiosis)

EDAMS (encephalo-duro-arterio-myo-synangiosis) surgery is a combination EDAS and EMS at the same time.

26.5.5 Omental Transposition Surgery

Omental transposition surgery is also another option for indirect way to establish revascularization in the brain by using omentum from the abdomen. The omentum is a special fat tissue that surrounds abdominal organs, and it spreads very fast to any part of the abdomen that needs support. It has rich blood supply. When it is placed on the surface of the cerebral cortex, it is expected that it will grow and spread very fast to supply the brain and improve the blood supply.

26.5.6 Multiple Burr Holes

Another option of indirect revascularization of the cortex is by doing multiple burr holes all over the skull and expecting that the scalp vessel will go through the burr hole and provide vascular supply to the cortex.

Patients with MMD although have occlusion of the internal carotid arteries, but usually the external carotid artery is patent. Surgical effort uses the external carotid artery to supply blood to ischemic cortex by either creating a direct or indirect revascularization bypass. A direct bypass usually require adequate superficial temporal artery (STA) at the ipsilateral side and then anastomosed directly to a distal M4 segment of middle cerebral artery (MCA). The indirect revascularization is performed by using a vascularized tissue that is also supplied by external carotid artery, including the dura, temporalis muscle, the STA itself, and even pericranium. The vascularized tissue is laid on the cortical surface and expect the new blood vessel will be formed and ingrowth toward the cortex. There is no good randomized study that compares the direct and indirect revascularization in terms of their safety and efficacy. The literature review also failed to reveal a difference in surgical morbidity or stroke rate (perioperative or long term) between the direct and indirect methods. Many institutions will perform direct revascularization for adults and indirect revascularization for children because of the smaller and more friable caliber of the vessels in children. However, there are many groups that perform indirect bypass for adult patients as well [15, 16]. According to Gordon Li et al., they recommend to perform direct bypass on all patients whenever possible, unless the STA or MCA is too small or friable. Direct revascularization surgery may provide an immediate increase in cortical blood flow and treat the ischemic cortex immediately. In the case with bilateral MMD, it is obvious to treat the symptomatic side first. If they are both asymptomatic, it is better to treat and revascularize the non-dominant hemisphere first because of higher incidence of transient neurologic symptoms following the surgery on dominant cortex.

The second surgery for the contralateral side is generally 1–4 weeks after the first surgery, unless there were significant complications after the first procedure.

26.5.7 Direct Revascularization

Prior to the surgery, it is important to assess the size of frontal and parietal branch of STA by using CT angiography or conventional angiography. The larger diameter branch is chosen as the donor vessel. The patient is positioned supine and the head is hold with head holder. The head is elevated above the heart and turned to the side, bringing the frontotemporal region uppermost in the field. Stimulating and recording electrodes are placed for monitoring of bilateral somatosensory evoked potentials (SSEP) and bilateral EEG. Cooling to approximately 33 °C is accomplished by either using cooling blanket and bladder irrigation or by putting IV catheter (InnerCool Therapies Philips, Andover, MA) into the inferior vena cava. In general, the InnerCool catheter is placed in the larger patients who are more difficult to cool and rewarm via surface techniques.

The course of the superficial temporal artery is plotted by using a Doppler probe. When parietal branch of STA is chosen as donor, the skin incision is planned over the artery along its course (Fig. 26.3). If the frontal branch is the donor, the inferior portion of the incision follows the STA, but as the artery tracks anterior to the hairline, the incision stays posterior behind the hairline for cosmetic purposes. After shaving the hair over the planned incision, prepare and drape the surgical area. The operating microscope is positioned and used for careful harvesting of the STA. A length of approximately 7 cm of STA together with a generous cuff of soft tissue to protect it is needed for the bypass (Fig. 26.4). Then the underlying temporalis fascia muscle is split and dissected from the frontotemporal bone. Burr holes are placed, the craniotomy bone flap is removed at frontotemporal area, and the dura is cut in a cruciate manner (Fig. 26.5).

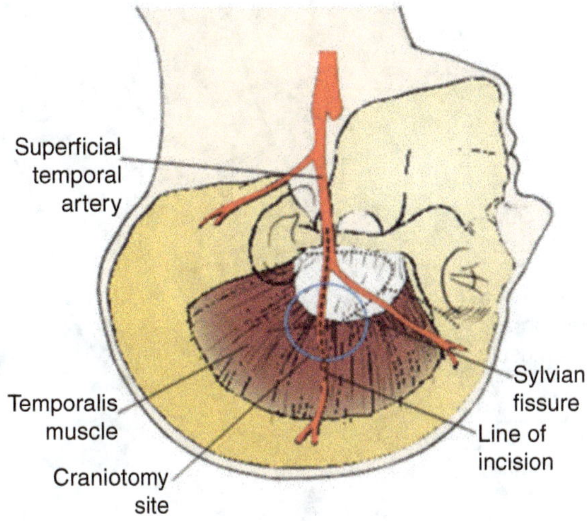

Fig. 26.3 The course of superficial temporal artery is mapped out using Doppler ultrasound, and skin incision is planned over the artery along its course

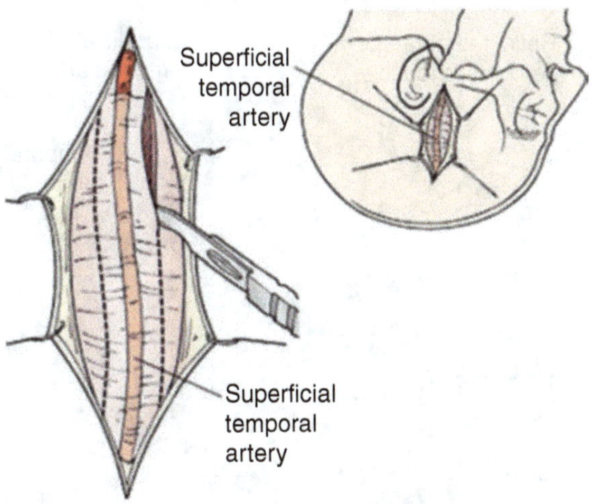

Fig. 26.4 Approximately 7 cm of STA with a generous cuff of soft tissue to protect is needed for the bypass. The artery and cuff are carefully dissected out using a combination of sharp dissection and cautery

Identification of a sufficiently large M4 segment of MCA (0.6 mm) emerging from Sylvian fissure is paramount for this procedure. The arachnoid overlying this cortical branch of the MCA is then microscopically opened. A 7 mm segment of M4 artery without branches is preferably chosen as the recipient, but any tiny branches arising from this segment can be coagulated and divided if necessary (Fig. 26.6). A jeweler-type bipolar is used. High-visibility background is placed under the M4 segment. Papaverine is intermittently instilled over the vessels to prevent

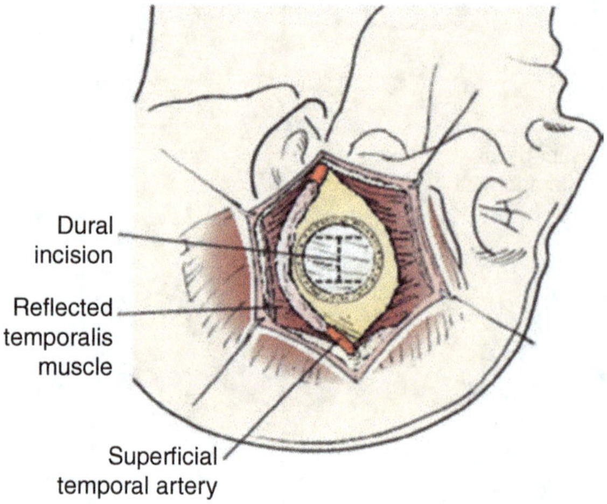

Fig. 26.5 The underlying temporalis fascia muscle is split and dissected from the frontotemporal bone. Burr holes are placed, the craniotomy bone flap is removed over the frontotemporal region, and the dura is opened in a cruciate manner

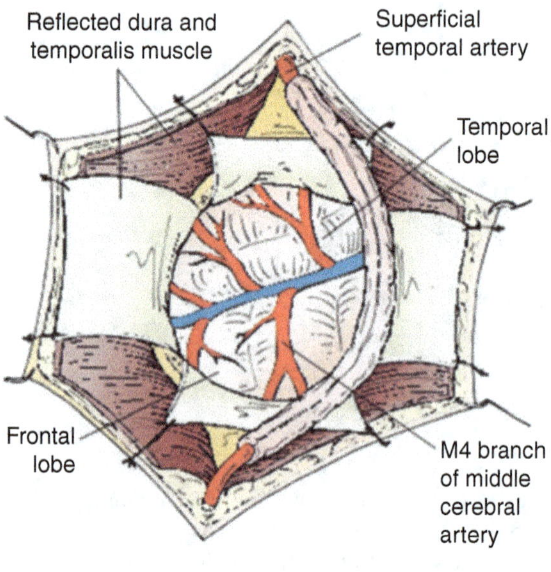

Fig. 26.6 Identification of a sufficiently large M4 branch of the MCA (0.6 mm) emerging from the Sylvian fissure is paramount for this procedure

spasm. Then the STA is temporarily occluded proximally and sectioned distally. The distal stump of the STA in the scalp is coagulated, and the STA is truncated to the proper length for anastomosis and fish mouthed. Temporary release of the proximal clip is performed to ensure excellent flow.

The artery is temporarily occluded again proximally and flushed with heparinized saline. Intravenous thiopental is given to induce burst suppression in the EEG. The mean arterial pressure is raised, and then the M4 MCA branch is temporarily occluded with Sugita aneurysm clips. An arteriotomy is made in the M4 branch, removing an elliptical portion of the superior wall, and irrigated with heparinized saline. Anastomosis between an end of STA and the side of the MCA segment is done with 10-0 interrupted suture (Fig. 26.7). The Sugita clips are then removed, restoring flow. Flow in all vessels is confirmed with the intraoperative Doppler. An intraoperative indocyanine green (ICG) angiogram is performed by injecting 2 ml of ICG dye intravenously and visualizing the graft with the near-infrared camera on the microscope.

If the anastomosis is done correctly, the ICG demonstrates wide patency of the graft with no stenosis and good filling of the pial vasculature. It is our practice to then lay the STA with its soft tissue cuff on the cortical surface to induce an indirect bypass as well as a direct one (Figs. 26.8 and 26.9). The dura is closed with 4-0 suture followed by synthetic dura, leaving an opening for the graft to enter without compromise. The bone is replaced using a plating system, also leaving an opening for the graft to enter unimpeded. The temporalis muscle and scalp are closed in several layers in the usual fashion. During the entire procedure, care is taken to keep the mean arterial pressure high normal for that patient and about ten points higher during the occlusion of the cortical MCA branch for adequate perfusion. Patients are maintained normocapnia during the entire operation to prevent vasoconstriction and ischemia from hyperventilation.

26.5.8 Indirect Revascularization

If the patient has a very small STA (<0.6 mm) or the vessel is too fragile for suture, then we perform an indirect revascularization (encephaloduroarteriosynangiosis (EDAS) or encephaloduromyosynangiosis (EDMS)). We have abandoned options such as free omental flap transplantation or pedicle omental flap transposition. In a similar fashion to the direct bypass procedure, patients are positioned and prepped, the

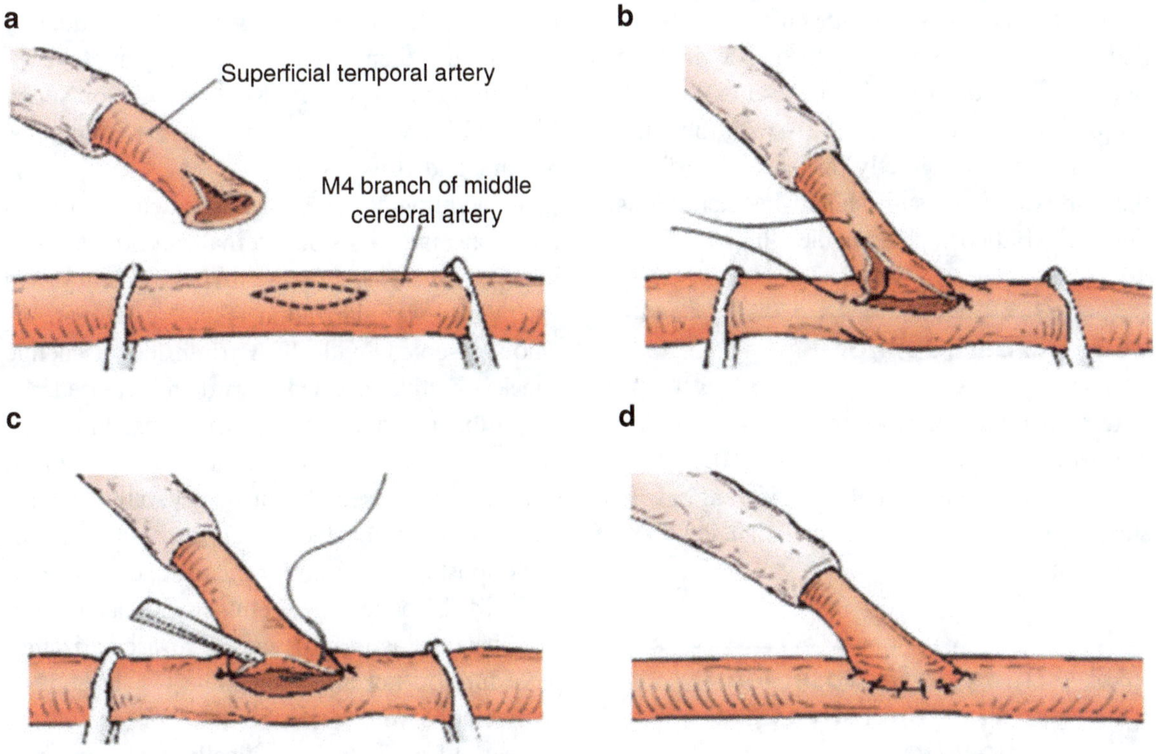

Fig. 26.7 (**a**) The superficial temporal artery is truncated to the proper length for anastomosis and fish mouthed. (**b**) An arteriotomy is made in the M4 branch, removing an elliptical portion of the superior wall. (**c** and **d**) An end-to-side anastomosis between the STA branch and the MCA branch is performed with 10-0 interrupted suture

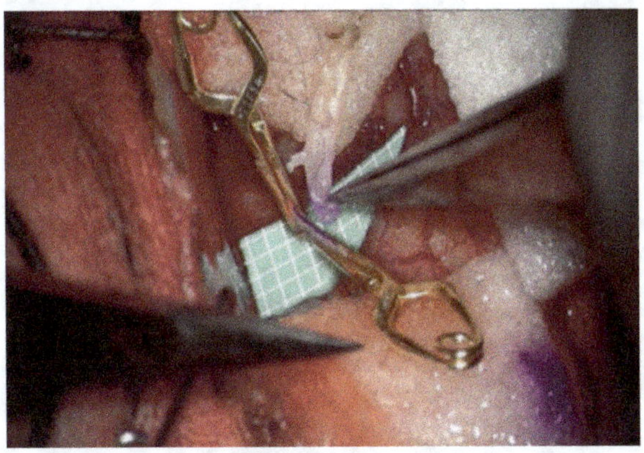

Fig. 26.8 Intraoperative photo of STA-MCA bypass procedure

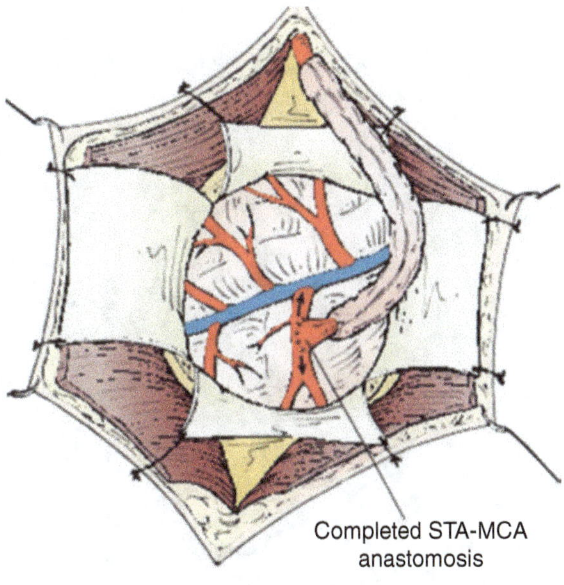

Fig. 26.9 Completed bypass showing the STA with its soft tissue cuff on the cortical surface to induce both an indirect and direct bypass

STA and generous soft tissue cuff are harvested, and the craniotomy is performed. The arachnoid overlying the deep sulci and fissures is microscopically opened, and the STA with the cuff of soft tissue is laid directly on the pial surface of the cortex. The closure should be meticulously done to avoid postoperative bleeding.

26.6 Expert Opinion

Although there are risks to direct and indirect revascularization procedures for MMD, according to data by several authors, they suggest that surgery is superior to medical management of these patients.

26.7 Things to Be Observed and Postoperative Care/Follow-Up

Patients are generally discharged after three to four hospital nights (the first night is spent in the intensive care unit). They are then evaluated clinically 1 week after each surgery and subsequently at 6 months, then 3 years, and finally at 10 years. It is important to perform MRI, SPECT, or Xenon CT and cerebral angiography at 6 months, 3 years, and 10 years.

In addition to internal carotid and vertebral injections, injections of external carotid artery are important to evaluate the bypass patency and extent of revascularization (Fig. 26.10). Patients who presented with TIA (transient ischemic attack) or stroke trended toward an increased risk of postoperative ischemic symptoms. Similarly, patients who presented with hemorrhage trended toward an increased risk of postoperative hemorrhage. Be aware that the MMD patient has a higher risk of postoperative stroke and death compared to a non-MMD patient. Sex, ethnicity, unilateral versus bilateral, age, and type of revascularization procedure do not affect outcome [7]. In another study, the 5-year risk of stroke or death was decreased from 65% in medically treated patients to 17% in surgically treated patients [15]. One study did fail to show a benefit of surgical treatment, but the authors reported an unusually high initial surgical morbidity and mortality [16].

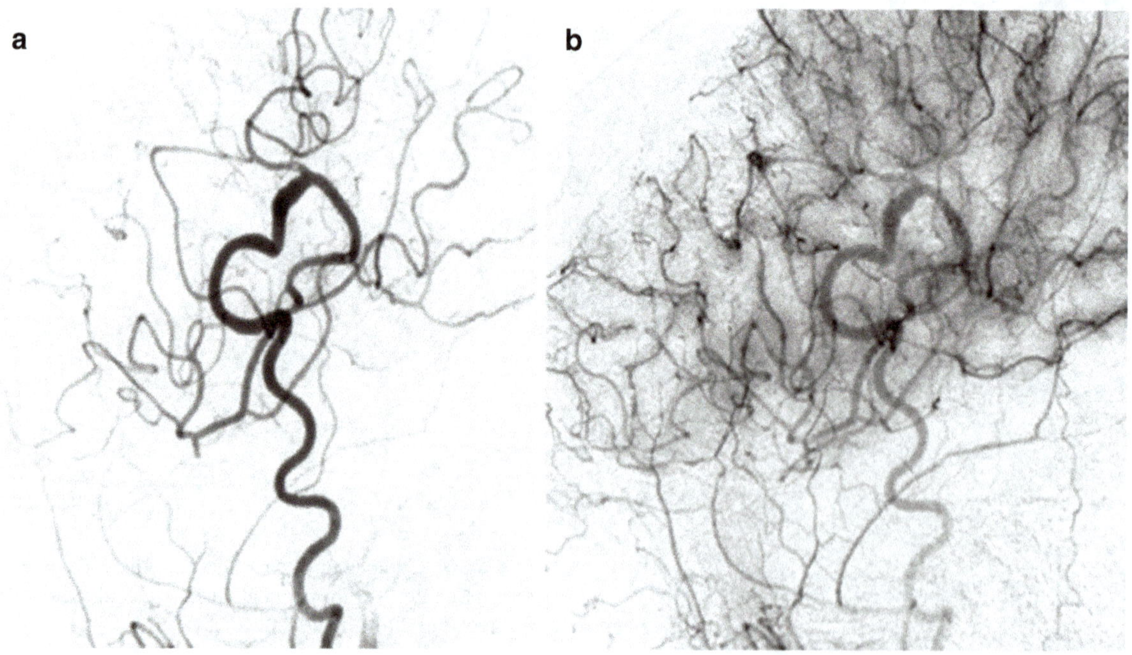

Fig. 26.10 (**a** and **b**) Left external carotid artery lateral injection demonstrating a patent superficial temporal artery to middle cerebral artery bypass supplying two thirds of the MCA territory

References

1. Fukui M. Guidelines for the diagnosis and treatment of spontaneous occlusion of the Circle of Willis ("Moyamoya" disease). Research Committee on Spontaneous Occlusion of the Circle of Willis (Moyamoya disease) of the Ministry of Health and Welfare, Japan. Clin Neurol Neurosurg. 1997;99(Suppl 2):S238–40.
2. Takeuchi K, Shimizu K. Hypoplasia of the bilateral internal carotid arteries. Brain Nerve. 1957;9: 37–43.
3. Hoffman HJ. Moyamoya disease and syndrome. Clin Neurol Neurosurg. 1997;99(Suppl 2):S39–44.
4. Baba T, Houkin K, Kuroda S. Novel epidemiological features of moya-moya disease. J Neurol Neurosurg Psychiatry. 2008;79:900–4.
5. Wakai K, Tamakoshi A, Ikezaki K, et al. Epidemiological features of moyamoya disease in Japan: findings from a nationwide survey. Clin Neurol Neurosurg. 1997;99(Suppl 2):S1–5.
6. Kuriyama S, Kusaka Y, Fujimura M, et al. Prevalence and clinic-epidemiological features of moyamoya disease in Japan: findings from a nationwide epidemiological survey. Stroke. 2008;39:42–7.
7. Guzman R, Lee M, Achrol A, et al. Clinical outcome after 450 revascularization procedures for moyamoya disease. J Neurosurg. 2009;111:927–35.
8. Olesen J, Friberg L, Olsen TS, et al. Ischaemia-induced (symptomatic) migraine attacks may be more frequent than migraine-induced ischemic insults. Brain. 1993;116(Pt 1):187–202.
9. Seol HJ, Wang KC, Kim SK, et al. Headache in pediatric moyamoya disease: review of 204 consecutive cases. J Neurosurg. 2005;103:439–42.
10. Achrol AS, Guzman R, Lee M, et al. Pathophysiology and genetic factors in moyamoya disease. Neurosurg Focus. 2009;26:E4.
11. Ikeda H, Sasaki T, Yoshimoto T, et al. Mapping of a familial moya-moya disease gene to chromosome 3p24.2-p26. Am J Hum Genet. 1999;64:533–7.
12. Inoue TK, Ikezaki K, Sasazuki T, et al. Linkage analysis of moyamoya disease on chromosome 6. J Child Neurol. 2000;15:179–82.
13. Sakurai K, Horiuchi Y, Ikeda H, et al. A novel susceptibility locus for moyamoya disease on chromosome 8q23. J Hum Genet. 2004;49:278–81.
14. Mineharu Y, Liu W, Inoue K, et al. Autosomal dominant moyamoya disease maps to chromosome 17q25.3. Neurology. 2008;70:2357–63.
15. Hallemeier CL, Rich KM, Grubb RL Jr, et al. Clinical features and out-come in North American adults with moyamoya phenomenon. Stroke. 2006;37:1490–6.
16. Kuroda S, Hashimoto N, Yoshimoto T, et al. Radiological findings, clinical course, and outcome in asymptomatic moyamoya disease: results of multicenter survey in Japan. Stroke. 2007;38: 1430–5.

27 Flow Arrest for Complex Intracranial Aneurysm Surgery by Using Adenosine

Xiangdong Wang, Yasuhiro Yamada, Tsukasa Kawase, and Yoko Kato

27.1 Introduction

The term complex intracranial aneurysms (CIAs) refers to aneurysm at a narrow and difficult location, difficult shape, and also giant size (aneurysm that is bigger than 25 mm in diameter) [1]. Giant aneurysms are more likely to bleed and present as subarachnoid hemorrhage, or sometimes they become partly thrombosed with ischemic brain causing mass effect with progressive symptoms or even death. Microsurgery and clip ligation can be challenging in CIAs because it is very difficult to have a panoramic view of the aneurysm, where sometimes the parent vessel is laid beneath the aneurysm, difficult to identify all branches and perforators, and also the surgical corridor could be very deep and narrow and surrounded by important neurovascular structures. During the clipping, it is important to make sure the aneurysm is well clipped to prevent injury from any perforator (Figs. 27.1, 27.2, and 27.3). Flow arrest can be induced by using adenosine; it will briefly reduce cerebral perfusion pressure

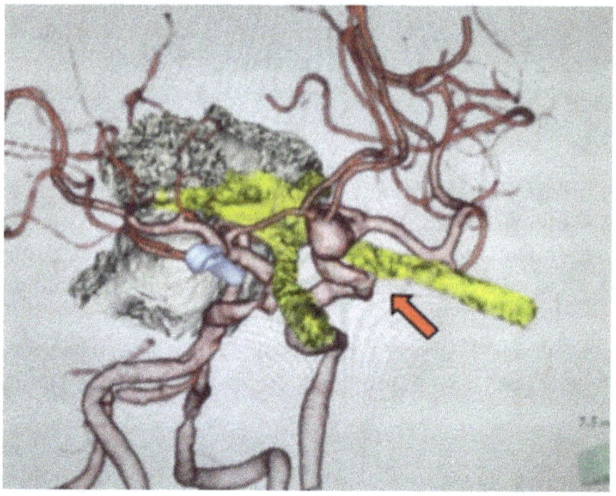

Fig. 27.1 Preoperative fusion images of CIAs

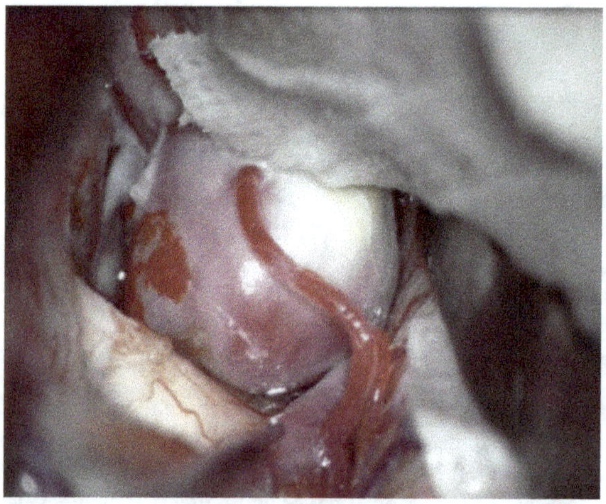

Fig. 27.2 Schematic representation of an A Com A aneurysm. The large mass does not allow circumferential dissection and visualization of the whole aneurysm, its branches, and perforators

X. Wang · Y. Yamada · T. Kawase
Department of Neurosurgery, Fujita Health University, Banbuntane Hotokukai Hospital, Nagoya city, Aichi, Japan
e-mail: kawasemi@hm8.aitai.ne.jp

Y. Kato (✉)
Department of Neurosurgery, Fujita Health University, Toyoake, Aichi, Japan
e-mail: kyoko@fujita-hu.ac.jp

J. July, E. J. Wahjoepramono (eds.), *Neurovascular Surgery*,
https://doi.org/10.1007/978-981-10-8950-3_27

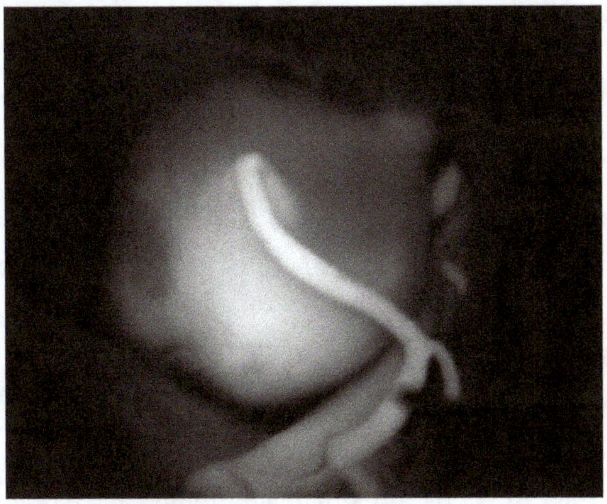

Fig. 27.3 Microsurgery-integrated indocyanine green video angiography (mICG-VA)

and the tension on aneurysm, thereby facilitating the clip ligation. The lenght of time while the flow arrest will provide the surgeon to work at the aneurysm and the parts surrounding it or even reduce the bleed if it was ruptured during dissection. It will provide the time interval for the surgeon to be able to secure the neck of the aneurysm. The adenosine is working by inducing the transient asystole for a few minutes.

There are 231 cases of intracranial aneurysms which used adenosine-induced flow arrest during microsurgery and clip ligation from 1999 to 2016 (Bebawy JF et al. have three published papers; there are some repeated cases in these three papers) [2].

27.2 Adenosine-Induced Transient Asystole

The adenosine is a nucleoside analog that can reduce the heartbeat and lengthen the electric conduction at the atrioventricular node. Adenosine will bind A1 receptors in the myocard, reducing adenylate cyclase activity and reducing intracellular cyclic adenosine monophosphate (c-AMP). This will prevent calcium conductance and then shut down pacemaker activity. Adenosine has a half-life of 0.6–10 s, and it is quickly washed out from the circulation by uptake into erythrocytes and vascular endothelial cells. Following the bolus injection, the heart rate will decrease linearly with the amount of dose until total AV node block happened. The adenosine effect will be seen 10–20 s after the bolus injection. There is a linear relationship between the dose and the length of asystole, and it reaches a plateau between 40 and 60 s at 1 mg/kg body weight [3]. Going through the asystole, there will be a hypotension that may stay for up to 1 min. In practice, the adenosine is commonly used by the emergency physician or cardiologist to treat supraventricular tachycardia [4]. In the endovascular surgery, adenosine sometimes is used during endovascular aortic aneurysm repair [5, 6]and AVM embolization [7, 8].

27.3 Indications of Using Adenosine-Induced Flow Arrest for Complex Aneurysm

There are three earlier single-patient case reports during 1999–2007. The first case was reported by Groff et al. [9]; the clipping of basilar apex aneurysm was done successfully with three doses of adenosine and no complications. Nussbaum et al. [10] then reported the second case. Nussbaum and his team successfully managed the intraoperative rupture of an A Com A (anterior communicating artery) aneurysm by using adenosine bolus injection. Prior to this attempt, they have tried temporary proximal control and cottonoid tamponade, but they failed to achieve adequate hemostasis. In this case, the adenosine facilitates the successful clipping of the aneurysm. The patient recovered very well, with no deficits and no complications related to the use of adenosine. Heppner et al. [11] reported the third case; it is a giant basilar apex aneurysm. Proximal control at the basilar trunk failed to relax the dome to allow perforator visualization and clip placement. They finally decided to give three boluses of adenosine while performing the aneurysm clipping. Sadly, this case resulted in a poor outcome, but it was considered not related with the adenosine.

Recently, there are ten serial cases describing adenosine role in facilitating intracranial aneurysm clipping during 2010–2016.

For CIAs clip ligation, if the aneurysm size is giant, the surgeon often finds it difficult to apply proximal control such as the case with big aneurysm at ICA bifurcation when it turns to ACA and MCA [12, 13]. Many surgeons used to prepare the extracranial carotid vessel at the neck for proximal control to reduce the dome tension while clipping the aneurysm or manage the bleed if the premature rupture occurs. Nowadays, they also can combine by using balloon occlusion endovascularly and suction decompression or do the deep hypothermic circulatory arrest, but it only could be done at the hospital with complete facility [14, 15]. Such combination of surgery may be associated with high morbidity rate that contributed from the dissection of friable arteries or distal arterial embolic occlusion due to endovascular manipulation. The other method is using cardiopulmonary bypass to facilitate clipping of difficult aneurysm, but there are risks of complication related to the bypass procedure such as arterial injury at the puncture site, emboli, and coagulopathy causing high number of postoperative intracranial hematomas [16]. If the proximal control is unfeasible for the case, then the use of adenosine may induce a short-time deep systemic hypotension with flow arrest to the parent artery [9, 11, 17]. The studies have shown that 57 (24.7%) of 231 patients got adenosine during posterior circulation clipping, which include 25(10.8%) basilar artery aneurysm and 29(12.55%) unsorted posterior circulation aneurysm. This supports the fact that the surgeries in this area are generally more difficult, with deep and narrow corridor; thus they are technically more challenging [3, 9, 11, 18, 19] .

Some studies [3, 9, 11, 19, 20] have pointed out that proximal control by using temporary clip remains the gold standard. The use of adenosine should be an adjunct and optional, while it's necessary during the surgery, it should not be a replacement of the temporary clip occlusion.

27.4 Adenosine-Induced Flow Arrest

Since the first successful use of adenosine to facilitate the clipping of difficult unruptured basilar apex aneurysm by Groff et al. [9], it has gained its popularity among neurosurgeons who were trying to do the complex aneurysm surgery.

Early surgery after the aneurysm rupture may have a higher incidence of premature rupture prior to clipping, and the surgical field sometimes so dirty by the subarachnoid blood causes difficulty to get the proximal and distal of the parent vessel. When the premature rupture happened, it is useful if the surgeon can get the blood to stop briefly and work fast to dissect the parent artery for the proximal control. The adenosine may provide long enough time to allow definitive clipping or readjust the clip position on the rupture site or trapping aneurysm with temporary clips.

27.5 Patient Selection

Adenosine is contraindicated for the patient with severe (>80%) left main coronary artery stenosis, severe multivessel disease (three vessels or grafts with >80% stenosis), AV block (sick sinus syndrome), or who is using pacemakers. It is also contraindicated to severe asthma, symptomatic asthma, and active perioperative wheezing due to the risk of bronchoconstriction.

Patient have to be carefully examined prior to surgery, including screen for cardiac function and coronary artery disease, cardiac valve, any irregular heartbeat, and cardiac conduction abnormalities.

27.6 Dose of Adenosine

There is no consensus yet about the optimal dose of adenosine during surgery. Luostarien et al. reported their first 16 patients with adenosine and demonstrated its safety and efficacy during surgery for ruptured intracranial aneurysm [21]. Of these 16 patients, 12 patients got 1 bolus, and 4 patients received multiple bolus. Median dose for a single injection was 12 mg (6–18), and the median total dose for multiple injections was 27 mg (18–89). Ten minutes after adenosine administration, all patients were hemodynamically stable, and 13 required vasoactive drugs during the procedure.

In terms of the dose, because individual responses to adenosine vary, different patients may need different doses of adenosine [21].We recommend we should establish an individual dose-response relationship for each patient by injecting escalating doses of adenosine.

27.6.1 Advantages of Adenosine-Induced Transient Asystole

1. When the blood flow stops temporarily to the parent artery, it helps in reducing tension in aneurysm and facilitating aneurysm dissection, minimizes premature rupture risk, and provides safe clip placement.
2. Adenosine has a short half-life and the circulation will be back to normal.
3. Adenosine can be given repeatedly after the patient recovers from the first dose.

27.7 Potential Risks: Complications of Adenosine-Induced Transient Asystole

There is 2.6% incidence of transient irregular heartbeat during recovery period [2]. One of them required intraoperative amiodarone injection to convert to sinus rhythm [3]. Troponin 1 elevation has been reported with an incidence of 1.73% [3, 19]; all of them are clinically asymptomatic in the postoperative care unit.

The adenosine is quickly metabolized and excreted from the body, but multiple bolus injection has been associated with a prolonged hypotension; it was reported that the multiple injection is used to control the premature aneurysm rupture [2]. The general agreement is to wait for complete hemodynamic return to get back to normal before giving another bolus injection.

27.8 Expert Opinion

There is still no general consensus about adenosine dose and how fast it should be given in every bolus injection. It is best to always prepare all necessary checks for the patient that is going to have complex aneurysm surgery. It includes the coronary vessel, heart conductivity study, its valve, and other comorbid condition such as asthma. It is very important if the surgeon is going to use the adenosine if other efforts for proximal control fail. Authors recommend that adenosine should be available all the time in the operating room and it should be used judiciously if the proximal control fails, is unsafe, or is difficult.

References

1. Hanel RA, Spetzler RF. Surgical treatment of complex intracranial aneurysms. Neurosurgery. 2008;62(6 Suppl 3):1289–97.
2. Guinn NR, McDonagh DL, Borel CO, et al. Adenosine-induced transient asystole for intracranial aneurysm surgery: a retrospective review. J Neurosurg Anesthesiol. 2011;23(1):35–40.
3. Bebawy JF, Gupta DK, Bendok BR, Hemmer LB, et al. Adenosine-induced flow arrest to facilitate intracranial aneurysm clip ligation: dose-response data and safety profile. Anesth Analg. 2010;110(5):1406–11.
4. Parker RB, McCollam PL. Adenosine in the episodic treatment of paroxysmal supraventricular tachycardia. Clin Pharm. 1990;9(4):261–71.
5. Kahn RA, Moskowitz DM, Marin ML, et al. Safety and efficacy of high-dose adenosine-induced asystole during endovascular AAA repair. J Endovasc Ther. 2000;7(4):292–6.
6. Plaschke K, Boeckler D, Schumacher H, Martin E, Bardenheuer HJ. Adenosineinduced cardiac arrest and EEG changes in patients with thoracic aorta endovascular repair. Br J Anaesth. 2006;96(3):310–6.
7. Hashimoto T, YoungWL ABD, Joshi S, Ostapkovich ND, Pile-Spellman J. Adenosine-induced ventricular asystole to induce transient profound systemic hypotension in patients undergoing endovascular therapy: dose-response characteristics. Anesthesiology. 2000;93(4):998–1001.
8. Pile-Spellman J, Young WL, Joshi S, et al. Adenosine-induced cardiac pause for endovascular arteriovenous malformations: technical case report. Neurosurgery. 1999;44(4):881–6.
9. Groff MW, Adams DC, Kahn RA, Kumbar UM, Yang BY, Bederson JB. Adenosine-induced transient asystole for management of a basilar artery aneurysm. Case report. J Neurosurg. 1999;91:687–90.

10. Nussbaum ES, Sebring LA, Ostanny I, Nelson WB. Transient cardiac standstill induced by adenosine in the management of intraoperative aneurysmal rupture: technical case report. Neurosurgery. 2000;47:240–3.
11. Heppner PA, Ellegala DB, Robertson N, Nemergut E, Jaganathan J, Mee E. Basilar tip aneurysm-adenosine induced asystole for the treatment of a basilar tip aneurysm following failure of temporary clipping. Acta Neurochir. 2007;149:517–20.
12. Batjer HH, Kopitnik TA Jr, Giller CA, Samson DS. Surgical management of proximal carotid artery aneurysms. Clin Neurosurg. 1994;41:21–38.
13. Heros RC, Nelson PB, Ojemann RG, Crowell RM, DeBrun G. Large and giant paraclinoid aneurysms: surgical techniques,complications, and results. Neurosurgery. 1983;12:153–63.
14. Fulkerson DH, Horner TG, Payner TD, Leipzig TJ, Scott JA, DeNardo AJ, Redelman K, Goodman JM. Endovascular retrograde suction decompression as an adjunct to surgical treatment of ophthalmic aneurysms: analysis of risks and clinical outcomes. Neurosurgery. 2009;64:107–12.
15. Parkinson RJ, Bendok BR, Getch CC, Yashar P, Shaibani A, Ankenbrandt W, Awad IA, Batjer HH. Retrograde suction decompression of giant paraclinoid aneurysms using a No. 7 French balloon-containing guide catheter. Technical note. J Neurosurg. 2006;105:479–81.
16. Young WL, Lawton MT, Gupta DK, Hashimoto T. Anesthetic management of deep hypothermic circulatory arrest for cerebral aneurysm clipping. Anesthesiology. 2002;96:497–503.
17. Lagerkranser M, Bergstrand G, Gordon E, Irestedt L, Lindquist C, Stange K, Sollevi A. Cerebral blood flow and metabolism during adenosine-induced hypotension in patients undergoing cerebral aneurysm surgery. Acta Anaesthesiol Scand. 1989;33:15–20.
18. Khan SA, McDonagh DL, Adogwa O, Gokhale S, et al. Perioperative cardiac complications and 30-day mortality in patients undergoing intracranial aneurysmal surgery with adenosine-induced flow arrest: a retrospective comparative study. Neurosurgery. 2014;74(3):267–71.
19. Bendok BR, Gupta DK, Rahme RJ, Eddleman CS, et al. Adenosine for temporary flow arrest during intracranial aneurysm surgery: a single-center retrospective review. Neurosurgery. 2011;69(4):815–20.
20. Bebawy JF, Zeeni C, Sharma S, Kim ES, et al. Adenosine-induced flow arrest to facilitate intracranial aneurysm clip ligation does not worsen neurologic outcome. Anesth Analg. 2013;117(5):1205–10.
21. Luostarinen T, Takala RS, Niemi TT, Katila AJ, et al. Adenosine-induced cardiac arrest during intraoperative cerebral aneurysm rupture. World Neurosurg. 2010;73(2):79–83.

28 Spinal Arteriovenous Malformations

Antonio López González, Mardjono Tjahjadi, Andrés Muñoz Nuñez, and Francisco Javier Márquez Rivas

28.1 Sign and Symptoms

Clinical signs and symptoms of spinal arteriovenous malformation (AVM) have different characteristics according to the type of the AVM. Various classifications have been proposed for this complex lesion [1–3]; we use our own modified classification just to simplify our work-up discussion.

We divide the spinal arteriovenous (AV) malformations by their fistula or nidus locations into dural, perimedullary, and intramedullary type and by fistulas or true malformations. Authors identify the dural AV fistulas (dAVF) (Fig. 28.1), perimedullary AV fistulas (AVF) (Fig. 28.2), and spinal cord true AV malformation (AVM) that is either juvenile-type AVM or glomus-type AVM.

	dAVF [4]	Perimedullary [5]	Juvenile [6]	Glomus [7]
Feeder	Radiculomeningeal	Spinal artery	Multiple spinal arteries	Multiple spinal arteries
Nidus	Small, in the dura, close to nerve root	Direct shunt	Large; not well delineated; located inside the spinal cord within functional neural tissue	Well delineated; located at one single spinal cord segment without neural tissue inside
Drainage	Single radicular vein and then to perimedullary venous plexus	Perimedullary venous plexus	Giant venous ectasia	Veins draining to the perimedullary plexus can be identified

A. L. González · A. M. Nuñez · F. J. M. Rivas (✉)
Department of Neurosurgery, Virgen Macarena and Virgen del Rocío University Hospitals, Seville, Spain
e-mail: andresmunioz@hormail.com; jaca5@arrakis.es

M. Tjahjadi
Department of Neurosurgery, Helsinki University Central Hospital, Helsinki, Finland

J. July, E. J. Wahjoepramono (eds.), *Neurovascular Surgery*, https://doi.org/10.1007/978-981-10-8950-3_28

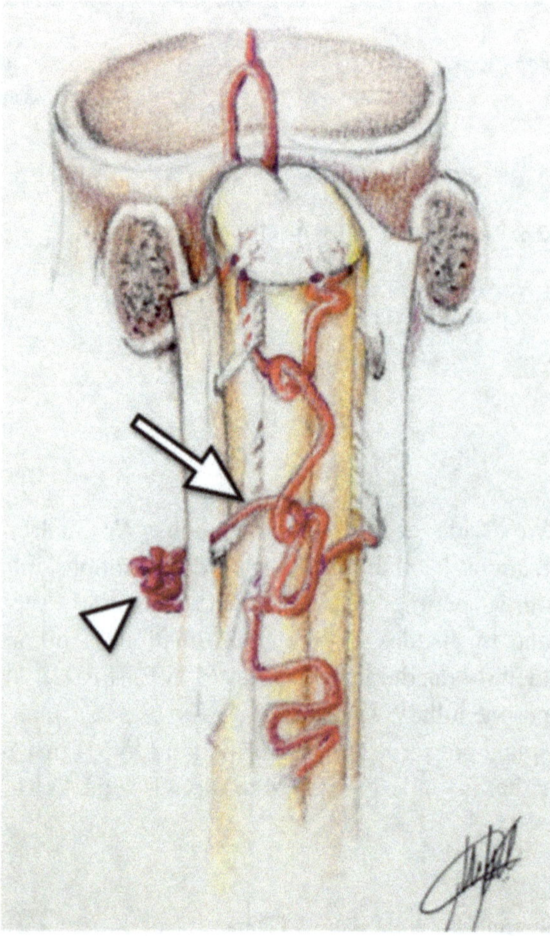

Fig. 28.1 Drawing showing a dAVF. Arrow indicates the fistulous vessel and the arrowhead the dural nidus over the nerve root

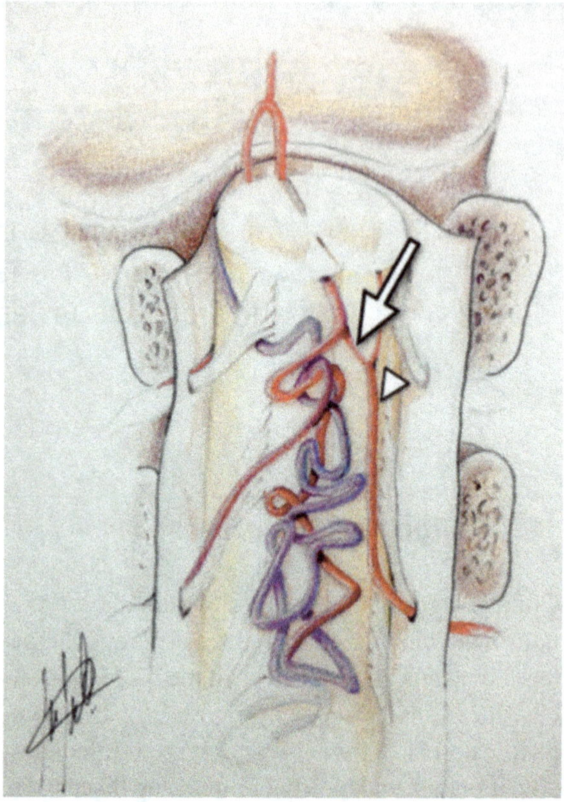

Fig. 28.2 Drawing showing a perimedullary AVF. Arrow indicates the fistulous vessel between a spinal artery and the venous plexus (*arrowhead*)

Most of the spinal AV malformations are found at the level of lower thoracic and thoracolumbar spine, and dural type is the most commonly found spinal AV malformation.

Patients who have dural type usually come to our service with complaint of slowly progressive myelopathy, and many of them had a long history of intermittent myelopathy previously. The myelopathy is caused by either direct mechanical compression of the spinal cord by the engorging vein or by the disturbance of spinal blood flow that resulted in spinal cord ischemia. In the clinical presentation, motor weakness is the most common symptom, followed by paresthesia and sphincter disturbances. Pain and acute onset of myelopathy are relatively seldom for this spinal AV malformation type. Perimedullary and intramedullary type may present as an acute onset of back pain or myelopathy. The pathogenesis is believed to be the ruptured of the nidus that caused subarachnoid hemorrhage or even intramedullary hemorrhage. Meningeal irritation signs might be found in the clinical presentation. But in a low-flow fistula or malformation, the symptoms can develop slowly and give a similar pathogenesis and clinical characteristic to the dural type [8, 9].

28.2 Investigation [4, 10–12]

Most of the spinal AV malformations are discovered by an MRI/MRA. But it is the selective DSA (digital subtraction angiography) that remains gold standard to identify the number, morphology, exact location, and dynamics of the feeders, nidus, and drainages of the malformation.

28.2.1 Magnetic Resonance Imaging

The T2WI MRI of the spinal cord may show diffuse hyperintense signal at the central area representing edema of the spinal cord. This lesion is possibly accompanied by the hypointense signal that occurs more likely at dorsal surface of the cord. These hypointense signals represent the congested perimedullary venous plexus (Fig. 28.3).

On T1-weighted images, the hypointense and swollen spinal cord is a common finding. Infusion of the contrast agent may show diffuse enhancement represents the chronic congested veins with a breakdown of a spinal cord-blood barrier.

MRA may provide benefit if it could show the suspicious level of the fistula associated with the vertebral level, and then this information can accelerate the selective DSA study.

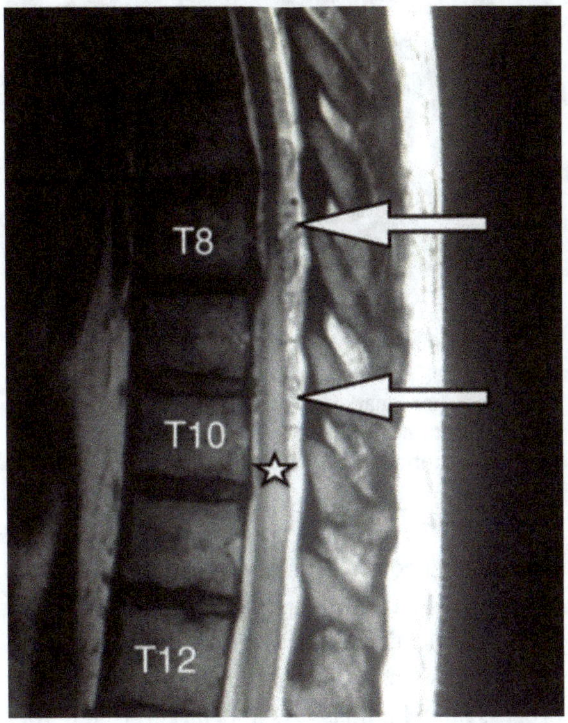

Fig. 28.3 Spine T2-weighted MRI. Sagittal view. Arrows point at hypointense signal areas at the dorsal surface of the cord. These hypointense signals represent the congested perimedullary venous plexus. The star is placed in a diffuse hyperintense signal at the central area of the spinal cord representing edema and radiological myelopathy

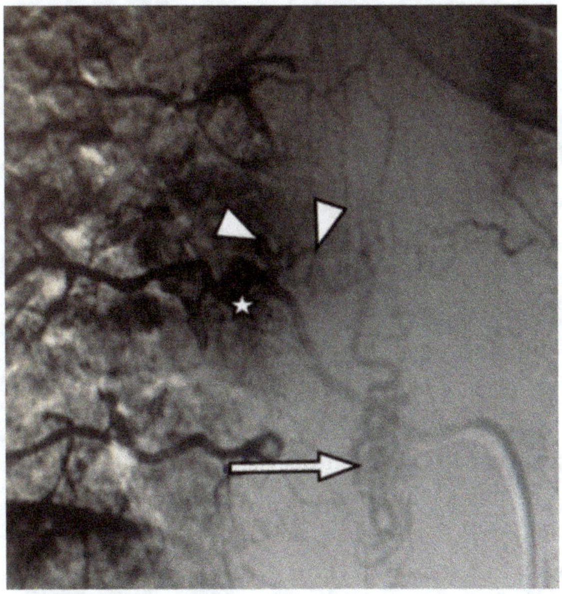

Fig. 28.4 Anteroposterior view of DSA showing a dAVF. The shunt vessel is marked by arrowheads and the engorged venous plexus by the arrow. A star is placed close to the dural nidus

28.2.2 Digital Subtraction Angiography

DSA becomes the treatment of choice because of the feasibility of this technique to study in the angioarchitecture of the vessels within or surrounding the lesion. Moreover DSA also gives valuable information about the flow dynamic of the lesions; therefore it can be an important instrument for selection of the treatment modalities (Fig. 28.4).

28.3 Preoperative Preparation

The patient must be preoperatively evaluated in a similar way to any other neurosurgical procedures. As surgery for this case is an elective procedure, the patient's general condition should be optimalized. The biochemical analysis and blood and coagulation studies must be evaluated and corrected if necessary prior to the surgery. Two blood bags must be reserved according to the patient's blood group. Any antiplatelet or anticoagulant drug must be stopped, and its effects must be reversed.

Intraoperative neurophysiological monitoring is not necessary in most of the cases, and it is reserved only for cavernomas and intramedullary AVMs.

Assessment of the exact location of the malformation is crucial for the successful procedure. Careful evaluation of MRI or DSA images is mandatory to know the exact level of the lesion. Marking the location of the skin incision in some situations can be tricky, especially when the lesion is located at the middle level of the back. Utilization of preoperative fluoroscopy is recommended to make a proper skin incision marking. The lateral fluoroscopy view is used by identifying the L5–S1 space, and the spine level can be counted cranially. The anteroposterior view helps us to identify the last rib and T12. This procedure can be done 1 day or several hours prior to the surgery, and to avoid any inaccuracy marking, we ask an interventional CT radiologist to draw the location of the lesion at the patient's skin and fix it with a single staple.

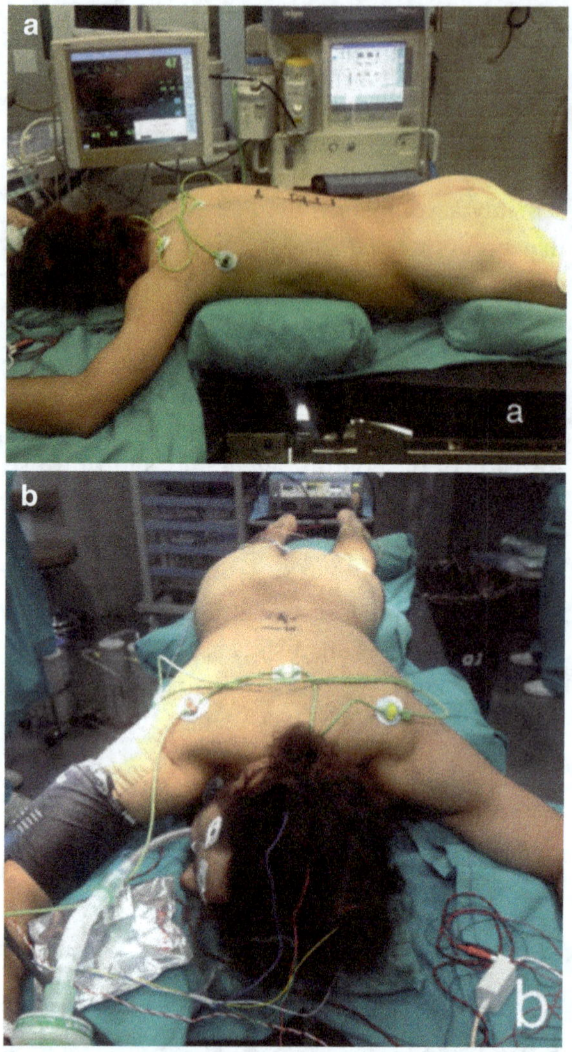

Fig. 28.5 (**a**) Lateral view of intraoperative patient's position. In this case, the chest and hips are placed over soft supports. The arms are over armrests. The incision has already been marked in the midline. (**b**) Cranial view. The head is turned right, and electrodes for neurophysiological monitoring are placed in the scalp and legs

28.3.1 Positioning

Patient is placed in a prone position with over two chest rolls or a Wilson frame. For lesions located at the dorsal spine, the two arms rest over armrests; for lumbar lesions, we prefer the knee-chest position and, for cervical spine lesions, the Wilson frame and the head fixed by Mayfield three-pin frame with patient's arms fixed and held parallel to the body (Figs. 28.5 and 28.6).

28.3.2 Approach

Spinal cord AVMs need a bilateral laminectomy, laminoplasty, or unilateral laminectomy to reach the lesion.

Skin incision marking is made longitudinally in the midline, over the spinous process long enough to get a good exposure of the spinal laminas below which the vascular lesion is. The site of skin incision is infiltrated with a mixture of ropivacaine and lidocaine combined with adrenaline. Skin incision is made with a scalpel no. 21; the subcutaneous layers are divided through the midline using the monopolar diathermy set at 50.

If the vascular lesion is a dAVF, we only need to dissect the ipsilateral muscles from the spinous process and laminas. As the target is the root entry, a unilateral laminectomy is enough to reach the field. We can prevent muscle bleeding by doing the dissection just at the plane between the muscle and bone and using bipolar cauterization set at 50 (for Malis bipolar system; Codman, Raynham, MA, USA) when a bleeding vessel is detected. Achieving a good hemostasis will make

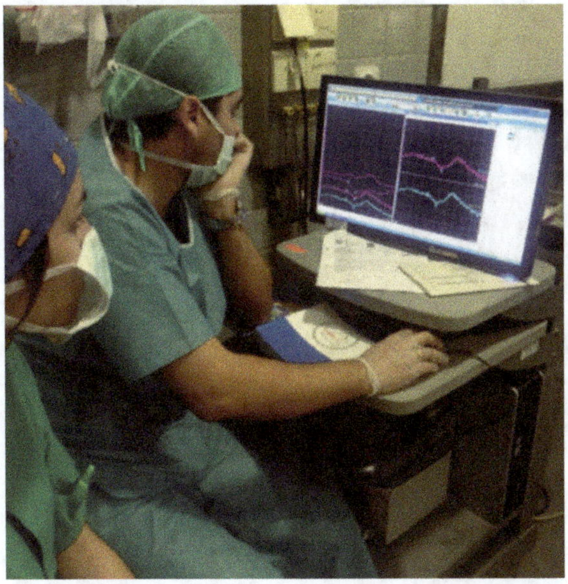

Fig. 28.6 The neurophysiologist is monitoring intraoperatively motor and somatosensory evoked potentials

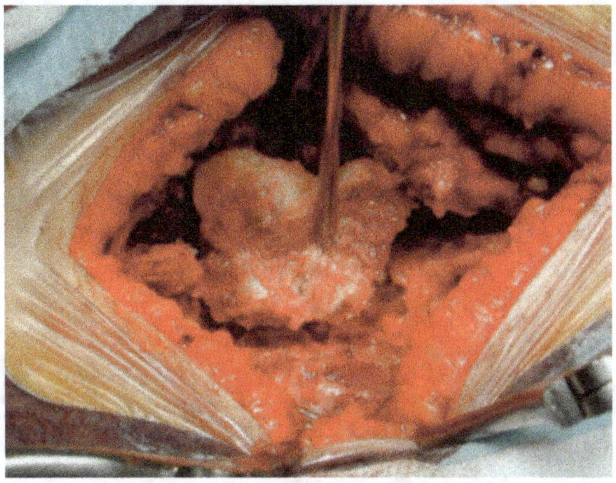

Fig. 28.7 Laminoplasty. The laminas are cut and elevated maintaining the supraspinous and interlaminar ligaments

surgery faster and easier. We may dissect the contralateral laminas partially for the easier placement of the muscle retractor.

It is important to retract the muscle not too tight to prevent the damage of the muscles that result in the postoperative back pain and increase the risk of infections. It is important to retract the muscle not too tight to prevent the muscle ischemia that may produce postoperative back pain and increase the risk of infections. If the lesion is a perimedullary AVF, a cavernoma, or a perimedullary or intramedullary AVM, a bilateral laminectomy, after bilateral muscle dissection, must be performed large enough to expose completely the malformation before the dura opening. For laminectomy, we use Beyer and Kerrison rongeurs.

In younger patients, a laminoplasty is an alternative. The procedure is done using the side-cut drill that is used in craniotomies. The laminas are cut and elevated maintaining the supraspinous and interlaminar ligaments (Fig. 28.7). After the spinal AVM removal, the laminas are placed into its location and fixed with titanium plates and screws.

After bone removal, good hemostasis must be achieved with bone wax over the bleeding bone and hemostatic agents such as Surgicel®, Helitene®, fibrin glue, or Tachosil® to stop the epidural venous bleeding.

The use of high-magnification operating microscope, powerful light source, and stereoscopic vision allows the neurosurgeon to use suitable delicate tools to operate on spinal cord lesions in an almost bloodless field. The microscope allows visualization and 3D appreciation of the relevant and detailed neuroanatomical structures [13].

28.4 Steps of the Surgery

The dura is necessarily observed carefully prior to the opening of dura, because the dura may firmly adhere to the draining vein or to the AVM itself. Adhesion is even more common in redo cases and prior episode of several bleedings and/or embolization.

In the midline, we prefer to perform a small cut in the dura with a scalpel blade no. 15. Then, we divide it longitudinally by pulling each dura edges back with two microforceps with teeth. This way of opening the dura minimizes the risk of cutting accidentally any superficial dilated vein with the tip of the sharp blade. The maneuver must be done in the midline for perimedullary AVFs, AVMs, and cavernomas, but if the approach has been performed through an ipsilateral laminectomy, the dura incision is done longitudinally in the middle of the dural area exposed.

The bilateral dural edges are tacked up by using 4/0 Safil® violet taper-point sutures. The tack-up stitches are used for two purposes: to expose widely the spinal cord and to stop oozing from the epidural space. Fibrin glue and surgical packing further enhance this effect. From this point on, the bipolar power setting is turned down to 20–25.

28.4.1 Dural and Perimedullary AV Fistula

If the patient suffers a spinal dAVF, our aim is to localize the exiting nerve root intradurally because the location of the fistula is expected near to the root.

Sometimes the anatomy is not clear at all at this point, and in order to ensure the correct fistulous vein, we do a small trick using the support of intraoperative video-angiography with indocyanine green (ICG). If the surgical microscope is equipped with infrared camera, after intravenous injection of ICG, the field of interest is illuminated with near-infrared light that shows real-time and dynamic angiographic images. Our trick is to compress the fistulous vein we suspect with a vascular temporary clip and then order the anesthesiologist to inject the indocyanine green of 0.2–0.5 mg/kg. As soon as we see the arterial phase, we release the temporary clip, and if the whole engorged perimedullary venous plexus fills immediately, it confirms that we compressed the feeding vessel of the fistula [14].

At this point, we coagulate the fistulous vein and divide it with microscissors (Fig. 28.8). To clip the fistulous vein with a vascular clip is also possible (Fig. 28.9). It is not necessary to localize the nerve root artery extradurally or remove the dural nidus. A new ICG video-angiography will show no filling or very slow filling of the venous plexus.

In the perimedullary AVFs, sometimes it is difficult to identify the fistula between perimedullary artery and venous plexus because the fistula may be hidden by the engorged venous plexus. In this situation, we must carefully identify the structures with microdissectors and perform an ICG video-angiography. When we have definitively identified the connection, we perform in the same way that in dAVFs, the vessel is coagulated and cut.

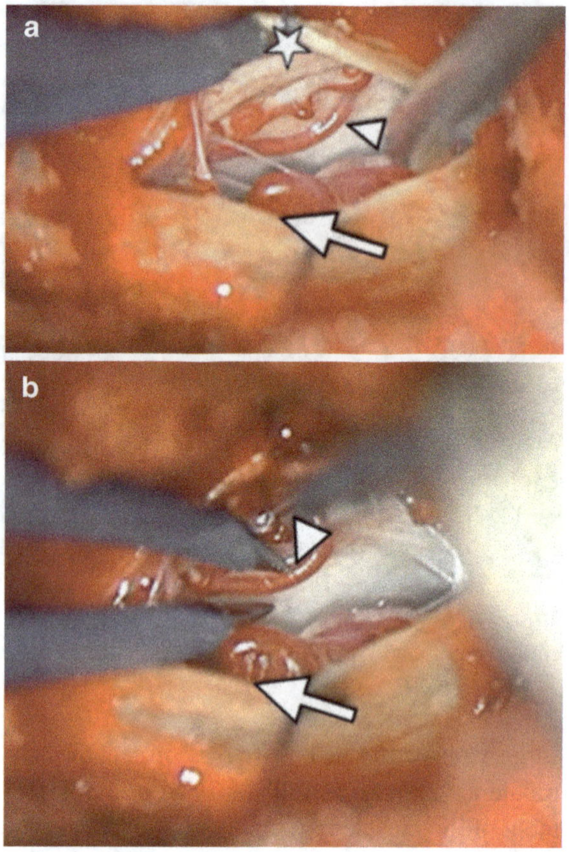

Fig. 28.8 (**a**) A dAVF under the operating microscope. After the dura is opened, the next structures can be identified: the nerve root (*star*), the fistulous vessel (*arrowhead*), and the engorged venous plexus (*arrow*). (**b**) The fistulous vessel is coagulated with bipolar forceps set at 20 (for Malis bipolar system; Codman, Raynham, MA, USA) before being cut with microscissors

28.4.2 Glomus AV Malformations

Only true spinal cord glomus-type AVMs that are located in the posterior horn can be managed surgically. Ventral AVMs or juvenile spinal AVMs at any location are extremely difficult or impossible to remove.

In the glomus-type AVMs, the midline dura opening must be done carefully because the previous subarachnoid hemorrhages at this level may promote adherences between the nidus, arachnoid, and dura mater.

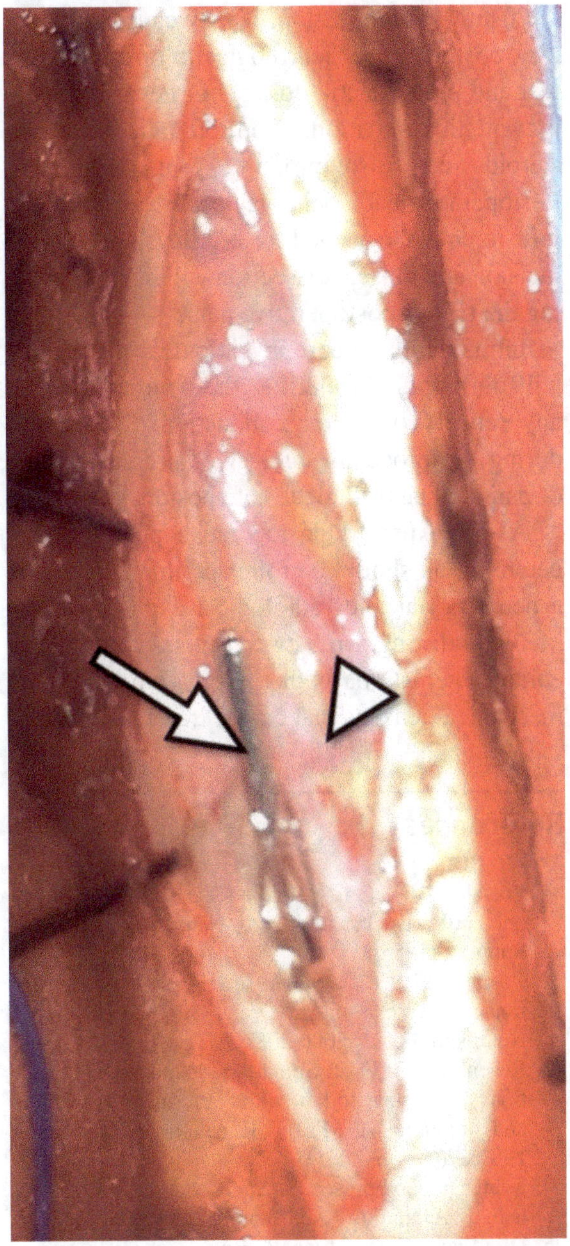

Fig. 28.9 A dAVF case. In this case, the neurosurgeon decided to clip the fistulous vessel with a definitive clip (*arrow*). After clipping, the venous plexus is less engorged (*arrowhead*)

After multiple dura tack-up stitches, the posterior horns of the spinal cord and the superficial AVM are exposed, and a diamond micro-knife is used to make pia mater incision at the border of nidus.

The correlation between angiography features of the AVM and the AVM itself in the operation field is extremely important to allow the early finding of the feeders and venous drainage. If the AVM was previously embolized, the particles inside the vessels can be visualized, and it makes the identification of feeder arteries easier. Normal medullary arteries (especially Adamkiewicz and anterior spinal artery) must be preserved. The dissection of the nidus from the gliotic medullary tissue must be very gentle, and it carries on by using bipolar forceps in the right hand and the suction in the left hand. Bipolar is not only used for cauterization but also as forceps. And the suction tube over a small cottonoid is used as a gentle retractor. The interruption of the feeding arteries is done using the micro-clipping or bipolar coagulation and cutting. When the nidus is totally dissected, bipolar cauterization to shrink the AVM makes its manipulation and final dissection easier. Only prior to the final AVM removal, the drainage veins are coagulated and cut. Abundant irrigation with saline solution and meticulous hemostasis should be achieved.

28.4.3 Spinal Cord Cavernomas

Surgical removal is possible for those spinal cord cavernomas which are located posteriorly or close to the midline. The gently opening of the posterior median sulcus allows to reach cavernomas placed in the midline or deep but adjacent to the posterior median sulcus. Fine dissection of the lesion with micro-instruments (in a similar way than for a well-delineated tumor) allows to remove it completely with low risk of bleeding or coagulation of any artery that supplies the spinal cord. It is important to achieve the gross resection because remnants may cause rebleeding and myelopathy.

For all the procedures described, final hemostasis is mandatory followed by waterproof dura closing in order to avoid postoperative linkage which would contribute to a longer postoperative period. To close the dura, we use 4/0 silk taper-point sutures. Epidural hemostasis is also important. We use bone wax for the bone and Surgicel®, Tachosil®, or fibrin glue for the epidural venous bleeding. If the approach has been made through a laminoplasty, the

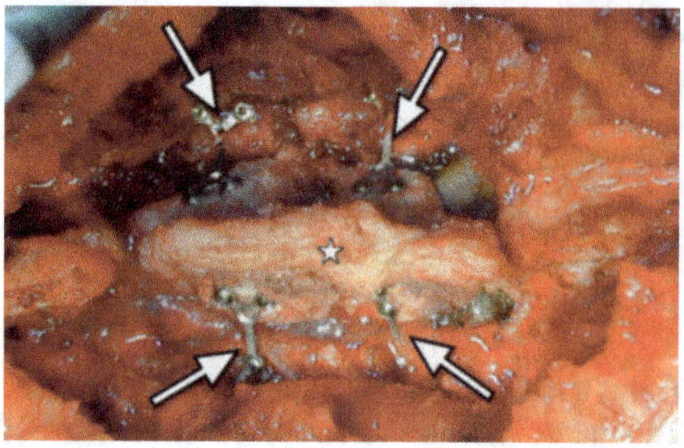

Fig. 28.10 If a laminoplasty is performed, the laminas (*star*) are placed into its original position and fixed by using miniplates (*arrows*)

laminas are replaced at this point and fixed with titanium miniplates (Fig. 28.10).

The muscle and fascia are closed with 0/0 Safil® violet cutting-point sutures and, finally, subcutaneous layers with 2/0 sutures.

28.5 Surgeon Plan to Handle the Complication

The most common complications after spinal cord surgeries are related to the closing. As it has been mentioned above, dura must be closed carefully in order to prevent CSF linkage. We always use tehsil and/or fibrin glue in order to achieve hemostasis but also to reinforce the dura closing. Laminoplasty itself, and the muscle and fascia properly closed as well, helps to prevent pseudomeningocele formation.

When a postoperative CSF leakage by the wound is detected, we order bed rest, external lumbar CSF drainage for 5 days, and prophylactic treatment with antibiotics. If the leakage still persists, a second surgical procedure is performed to identify the location of the defect and close it with stitches or sealants.

After a successful surgery, patient immediate neurological recovery is not expected. Stability of the symptoms and slow recovery are also signs of good results of the procedure. In some situations, especially in dural or perimedullary arteriovenous fistula cases, there is an increasing risk of perimedullary venous plexus thrombosis after the fistula disconnection. It may cause a temporary postoperative neurological worsening. Bed rest and prophylactic dosages of heparin help to prevent this situation. Prothrombotic effects of steroids can also promote vein thrombosis. Postoperative back pain may occur and analgesic infusion may be needed for 2–3 days. Proper skin incision and muscle dissection will help in reducing the risk of postoperative pain.

Intraoperative neurophysiological monitoring will be helpful in alerting the neurosurgeon of any sensory or motor conduction disturbances during the procedure and gives prognostication of patients' neurological state postoperatively.

A non-expected postoperative patient motor deterioration should be followed immediately by a neurological and radiological exploration. An MRI can distinguish between spinal cord edema, epidural hematoma with compression, and other mechanical reasons that can be treated surgically.

References

1. Spetzler RF, et al. Modified classification of spinal cord vascular lesions. J Neurosurg. 2002;96(2 Suppl):145–56.
2. Zozulya YP, et al. Spinal arteriovenous malformations: new classification and surgical treatment. Neurosurg Focus. 2006;20(5):E7.
3. Rosenblum B, et al. Spinal arteriovenous malformations: a comparison of dural arteriovenous fistulas and intradural AVM's in 81 patients. J Neurosurg. 1987;67(6):795–802.
4. Krings T, Geibprasert S. Spinal dural arteriovenous fistulas. AJNR Am J Neuroradiol. 2009;30(4):639–48.
5. Djindjian M, Djindjian R, Rey A, et al. Intradural extramedullary spinal arteriovenous malformation fed by the anterior spinal artery. Surg Neurol. 1977;8:85.
6. Berenstein A, Lasjaunia P. Endovascular treatment of spine and spinal cord lesions. Surgical neuroangiography, vol. 4. Heidelberg: Springer; 1992. p. 24–75.
7. Boström A, Krings T, Hans FJ, Schramm J, Thron AK, Gilsbach JM. Spinal glomus-type arteriovenous malformations: microsurgical treatment in 20 cases. J Neurosurg Spine. 2009;10(5):423–9.
8. Dumont AS, Oldfield EH. Spinal vascular malformations. In: Winn HR, editor. Youmans neurological surgery, vol. 4. Philadelphia: Elsevier; 2011. p. 4167–202.
9. Jellema K, et al. Spinal dural arteriovenous fistulas: clinical features in 80 patients. J Neurol Neurosurg Psychiatry. 2003;74(10):1438–40.

10. Saraf-Lavi E, et al. Detection of spinal dural arteriovenous fistulae with MR imaging and contrast-enhanced MR angiography: sensitivity, specificity, and prediction of vertebral level. AJNR Am J Neuroradiol. 2002;23(5):858–67.
11. Krings T, et al. Imaging in spinal vascular disease. Neuroimaging Clin N Am. 2007;17(1):57–72.
12. Toossi S, et al. Utility of MRI in spinal arteriovenous fistula. Neurology. 2012;79(1):25–30.
13. Lehecka M, Laakso A, Hernesniemi J, Çelik Ö. Helsinki microneurosurgery basics and tricks. 2011. p. 77–8.
14. Simal Julián JA, Miranda Lloret P, López González A, Evangelista Zamora R, Botella Asunción C. Indocyanine green videoangiography in negative: definition and usefulness in spinal dural arteriovenous fistulae. Eur Spine J. 2013;22(Suppl 3):S471–7.

29 Vasospasm Following Aneurysmal Subarachnoid Hemorrhage

Eduardo Vieira and Hildo Azevedo-Filho

29.1 Introduction

Majority of morbidity and mortality due to aneurysmal subarachnoid hemorrhage (aSAH) is secondary to cerebral ischemia. Classically, the angiographic arterial narrowing following aSAH has been termed as angiographic vasospasm, which may or may not lead to clinical manifestations and cerebral ischemia, in which case it would be called symptomatic vasospasm. This concept has recently been questioned. Not always angiographic vasospasm leads to cerebral ischemia, which, in turn, may occur in a territory different from the one irrigated by the narrowed artery or even in the absence of any angiographic vasospasm, i.e., cerebral ischemia that occurs late (days after aSAH) cannot be attributed solely to the arterial narrowing seen on angiography [1]. Currently, the term "delayed cerebral ischemia" (DCI) has been proposed to replace the previously used "symptomatic vasospasm." The clinician should be able to recognize and differentiate the radiological vasospasm from the clinical worsening secondary to DCI, whose etiology is multifactorial and includes angiographic arterial narrowing (Fig. 29.1). Alternative mechanisms have been proposed and include microvascular spasm and failure of cerebral blood flow (CBF) autoregulation, microthrombosis and microembolism, cortical spreading depolarization and ischemia, and delayed neuronal apoptosis resulting from acute brain injury. A more extensive review of the pathophysiology of DCI is out of the scope of this review.

DCI is a diagnosis of exclusion. When there is neurological deterioration, the diagnosis of DCI can only be established when causes like hydrocephalus, hyponatremia, infection, and bleeding are ruled out, and the introduction of hypertensive therapy or endovascular treatment leads to clinical improvement. In the next sessions, we will discuss about the risk factors, prevention, monitoring, and treatment of DCI.

29.2 Risk Factors

The hemoglobin (Hb) in subarachnoid space is a very important factor that triggers vasospasm and DCI. Hb is extremely toxic in the subarachnoid space leading to the rapid activation of cellular adhesion molecules (CAMs) on luminal surface of endothelial cells, enabling macrophages and neutrophils to penetrate into subarachnoid space, where they will phagocytize RBCs and free Hb. After this process, however, macrophages and neutrophils are trapped in the subarachnoid space due to the lack of lymphatic drainage in CNS (central nervous system) and to the difficulty in CSF drainage resulting from aSAH. Between

E. Vieira (✉) · H. Azevedo-Filho
Department of Neurological Surgery, Hospital da Restauracao, Recife, Brazil

J. July, E. J. Wahjoepramono (eds.), *Neurovascular Surgery*,
https://doi.org/10.1007/978-981-10-8950-3_29

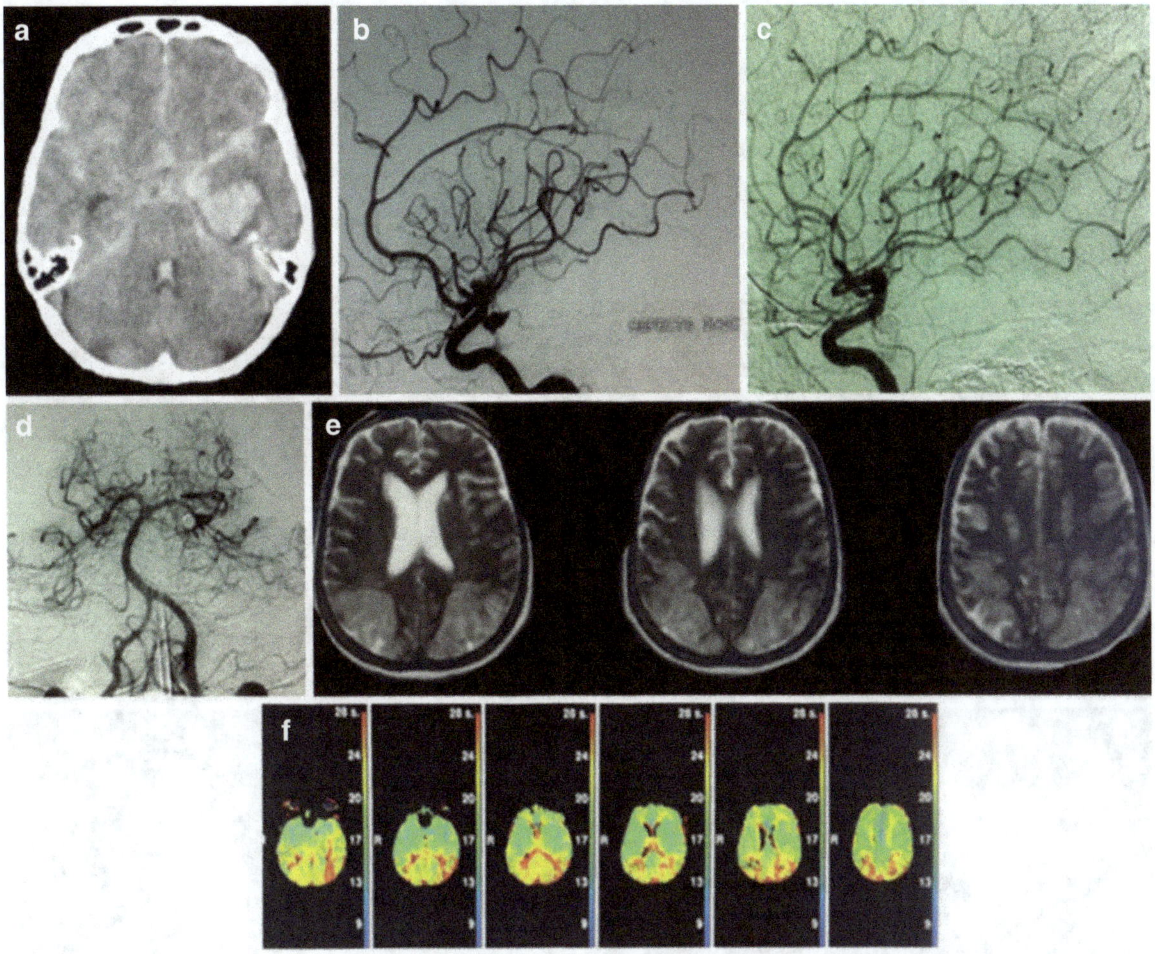

Fig. 29.1 This 72-year-old female patient with a typical history of sudden headache associated with disorientation (HH III) was admitted to hospital. (**a**) CT scan showed a Fisher III with medial temporal hematoma. (**b**) Angiography performed 24 h after admission confirmed an ICA-PCom aneurysm, which was coiled. The patient did well until the ninth day after bleeding, when she became drowsy and unresponsive. (**c**) and (**d**) Angiography performed on the tenth day after bleeding did not reveal vasospasm, and hypertensive therapy was maintained. (**e**) MRI showed ischemic areas predominantly in the territory of posterior cerebral arteries. (**f**) Perfusion study revealed a decreased CBF and CVF, consistent with irreversible ischemia. The cause of DCI is multifactorial, although it's associated with vasospasm, it can occur in the absence of angiographic vasospasm

2 and 4 days, these cells die and disintegrate, releasing intracellular endothelin and free oxygen radicals, leading to vasoconstriction and arteriopathy. That said, it is easy to realize that key factor for DCI is quantity of blood that stays in subarachnoid space.

Quantity of blood in subarachnoid space can be measured by cranial CT and based on this measurement; scales for predicting the possibility of vasospasm were developed. The most widespread and used is the one proposed by Fisher et al. (Table 29.1) [2]. Analyzing this scale, one can notice that patients at highest chance to have vasospasm and DCI are those classified as grade 3, and within this group, there is a wide possible range in quantity of blood present in subarachnoid space, creating a vital variation in probability of developing DCI and vasospasm in patients of the same group of the scale (Fig. 29.2), i.e., the Fisher scale fails to identify those patients at highest risk of developing DCI. Wilson et al. proposed a new scale (BNI scale) (Table 29.1) where the thickness of the clot present in the subarachnoid space was evaluated,

Table 29.1 Comparison between Fisher and BNI scales

Scale	Grade 1	Grade 2	Grade 3	Grade 4	Grade 5
Fisher	No blood	Clot less than 1 mm thick	Clot more than 1 mm thick	Grade 1 or 2 and associated intracerebral hematoma or hemoventricle	–
BNI	No blood	Clot less than 5 mm thick	Clot 5–10 mm thick	Clot 10–15 mm thick	Clot more than 15 mm thick

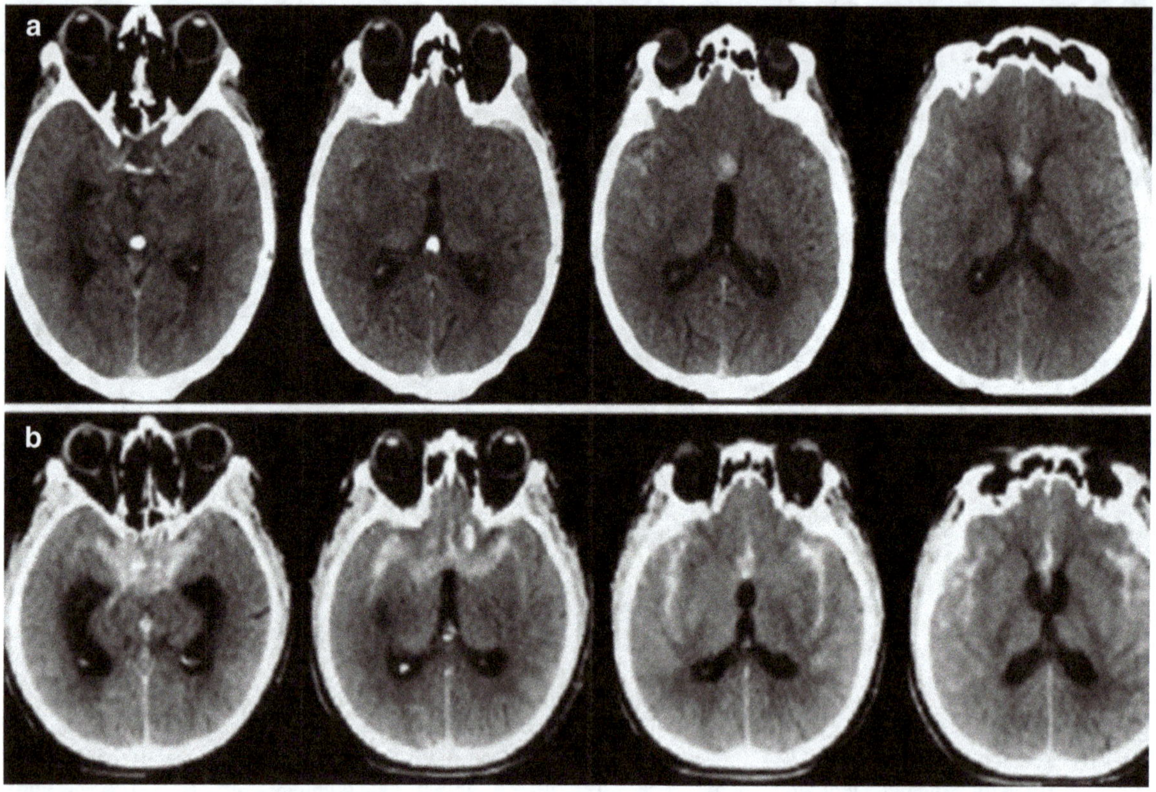

Fig. 29.2 Two patients (A and B) with a Fisher grade 3 aSAH. There is a significant difference between the volumes of blood present in the subarachnoid space between these two patients. Although classified within the same subgroup, patient B has a greater chance of developing vasospasm and DCI with a consequent poor outcome

stratifying those patients grouped as grade 3 in Fisher scale and showing that the size of the thickness of the clot in subarachnoid space is directly proportional to risk of vasospasm and DCI (Table 29.2) [3].

Other risk factors for having the vasospasm and DCI are Hunt-Hess grades 4 and 5, history of hypertension, smoking, early angiographic vasospasm, and young age (<35 years) [4–6]. Hypovolemia is an important and avoidable risk factor that can occur due to cerebral salt-wasting syndrome (CSWS) and should be avoided at all costs.

29.3 Prevention

One of the most important factors in the prevention of DCI is to maintain normovolemia. It is important to emphasize, however, that there is no space for prophylactic hypervolemic therapy, as it does not result in increased CBF nor in better clinical results [7].

The administration of nimodipine, a calcium channel blocker, for 21 days, starting from the moment of admission is probably the only class I recommendation on most recent guiding principle for the management of aSAH from AHA/

Table 29.2 Differences in the incidence of DCI between the BNI and Fisher scales in 218 patients

Fisher scale			BNI scale	
DCI (%)	Distribution (%)	Grade	Distribution (%)	DCI (%)
0	0	**1**	3.7	0
15	6	**2**	33	13
23	83.5	**3**	44.5	22
6	7.3	**4**	12.4	30
–	–	**5**	6.4	50

Using the classification of Fisher, 83.5% of patients are classified as grade 3, and within this subgroup, the greater the thickness of the clot on the CT scan, the greater the chance of DCI

ASA [8]. The drug should be administered orally with 60 mg that is given every 4 h, with a decrease in the relative risk (RR) for DCI of 18% (95% CI = 7–28%) and a number necessary to treat (NNT) of 13 [9, 10]. It is important to emphasize that there is no benefit if the drug is started more than 72 h after bleeding. Importantly, the medication does not prevent vasospasm. It is believed that nimodipine acts through neuroprotective mechanisms, stabilizing cell membranes, decreasing the risk of DCI, and improving patients' outcomes.

Endothelin is a potent vasoconstrictor peptide, mediator of cerebral vasospasm. It is formed through a wide diversity of cells, such as leukocytes and macrophages in the CSF as described above. The use of the inhibitor of endothelin clazosentan was evaluated in different studies.

The results showed that the drug reduces the incidence of angiographic vasospasm in a dose-dependent manner, with no influence, however, on the incidence of DCI and morbidity or mortality [11–14]. This clinical-radiological dissociation is one more data to support the theory that vasospasm cannot, solely, be responsible for DCI.

Statins and magnesium sulfate have been proposed for the prevention of vasospasm and DCI. Two randomized controlled trials (RCTs), the STASH study [15], for statins, and the MASH-2 study [16], for magnesium sulfate, showed that the use of these drugs is of no benefit on the prophylaxis of DCI. Although there is no indication of starting, patients who already use statins may continue the medication after aSAH.

29.4 Monitoring and Diagnosis

The best way to assess and monitor a patient at risk of vasospasm and DCI is through seriated clinical examinations. If there are a decrease level of consciousness and also an onset of new focal deficits, it should prompt investigation in order to exclude hydrocephalus, rebleeding, infection, and hyponatremia. If these entities are all excluded, the diagnosis of DCI is made, and treatment should be instituted as soon as possible.

Critical patients, especially those who already present in coma, are harder to monitor and to evaluate. Because of its noninvasiveness and wide availability, transcranial Doppler ultrasonography (TCD) is the most commonly employed auxiliary method. Although it has high specificity, it lacks sensibility for the development of DCI, especially for territories other than the middle cerebral artery (MCA) [17]. One should never rely solely on TCD to rule out vasospasm and DCI.

In these cases, other auxiliary methods that can be employed are the CT angiography (CTA) and CT perfusion. The CTA has excellent accuracy (98–100%) for severe vasospasm (narrowing>50%) when compared to digital subtraction angiography (DSA) but loses sensitivity in mild to moderate vasospasm (57–85%). CT perfusion complements CT angiography demonstrating perfusion abnormalities, even in the absence of proximal vasospasm. Three parameters are calculated, which, if considered together, can guide the treatment of vasospasm and DCI in critically ill patients:

- Mean transit time (MTT) is the average length of transit time for blood that is located in particular area of the brain. It is defined in seconds.
- Cerebral blood volume (CBV) is the whole blood volume that stays in a certain volume of the brain, which is usually measured in ml/100 g.
- Cerebral blood flow (CBF) is the volume of blood that flows in a certain volume of the brain, which is usually measured in ml/100 g/min.

Table 29.3 Variables to be observed on CT perfusion and treatment to be adopted

MTT	CBV	CBF	Meaning	Treatment
↑	↔ or ↑	↔	Perfusion abnormality adequately compensated by cerebral autoregulation	Close observation
↑	↔ or ↑	↓	Perfusion abnormality with reversible cerebral ischemia (penumbra)	Hypertensive and/or endovascular
↑	↓	↓	Perfusion abnormality with irreversible cerebral ischemia	Not indicated

The MTT is the most sensitive parameter for DCI and vasospasm and should be the first to be evaluated when analyzing the CT perfusion. Increase in MTT demands strict observation of CBV and CBF (Table 29.3) [18]. MRI with diffusion and perfusion sequences is also a good alternative but more expensive, time-consuming, and less available. Although DSA is still defined as a gold standard auxiliary method for diagnosis of vasospasm, its use must be reserved when endovascular treatment of DCI is considered.

29.5 Treatment

Once the diagnosis of DCI is confirmed, appropriate therapy should be started promptly. Classically, the first-line treatment has been the triple-H treatment which includes hypertension, hemodilution, and hypervolemia. Initial goal should be to raise the mean arterial pressure (MAP) by 20% from baseline. If this measure fails, sequential increases of 10% are induced until clinical response is achieved (with a limit of 220 mmHg and 120 mmHg for systolic and diastolic blood pressure, respectively). During this hypertensive therapy, close monitoring of cardiac function is necessary, especially in elderly or high Hunt-Hess grade patients, because they are at greater risk of cardiomyopathy related to aSAH. If, after 6–12 h of triple-H therapy, there is no clinical improvement, then endovascular therapy is indicated.

Recently, the utility of each component from triple-H treatment has been evaluated. Of the three components, the more beneficial one is hypertension, which acts in increasing oxygenation and CBF. Hypervolemia and hemodilution may increase the CBF but have been associated with decreased cerebral tissue oxygenation (PtiO2) [19, 20]. This effect seems to be associated with a decrease in Hb levels caused by hemodilution. During triple-H therapy, hemoglobin concentration should be monitored and should not fall below 9–10 g/dl. In critically ill patients, ideally PtiO2 should be monitored.

Once indicated, endovascular therapy should be performed as soon as possible. Balloon angioplasty is the preferred method and should be used whenever feasible. Usually it is reserved for proximal vasospasm, including supraclinoid ICA, proximal ACA (mainly A1), proximal MCA (M1, M2), vertebral artery (VA), basilar artery (BA), and proximal PCA (P1, P2). Early angiographic studies (baseline) must be assessed before proceeding with angioplasty in order to avoid dilatation of a hypoplastic vessel. Angioplasty at the location of recent clipping of a ruptured aneurysm is not safe and carries high risk of vessel rupture [21]. Intra-arterial infusion of vasodilators (papaverine, milrinone, or, preferably, nimodipine which is a calcium channel blockers) has a modest and ephemeral benefit and should be used in conjunction with balloon angioplasty or in the case of distal vasospasm, in which case angioplasty is not feasible.

References

1. Brown RJ, Kumar A, Dhar R, et al. The relationship between delayed infarcts and angiographic vasospasm after aneurysmal subarachnoid hemorrhage. Neurosurgery. 2013;72(5):702–7.
2. Fisher CM, Kistler JP, Davis JM. Relation of cerebral vasospasm to subarachnoid hemorrhage visualized by computerized tomographic scanning. Neurosurgery. 1980;6:1–9.
3. Wilson DA, Nakaji P, Abla AA, et al. A simple and quantitative method to predict symptomatic vasospasm after subarachnoid hemorrhage based on

computer tomography: beyond the Fisher scale. Neurosurgery. 2012;4:721.
4. Frontera JA, Claassen J, Schmidt JM, et al. Prediction of symptomatic vasospasm after subarachnoid hemorrhage: the modified fisher scale. Neurosurgery. 2006;59:21–7.
5. Rabb CH, Tang G, Chin LS, et al. A statistical analysis of factors related to symptomatic cerebral vasospasm. Acta Neurochir. 1994;127:27–31.
6. Lasner TM, Weil RJ, Riina HA, et al. Cigarette smoking-induced increase in the risk of symptomatic vasospasm after aneurysmal subarachnoid hemorrhage. J Neurosurg. 1997;87(3):381–4.
7. Lennihan L, Mayer SA, Fink ME, et al. Effect of hypervolemic therapy on cerebral blood flow after subarachnoid hemorrhage: a randomized controlled trial. Stroke. 2000;31:383–91.
8. Connolly ES, Rabinstein AA, Carhuapoma JR, et al. Guidelines for the management of aneurysmal subarachnoid hemorrhage: a guideline for healthcare professionals from the American Heart Association/American Stroke Association. Stroke. 2012;43:1711–37.
9. Pickard JD, Murray GD, Illingworth R, et al. Effect of oral nimodipine on cerebral infarction and outcome after subarachnoid haemorrhage: British aneurysm nimodipine trial. BMJ. 1989;298:636–42.
10. Rinkel GJE, Feigin VL, Algra A, et al. Calcium antagonists for aneurysmal subarachnoid haemorrhage. Cochrane Database Syst Rev. 2005;(1):CD000277.
11. MacDonald RL, Kassell NF, Mayer S, et al. Clazosentan to overcome neurological ischemia and infarction occurring after subarachnoid hemorrhage (CONSCIOUS-1): randomized, double-blind, placebo-controlled phase 2 dose-finding trial. Stroke. 2008;39(11):3015–21.
12. MacDonald RL, Higashida RT, Keller E, et al. Clazosentan, an endothelin receptor antagonist, in patients with aneurysmal subarachnoid haemorrhage undergoing surgical clipping: a randomised, double-blind, placebo-controlled phase 3 trial (CONSCIOUS-2). Lancet Neurol. 2011;10(7):618–25.
13. MacDonald RL, Higashida RT, Keller E, et al. Randomized trial of clazosentan in patients with aneurysmal subarachnoid hemorrhage undergoing endovascular coiling. Stroke. 2012;43(6):1463–9.
14. Vergouwen MD, Algra A, Rinkel GJ. Endothelin receptor antagonists for aneurysmal subarachnoid hemorrhage: a systematic review and metaanalysis update. Stroke. 2012;43(10):2671–6.
15. Kirkpatrick PJ, Tuner CL, Smith C, Hutchinson PJ, Murray GD. Simvastatin in aneurysmal subarachnoid haemorrhage (STASH): a multicenter randomized phase 3 trial. Lancet Neurol. 2014;13(7):666–75.
16. Dorhout Mees SM, Algra A, Vandertop WP, et al. Magnesium for aneurysmal subarachnoid haemorrhage (MASH-2): a randomised placebo-controlled trial. Lancet. 2012;380(9836):44–9.
17. Lysakowski C, Walder B, Costanza MC, et al. Transcranial Doppler versus angiography in patients with vasospasm due to a ruptured cerebral aneurysm: a systematic review. Stroke. 2001;32:2292–8.
18. Binaghi S, Colleoni ML, Maeder P, et al. CT angiography and perfusion CT in cerebral vasospasm after subarachnoid hemorrhage. AJNR Am J Neuroradiol. 2007;28(4):750–8.
19. Dankbaar JW, Slooter AJ, Rinkel GJ, et al. Effect of different components of triple-H therapy on cerebral perfusion in patients with aneurysmal subarachnoid haemorrhage: a systematic review. Crit Care. 2010;14(1):R23.
20. Raabe A, Beck J, Keller M, et al. Relative importance of hypertension compared with hypervolemia for increasing cerebral oxygenation in patients with cerebral vasospasm after subarachnoid hemorrhage. J Neurosurg. 2005;103(6):974–81.
21. Linskey ME, Horton JA, Rao GR, et al. Fatal rupture of the intracranial carotid artery during transluminal angioplasty for vasospasm induced by subarachnoid hemorrhage. Case report. J Neurosurg. 1991;74(6):985–90.

30 Retractorless Surgery of Vascular Lesions

Thomas Kretschmer, Christian Heinen, and Thomas Schmidt

30.1 Introduction

The introduction of the operating microscope enabled modern neurosurgery. For usually deep-seated vascular lesions and confining, overhanging brain parenchyma walls, self-retaining retractors were necessary to enable open and safe dissection corridors. However, retractors also exert secondary pressure effects and can limit the degree of manual freedom [1].

Since longer a rigid retractor-free technique for cerebral surgery in general and cerebrovascular pathology in particular has been propagated. Professor Yasargil's published comment on Kivisaari et al.'s 2000 paper on sequelae of retractor use [2] merits reiteration: "most prominent finding supports that one-third (36%) of the patients is related with brain retractor. All effort to reduce the use of brain retractor such as wide splitting of the sylvian fissure, release the CSF from the basal cisterns, and the use of mannitol, should be done with also the attention to appreciate all arteries and veins during dissection."

Despite lower surgical case rates after publication and unjustified generalization of the ISAT 2002 results [3], cerebrovascular surgery developed substantially and in proficient hands at many centers changed toward considerably more focused, efficient, and extremely tissue sparing surgery [4]. As was put forward by the Spetzler group discussion, the 3-year BRAT results have also pointed out that if the surgeon avoids using the rigid retraction during complex aneurysm surgery, it will avoid adjacent brain injury [4].

To date a growing community of neurosurgeons thus adopted a retractorless dissection technique by making full use of neurosurgeries' current armamentarium, merging all the long known knowledge and tricks with the tools of modern microsurgery. Implementation of a bimanual dissection technique without rigid fixation but rather intensive use of microscope mouthpiece and foot control enables us to work within very confined spaces perfectly safe.

30.2 Brain Retraction

Brain retraction can produce high local pressure on the brain and then reduce the blood flow locally, and some surgeon said that the retractor could hide the anatomy under the retractor. If the brain swelling, sometimes the retractor also directly injures and sometimes cut through the brain. Narrow rigid retractor blades on already edematous tissue lead to even higher tissue pressures (e.g., incising retractor edges). Brain retraction for several minutes to hours can exert permanent pressure effects. Some of these effects can be demonstrated on post-op MRI [5]: high

T. Kretschmer (✉) · C. Heinen · T. Schmidt
Department of Neurosurgery, Evangelisches Krankenhaus Oldenburg, Oldenburg, Germany

J. July, E. J. Wahjoepramono (eds.), *Neurovascular Surgery*,
https://doi.org/10.1007/978-981-10-8950-3_30

signal was demonstrated in one-third of clipped aneurysm cases during follow-up (36/101 cases). They were located at the basal frontotemporal area of the approach in aneurysm clippings of the anterior circulation. These signals could be traced 2–6 years after surgery and thus were interpreted as signs of damage.

30.3 With Fixed Retractors

Working with self-retaining, rigid retractors enables and favors a different style of dissection and is possible without the use of a microscope mouthpiece. The retractors not only create an open view on the exposed pathology but also free the hands to easily move out of the operative site to adjust for zoom, focus, or microscope head-piece position or receive and change instruments. A set retractor usually opens a funnel-shaped straight corridor from the surface to the depth to allow for an unimpeded view to the bottom of the created corridor. During the course of surgery, retractors are frequently reset. Long-standing brain retraction or retraction on swollen or "red and angry" brain can induce direct and instantly visible parenchyma damage. Expert microsurgeons make a point that proper retractor setting never exerts pressure but only is placed on the brain surface as shelter.

30.4 Without Fixed Retractors

In principle of retractorless surgery, dynamic and constantly alternating mini-retraction is applied by the microinstruments to proceed along natural sulcal and fissural trails until the pathology is reached. So, in its true sense, surgery is not retraction-free but free of fixed retraction. Craniotomies are planned in a way to create corridors by gravity even before dissection starts. The combined measures of optimal positioning, "custom-tailored" focused craniotomy with drilling on the cranial base side, adequate anesthesia for slack brain, and CSF drainage via the cisterns plus meticulous bloodless dissection most of the time opens a dissection corridor that will stay open on its own without additional measures (see figures for approach examples). So, there is no need to pull parenchyma out of the way. The created dissection corridors remain open. We are sure that anyone who made a "successful" transition from the use of fixed retraction to retractorless also experienced that his way to handle brain and vessels developed in equal measure, as the need for more effective movement arises, and back and forth movements are discouraged.

30.5 Elements

30.5.1 Operative Field (Fig. 30.1)

The surgeons' hands need to be unrestricted and free at all times.

For this the operative field should be tidy and not overcrowded by appliances, tubing, and cables. We prefer to have nothing in the field that could potentially interfere with our hands. Everything not on the side opposite to the surgeon like a Leyla bar is attached to two adjustable rods attached to the head clamp (Mayfield system). We prefer to set up the rods like a frame around the head resembling a tilted V. This V-frame is positioned far below the plane of craniotomy to ensure that the attached soft tissue hooks can be kept low profile and are not spanned out above the craniotomy. Everything

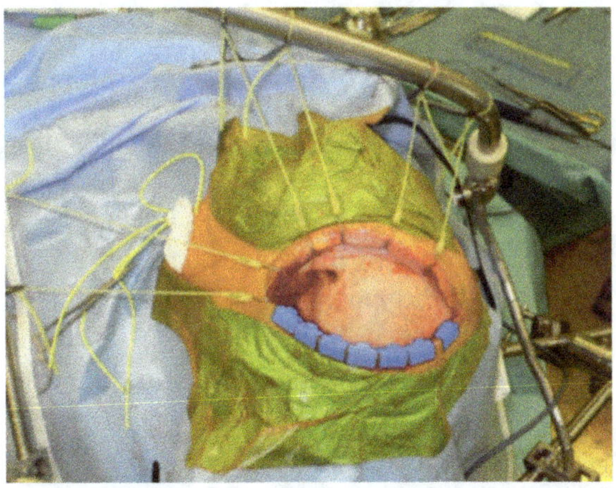

Fig. 30.1 Operative field. The field needs to be set up tidy and kept absolutely clean, and any clutter from cables and extensions should be avoided to keep the space above the craniotomy clear for unrestricted movement of hands

else attached to the rods will also be fixed in such a manner. With Sugita frames, the system as such implements a ring that is placed following the same principles.

30.5.2 Microscope

The use of a microscope is precondition to modern neurosurgery: retractorless neurosurgery relates to intracranial neurosurgery during the microscopic phase of surgery. Retractorless neurosurgery is dependent on microscopes that can be operated with a mouthpiece. It is not possible to perform retractorless microsurgery with microscopes that exclusively need to be repositioned manually. The microscope needs to be especially well balanced if it is worked with a mouthpiece in order to prevent annoying micro-oscillation after release and engagement of brakes via the mouthpiece.

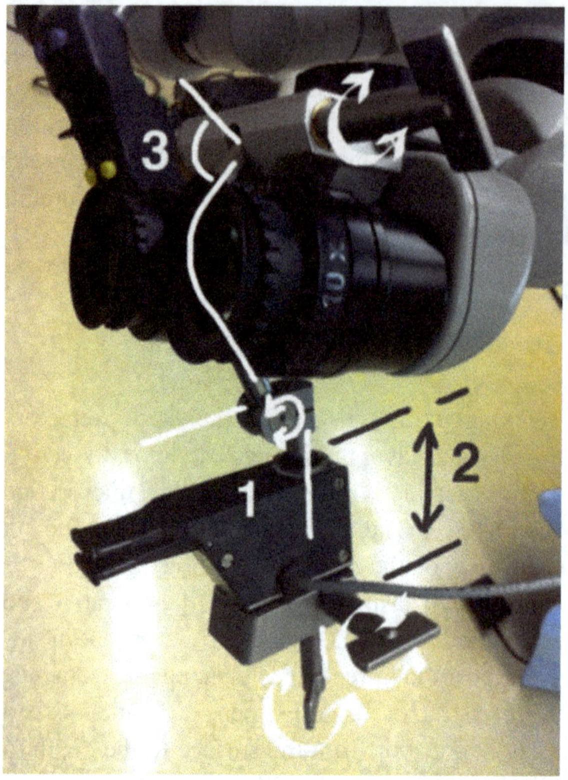

Fig. 30.2 Mouthpiece. Mastering use of the mouthpiece is absolute key to retractorless surgery. A first step is to be able to properly position it in the mouth to not interfere with the accustomed head and eye lens position. Therefore, it can be adapted by changing its position in two planes. The joints marked at 1 and 3 enable movement in an axial plane to bring the piece forward into the mouth. Number 2 marks possible vertical movement. The three screws are loosened, head and eyes are brought in the operative position, and then the mouthpiece is guided into the mouth in a way that the lips can have close contact with the mouthpiece blades

30.5.3 Mouthpiece (Fig. 30.2)

The proper position of the mouthpiece needs to be individually adjusted for every surgeon, and even for every surgeon individually for every case, as the main direction and angle of the microscope head will depend on the approach used. So, for posterior fossa surgery, a far steeper angle in the sagittal plane is used in comparison to the alignment for a supratentorial convexity process.

For adjusting the mouthpiece, the microscope head is brought in the anticipated direction, the pupillary distance is set on the oculars, and the head and eyes are brought in the surgeon's usual position. Then all three locking screws are opened, and the mouthpiece is introduced in the mouth, with contact of the upper plate to the upper teeth and lip; the microscope head brakes are disengaged when the lower mouthpiece plate is released by gentle pressure of the lower lip. By holding the released position with the lower lip, the microscope head will float, if the microscope has been properly balanced (as opposed to pull in one direction if not balanced). Now, it is possible to steer the microscope with the mouth in three planes. Thus, it can be steered to easily follow the focus point of dissection. By slightly changing the distance of the microscope in relation to the surgical plane, the focus can be adapted and fine-tuned without having to use the focus button of the microscope/foot paddle constantly. By using this technique for subtle focus adaption, the focus change by microscope handle or foot paddle will be only necessary for larger focus changes. Once used to this tool, the involved maneuvers pass off completely "subcortical." This becomes the surgeon's major tool to prevent frequent in and out maneuvers of the surgeons' hands out of the surgical site. It is precondition to establish a real flow of movements and improves surgical efficiency immensely, since every movement and instrument maneuver lead to advance dissection one step further without being interrupted by frequent adaption movements. The other merit is true bimanual work in the sense of alternating the "leading" hand (if there is one) in dependence on suitability of current position and not freedom of hand. Coarser adjustments of the microscope by movement via microscope head handles are disengaged and only necessary less frequently. Most coarse adjustments can be executed with a foot pedal (zoom-focus-position of microscope head).

30.5.4 Foot Pedal (Fig. 30.3)

The foot pedal has at least two rocker-like pedals that are used for bidirectional zoom and focus. Usually on the pedal frame, there are additional knobs that can be individually set for other functions (photo documentation, light adjustment, video start/stop). There are foot pedals that have an integrated joystick that allows for stepless adjustment of the microscope head in all planes. In interplay with an armrest chair, a wireless pedal avoids cable clutter at the surgeons' feet and eases change of chair position.

30.5.5 Chair or Other Means of Armrest (Fig. 30.4)

Resting the forearms or at least the hand by contact of the small finger on the surface to stabilize the hand is a basic microsurgical principle. It eases and enables precise finger and instrument movements. Appropriate chairs with mounted armrests can be used independent from patient positioning and method of head fixation. There are many useful models, depending on the individual preferences.

Several points with regard to positioning of the surgeon are crucial to aid microsurgery as

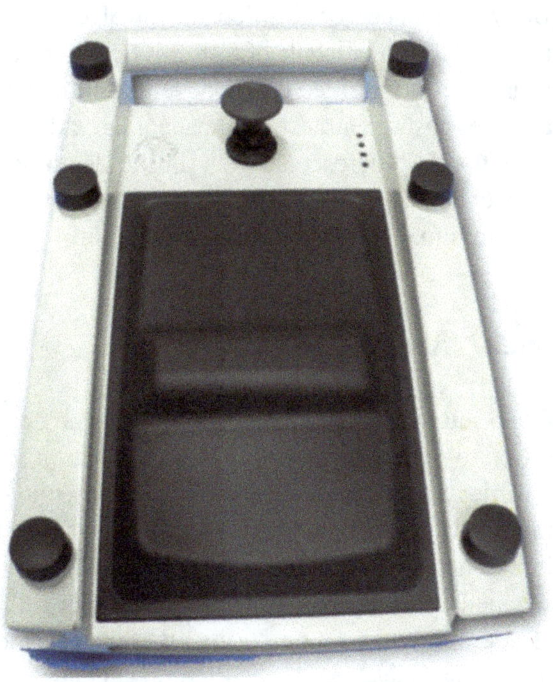

Fig. 30.3 Foot pedal. Foot pedals can serve multiple functions with freely selectable function allocation to several knobs (e.g., photo, video on/off, ±light, ICG on/off). The joystick steers the microscope head; ±zoom and ±focus can be allocated to the left or right side. Wireless function transmission avoids cable clutter

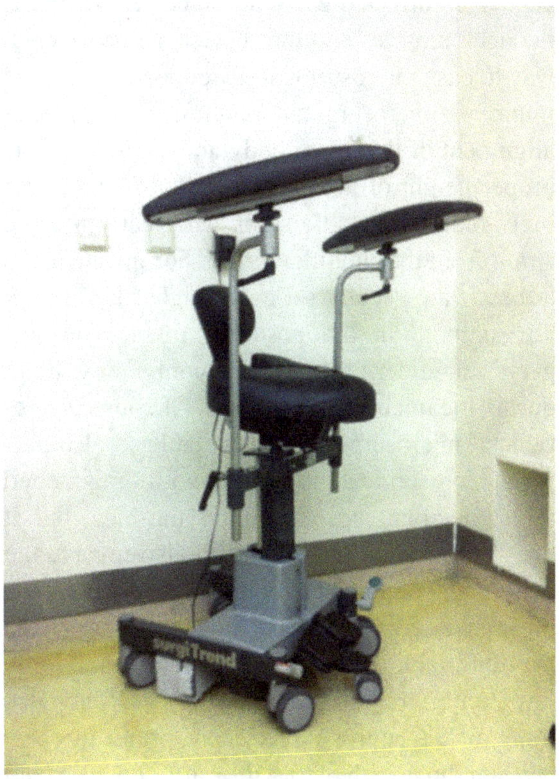

Fig. 30.4 Armrest and chair. Chair and armrests should be adjustable in every plane and height to accustom for all possible surgeon and patient positions. Useful is a function that enables to move the armrests backward and forward. The base should not protrude too much forward in order to avoid interference with foot pedals

such, and long, concentrated microsurgical work in particular, as well as to improve security of risky maneuvers. The precondition of rested forearms is easier to achieve in a setting where the surgeon works on the surface of an extremity (e.g., reconstructive microsurgical hand surgery, where you can place and rest your hand on an arm table or microsurgical work at the surface of the head). It is not so easy, however, to achieve if working under uncomfortable angles in the depth of the neurocranium. To spend some time to think about the adequate position of the surgeon is absolutely helpful and required to perform long-standing retractorless microsurgical work. It should be comfortable enough to allow for long dissection, it should enable to rest the forearms without compromise, and it should not interfere at all with the head clamp and its extensions. Neurosurgeons tend to bend their neck forward and take up a swan neck posture. This is a small detail that probably only can be prevented if corrected early in the career; it strains the neck muscles and the cervical spine. A great way to ease microsurgical dissection as such and improve microsurgical endurance is proper alignment of the upper body and shoulders. The proper height of flexible armrests of an accordingly multi-adjustable stool can greatly remove strain from the shoulder girdle. For instance, the armrests are usually set much higher if working retrosigmoid in the posterior fossa. The surgeon's shoulder girdle should not be tense at all during the microsurgical phase. Of course, experienced microsurgeons will be able to also perform microsurgical movements with straightened arms, involving also shoulder muscles; but it does not make a lot of sense to also involve the deltoid and trapezius in microsurgery if it can be prevented (e.g., doing CP angle surgery in an uncomfortable position below the craniotomy level with straight arms to reach far enough). Some of the neurosurgical icons prefer to operate standing with a flexible arm board stand because they will be fast enough to not require a sitting position and rather prefer to be able to frequently change their own standing position in relation to the patient. The principle still remains the same. A standing position, however, excludes comfortable simultaneous use of two or more foot pedal-driven devices (multifunction foot pedal, bipolar, ultrasonic aspirator). When a pedal is used standing, the surgeon completely bears his weight on one leg for the time using the pedal. This can be bothersome, when you make continuous use of one or two pedal devices.

30.5.6 Cisterns

The ability to open cisterns fast and tissue sparing is pivotal to open a microsurgical dissection corridor at the beginning of the microsurgical phase of surgery.

Knowledge of appropriate measures to reach the decisive neighboring cistern shortly after craniotomy is thus very important. Reaching the cistern very early is largely connected to precise placement of craniotomy and measures for slack brain to avoid undue pressure on brain parenchyma in order to reach deep.

Additional space is gained by reducing the bone right after craniotomy, before dural opening. Bony eminences or the floor of involved skull base and the inner tabula of respective craniotomy rims are neatly drilled down. Several millimeters at the exposure entrance can make a large difference for the microscopic view in the depth and frequently enable to reach a cistern with no or only minimal and short retraction of brain.

30.5.7 Anesthesiology

Good interaction with anesthesiology is precondition to reach the necessary brain relaxation for effortless opening of surgical corridors without the use of fixed retraction. We like to start fast infusion of mannitol after the patient has been prepped and draped to reach its full effect right after craniotomy. Among many other factors, the following anesthesiological competencies are quite essential:

- Awareness for the kind of surgery undertaken.
- Awareness of pathology.
- Awareness of cerebral condition.

- Awareness of possible hazardous complications and resultant need for instant and adequate response.
- Appropriate maneuvers to slacken the brain.
- Experience with induction of measures to increase brain tolerance to ischemia from intentional temporary clipping of major branches.

As for drugs:

- Mannitol to dehydrate brain tissue (1 g/kg).
- Decadron to minimize edema from pressure effects or other mechanical injuries depending on the individual pathology.
- ICG application.
- Systemic adenosine administration for emergency cardiac standstill.

30.5.8 Instruments Used

There are no magic instruments; it is the handling of them. All the usual microinstruments can be used. Some instruments like clip appliers have been especially designed for keyhole approaches with long, narrow shafts and modified clip mechanisms. Lighted instrument tips are the current novelty. A major tool remains the suction device. There is great variance in terms of shape, length, tip design, and fenestration for suction strength regulation.

The sucker is by far more than a mere suction device, and its full potential as dynamic macro- and microretractor, tissue dissector, and tissue aspirator is to be discovered. Its potential for stepless suction force control needs to be mastered. Precise control of suction force with the thumb over the opening is absolute key (rolling the thumb back and forward over the fenestration). We prefer a keyhole-teardrop-shaped opening to a circular one as it allows for fine-tuned suction control, especially for cerebrovascular work.

The merit of special instruments as such is completely overrated, as we think every surgeon needs to find out and decide on some basic microinstruments that allow him to manage the bulk of his microsurgical work. Permanent use of, and getting used to, the same instruments is the real key. Consequently, our basic trays might appear quite reduced, and are not stuffed with instruments. We rather open separate instruments according to real need for them (e.g., special curette, plate knife, fish-hooked knife). However, it greatly helps to not wait for instruments, which have to be frequently cleaned during surgery (e.g., bipolar forceps). So, it might make sense to have several of the same type on the table, to not stop the surgical flow abruptly because an instrument is cleaned. In fact, if you work retractorless, and especially during a demanding microsurgical phase, it is quite bothersome, tiring, and also dangerous if you frequently were to wait with an outreached arm for an instrument while being completely focused to the pathology and, at the same time, holding a vessel or part of the brain with your dynamic retraction device at the other hand.

Only very few surgeons are ambidextrous in its true sense, and most of them still will have a more dominant (e.g., mainly cutting) hand. However, if working retractorless, it is very useful if the surgeon is not dependent on using a microscissors or knife exclusively with his dominant hand. A good surgical flow can then be established if a structure that needs to be held, retracted, or cut is handled in that way at the moment where this becomes clear without any more time delay by changing hand. Going back and forth before execution of a maneuver is not efficient (e.g., realize adhesion that just became visible by slight microretraction of tissue needs to be cut, letting loose again, look again, reconfirm several times, and then execute the maneuver). It is obvious that the hand that is the easiest to perform a certain maneuver might be on the right or left in dependence on the hand that performs the microretraction maneuver at the moment.

Think of:

- Removing the bone or sacrifice the skull base bone rather than the brain.
- Using one of the hands as dynamic suction and alternating to the other side so the surgeon may avoid the need of retractor.
- Sucker tip retraction—As microretraction.
- Sucker shaft retraction—As macroretraction.
- Microscissors and bipolar shafts that also allow for soft retraction and temporarily can retract their side of the dissection funnel.

- Microretraction with instrument tips.
- Use all the fingers efficiently including the use of the thumb to control fenestration.

30.6 Advantages of Retractorless Dissection Technique

In combination with the mentioned techniques, we see the following advantages of a retractor-free dissection technique:

- More thought on approach planning, positioning, and trajectory.
- Free surgical field.
- Concentration on manual maneuvers and approach tactics.
- Forced use of mouthpiece and foot pedal, therefore more freedom of hands and less unnecessary in and out maneuvers of the hands.
- No manual readjustment of zoom, focus, and microscope head alignment.
- Thus, improved surgical flow by omission of redundant movements and readjustments.
- Overall streamlined (efficient and effective) surgery.
- Less collateral damage.

30.7 Learning and Transition

Retractorless surgery goes completely along with the principles of "safe and simple surgery" outlined by Hernesniemi and the Helsinki group [6]. The novice should learn the technique and basic principles during surgery by assisting an expert that is willing to point out the elements. Adopting the necessary techniques will be a gradual approach from easier to increasingly complex pathology. To always have fixed retractors mounted and ready to use is a good practice to not put the patient at risk should a situation occur where the surgeon was more confident with a retractor in place; plus, it helps to improve one's own confidence, as no time is lost should the need for fixed retraction arise.

Naturally it is easier to begin working on superficial pathology that is not covered by parenchyma. Good positioning uses gravity to move a lobe caudally in order to open up a corridor (e.g., pathology side facing downward). Less instruments will be used more and more intensely allocating them more than one function. So, dynamic retraction is possible with the shaft of an instrument for more macroscopic shift of tissue or in a true microsurgical manner by using the instrument's tip. For instance, one will find that a scissor is not restricted to the use of cutting tissue.

A completely clean operative field with only low-profile attachments, restriction to fewer instruments, less cotton patties (one displayed at the instrument trajectory is usually enough), and less of anything obstructing the view is key to increased maneuverability in the operative corridor especially so for cerebrovascular surgery with the need for clip application. Even with a fixed retractor technique, creation of a "cottonoma" around the pathology never is a good idea.

It is easier to protect uncovered tissue. To focus on deep-seated areas implies the use of a high (or the highest) zoom factor. At the same time, superficial tissue that is not in focus must not be put at risk or maltreated by untoward instrument contact and pressure (e.g., instrument shafts).

Precise and bloodless arachnoid and sulcal opening by different means and maneuvers is key to open spaces that will unfold into dissection corridors.

The "water dissection technique" is a great way to open closed space perfectly clean and tissue-protecting [7].

30.8 Suggestion to Avoid Complication

- Be aware of attempting a complete retractorless approach on your own if you are technically not ready yet.
- Be aware of false ambition, in a situation, where a retractor would enhance your surgery and simply put would be the better choice for the patient's brain.
- Be aware of created dissection corridors that do not allow for sufficient view. "Sufficient view" is quite relative and depends to a part also on already existing expertise.
- Be aware of making compromises to work retractorless.

- Retractorless dissection technique alone does not do the trick; it is the involved tissue sparing and bloodless clean and very meticulous necessary technique that is necessary for work without the use of a fixed retractor that will lead to a save, more focused, and fast tissue sparing flow of surgery.

30.8.1 Vascular Pathology with Higher Likelihood to Need Fixed Retraction Within Transition Process

- MCA—Depending on Sylvian fissure configuration and opening, brain edema and atrophy will require temporary fixed retraction for the non-experienced to prevent the lobes falling back into the dissection corridor.
- AComA aneurysms—Will be difficult to do without fixed retraction and mini-craniotomy if not already experienced with retractorless dissection technique.

30.9 Approach Examples

The figure series shows examples of created dissection corridors for different vascular pathology and approaches.

30.9.1 Anterior Circulation

30.9.1.1 Lateral Supraorbital (Fig. 30.5)

This is our preferred approach for anterior circulation pathology. A craniotomy cut flush to the

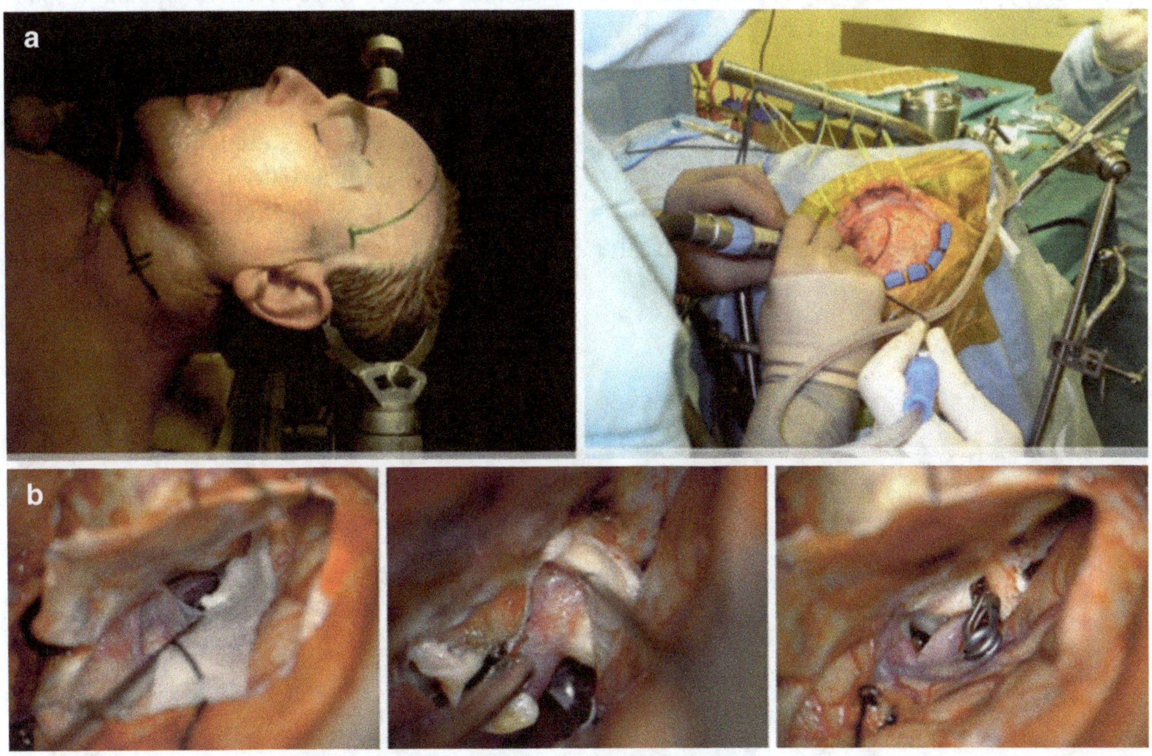

Fig. 30.5 Lateral supraorbital approach. (**a**) Positioning and incision for ophthalmic artery aneurysm on the left side with head elevated and reclined only mildly turned to the right with additional skin mark for exposure of carotid artery for proximal control (*left image*). Right craniotomy with free surgical field and attachment bars far below surgical plane to enable free hand movements (*right image*). (**b**) Left—surgical corridor right after cistern has been opened without additional retraction due to craniotomy cut flush with frontal floor and dura pulled over the bone. Middle—exposure of ICA (sucker on artery), optic nerve lifted with dissector, below and left of dissector ophthalmic artery, below and right of dissector the calcified aneurysm. Partially drilled anterior clinoid process in front and left of suction with mobilized dural lip in left corner. External dural ring already opened and optic canal partially unroofed to allow for secure optic nerve mobilization. Right—surgical site with aneurysm clipped, dural flap folded back

cranial base, and a reflected dura pulled well over this base, opens a subfrontal corridor even before the optic cistern is opened. It is thus very easy to open the cistern right from the beginning without placement of a retractor.

30.9.1.2 Sylvian Fissure (Fig. 30.6)

Doing the opening of Sylvian fissure with full focus and fast, is a very important dissection module [8–10]. It is important to have a good orientation to not choose the wrong trajectory and get lost in the fissure. Taking into account the position of the patient head in relation to the floor (angled down) is key to not move to along the wrong trajectory. Flushing the fissure with saline intermittently to open it up is a great way to help dissection (water dissection technique after Toth; see above).

30.9.1.3 Interhemispheric (Fig. 30.7)

ACA aneurysms are classically approached interhemispherically. A corridor can be created no matter if the head is in neutral or in 90° turned position. For this we do not see the need for additional lumbar drainage. The depicted example of a large thalamic cavernoma demonstrates how trajectory planning, use of navigation, and gravity can greatly help to create a minimal invasive but large (enough) corridor for removal of pathology in an eloquent area.

30.9.1.4 Subtemporal (Fig. 30.8)

Subtemporal work is manageable without retraction. Retractors placed subtemporally tend to create marked pressure effects even if placed extradural. Key to retractorless at this location is placement of a lumbar drain and ample CSF drainage (30–60 ml). This is the only approach, where we use routine lumbar drainage.

30.9.2 Posterior Circulation

30.9.2.1 Retrosigmoid Suboccipital (Fig. 30.9)

For retrosigmoid approaches we prefer the patient at supine position and the head turned slightly. After the cisterna magna has been opened, there is ample room to dissect. There is enough space to drill the petrous bone as shown or remove large pathology. Large pathology and frequent use of table repositioning are made in dependence on dissection trajectory (e.g., brain stem/cerebellum table is angled toward floor, toward tentorium table is angled up, and toward petrous bone table is rotated in longitudinal axis).

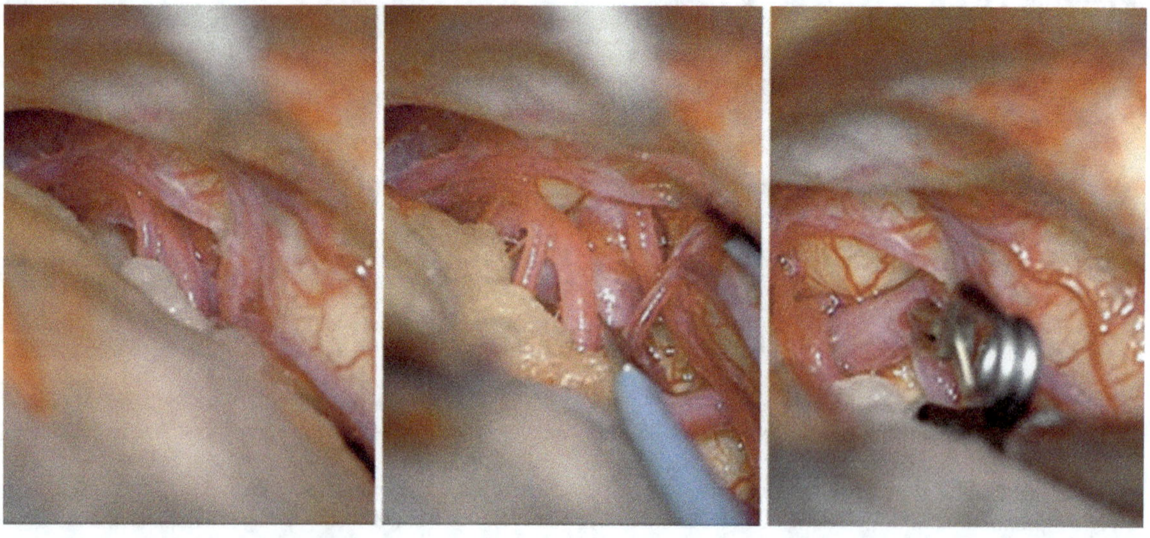

Fig. 30.6 Trans-Sylvian approach. Focused opening and clipping of left Sylvian fissure via lateral supraorbital approach for small, broad-based media aneurysm

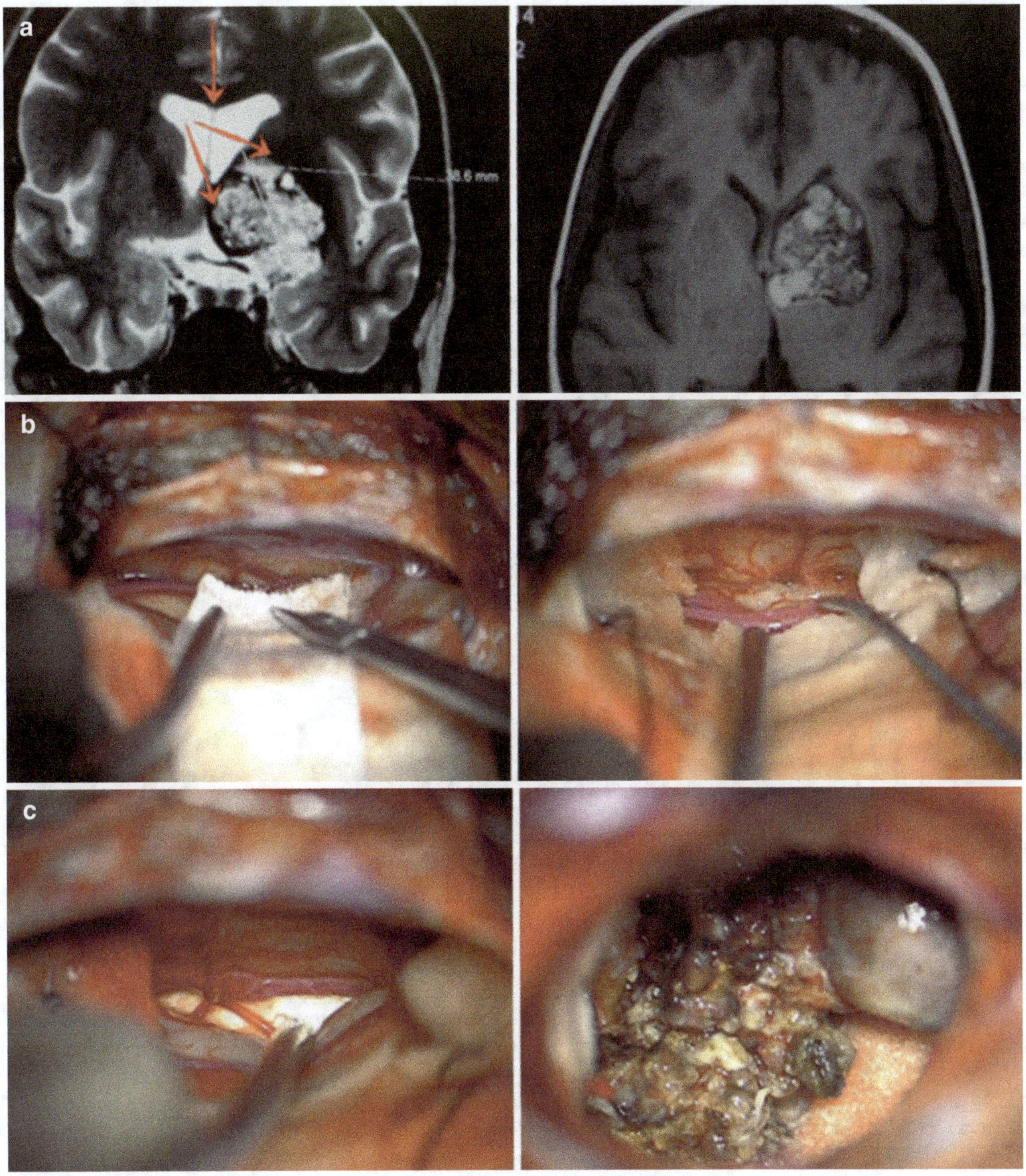

Fig. 30.7 Interhemispheric approach. Depicted is an interhemispheric approach with a contralateral transcallosal route for a basal ganglia cavernoma. (**a**) Left—coronal view of left basal ganglia cavernoma and interhemispheric-contralateral-transcallosal route in order to obtain a direct view on the cavernoma once the right frontal lobe recedes back by gravity. Right—axial view of cavernoma. (**b**) Left—patient is placed supine-semilateral, head is turned 45° with temporal squama parallel to floor and raised in order to erect the falx from a "parallel-to-floor" position to around 60° angled to floor. A mini-craniotomy traversing the sagittal sinus was fashioned. The dura can be seen pedicled into direction of the sagittal sinus and gently pulled back by dural stitches in order to allow a direct view to the falx. Adhesions have been released, and the right frontal lobe did already recede underneath the dura. Right—dissection already progressed deeper to below falx level, as can be seen by contralateral frontal lobe. (**c**) Left—glistening white of corpus callosum underneath suction tip. Right—partially dissected cavernoma after some coagulation for size shrinking, placed within ventricle depicting typical mulberry appearance. In order to reach different parts of this large process, the trajectory is systematically changed in dependence on part of cavernoma addressed. This is reached by changing patient/OR table and microscope head position alike (e.g., Trendelenburg/reversed Trendelenburg, rotation around longitudinal axis of patient)

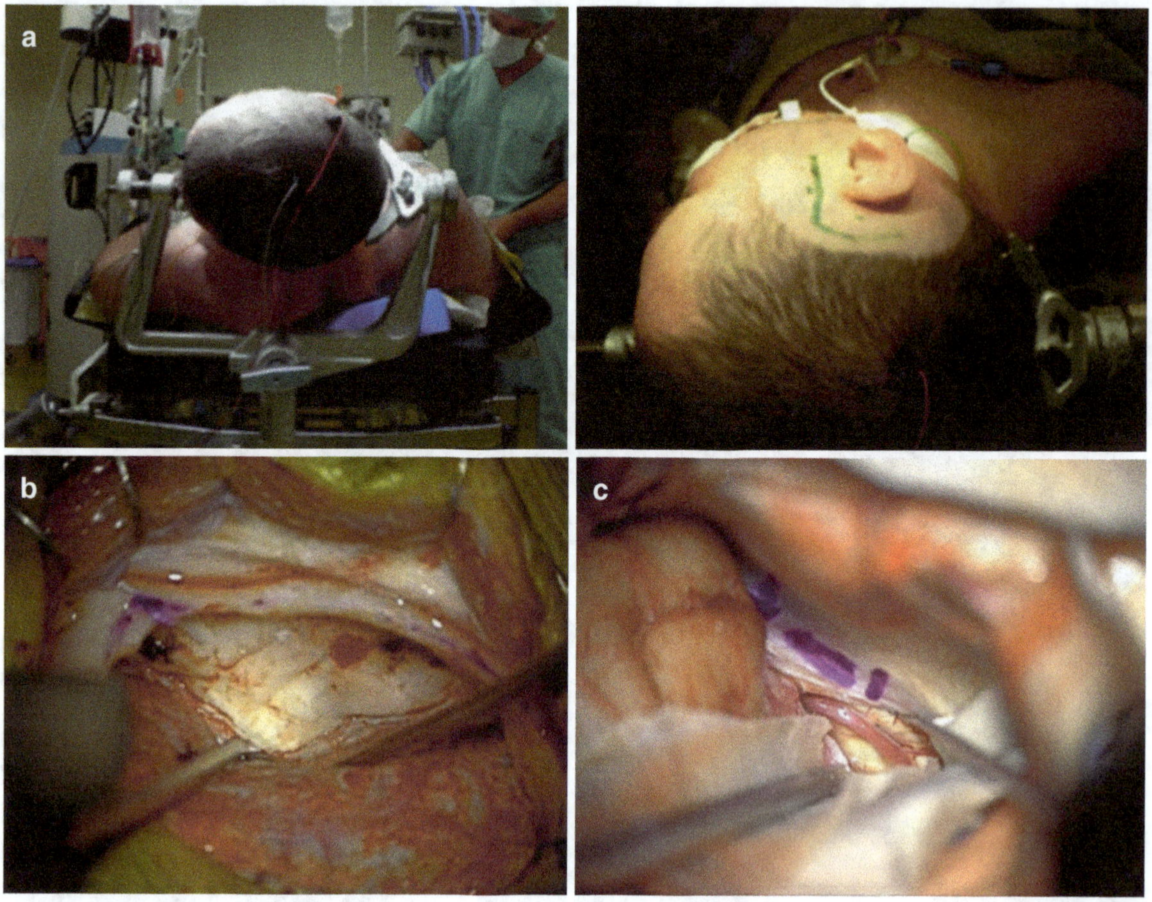

Fig. 30.8 Subtemporal approach. Easily, obtainable space in a subtemporal approach. Prerequisite is prior lumbar drainage. (**a**) Above—patient position with head elevated above heart level, temporal squama parallel to floor by placement of right shoulder bolster (*blue*) and turning the head 60–70° to the left. Below—hockey stick/L-shaped/straight skin incision mark; incisions are variable depending on planned shape of craniotomy (more horizontal width vs height) accentuating either vertical or horizontal part. (**b**) Extradural view on petrous bone exposing anterior and dorsal rim and beginning of petrosal tip without retraction, after proper positioning, drainage of 50 ml CSF, and low mini-craniotomy cut close to floor (on purpose not completely flush, for pathology approached in this case). (**c**) Subtemporal view on ponto-mesencephalic vein for extirpation of ponto-mesencephalic cavernoma. Narrow dark line above vein from middle to right arises from cavernoma gleaming through. Sucker on cotton patty placed on subtemporal cortex. Dissector on tentorial edge, tentorium marked with blue pen

30.10 Expert Opinion

A retractorless technique forces the surgeon to make full use of the known microsurgical techniques in a very meticulous way. At the same time, it opens the mind to avoid any unnecessary adjuncts of surgery and leads to a very target directed way of surgery circumventing unnecessary moves. Every surgical maneuver and movement should lead to a dissection progress. The surgeons' hands stay within the operative site, and frequent in and out movements of the hands are to be avoided.

As a result, the dissection progress of somebody used to work microsurgically without any retractor is usually very straightforward. Brute maneuvers need to be avoided at all times. Retractorless advancement only makes sense if it is less traumatic as compared to a continuously placed retractor. Overall it comes down to rigorously using the additional space that is given by opening the neighboring cisterns, gravity, and bone reduction. It raises the awareness for tissue control and avoids any additional adjuncts in the operative field. For example, surgeon put an unnecessary carpet of cotton patties, that interferes with clip application.

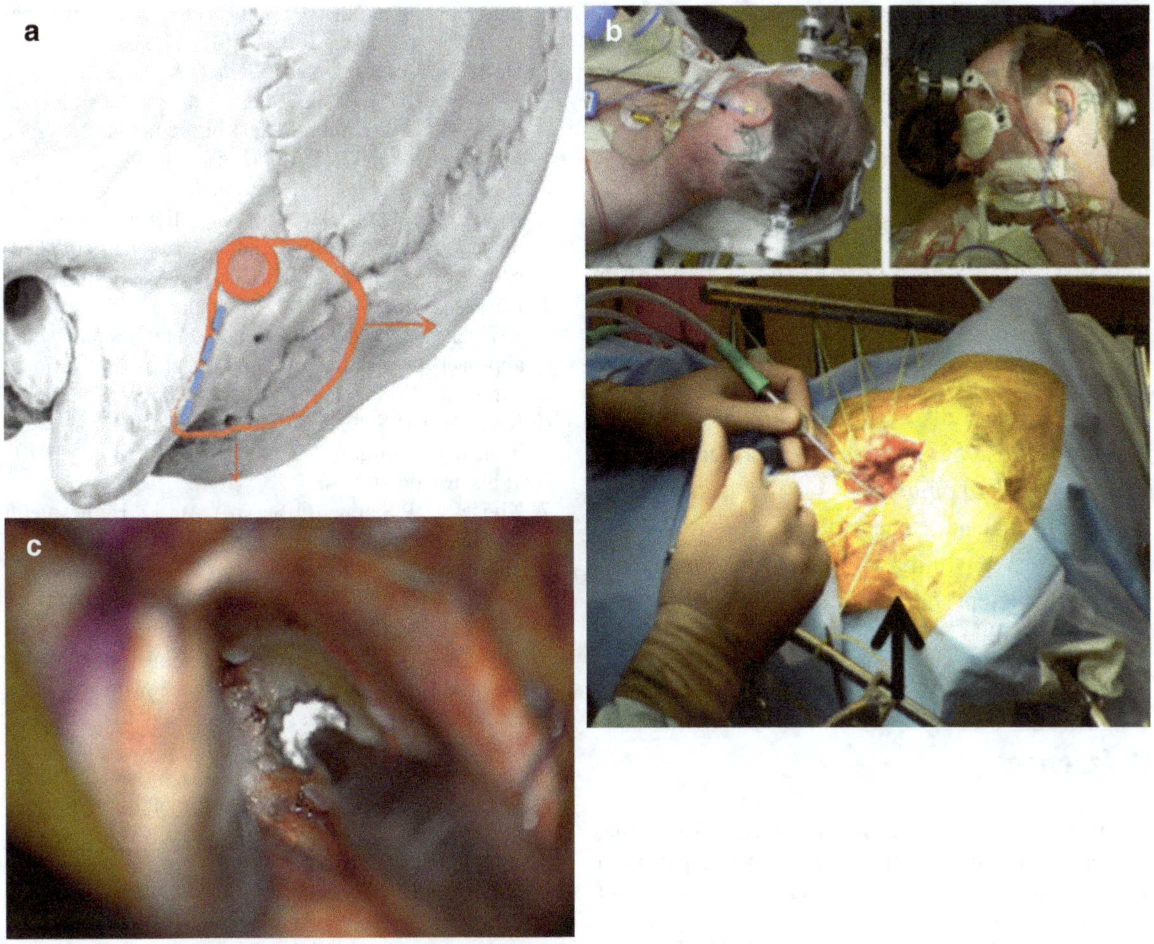

Fig. 30.9 Retrosigmoid approach. A retrosigmoid mini-craniotomy is depicted with patient at supine position, and the head is turned toward the contralateral side. Proper positioning and initial CSF drainage from the cisterna magna readily open a dissection corridor even with large posterior fossa pathology. Corridors are usually large enough to also enable for microsurgical drilling. (**a**) Drawing shows osteoplastic craniotomy with possible extensions (*arrows*) depending on pathology. We prefer a burr hole placed directly into the transverse-sigmoid angle, straddling normal dura to be able to envision sinus and dura. The burr hole placement is greatly helped by neuro-navigation. Curved line depicts craniotomy; straight line is created by craniotomy drill without covering shoe. This creates a tear-off edge. Along this line, we lever the bone flap out, in order to not risk a sinus tear. This technique is fast and prevents tedious drilling and at the same time minimizes bone loss. The bone flap is reinserted after dura closure and fixed with mini-plates and screws. (**b**) Positioning of patient with head elevated above heart level turned 60–70° and inclination toward the contralateral shoulder. C-shaped retroauricular incision. Arrow depicts position of surgeon once dura is opened. Dissection is downward (in contrast to a sitting or semi-sitting position). Forearms can easily be placed on an arm-rest with the surgeon remaining seated. (**c**) A magnified surgeon's view with this kind of retrosigmoid approach, which demonstrates how a conventional drill can be safely inserted to work on the petrous bone

The other real merit is to use mouth and feet for all the movements that usually would be done with the hands. A surgeon used to mouthpiece and foot control adjusts microscope head, focus, and zoom subcortically. An absolute pristine surgical field and removal of anything unnecessary are prerequisites. It surely helps to only use attachments that are low profile and do not interfere with the hands. Positioning and use of "gravity retraction" obtain new meaning.

Retractorless dissection can be adopted by making full use of all known neuromicrosurgical methods and principles.

The immanent necessities for retractorless neurosurgery pave the way for a far more effective and efficient and bloodless dissection technique that will be very tissue sparing.

References

1. Andrews RJ, Muto RP. Retraction brain ischaemia: cerebral blood flow, evoked potentials, hypotension and hyperventilation in a new animal model. Neurol Res. 1992;14(1):12–8.
2. Dashti R, Hernesniemi J, Niemelä M, Rinne J, Lehecka M, Shen H, et al. Microneurosurgical management of distal middle cerebral artery aneurysms. Surg Neurol. 2007;67(6):553–63.
3. Dashti R, Hernesniemi J, Niemelä M, Rinne J, Porras M, Lehecka M, et al. Microneurosurgical management of middle cerebral artery bifurcation aneurysms. Surg Neurol. 2007;67(5):441–56.
4. Dashti R, Rinne J, Hernesniemi J, Niemela M, Kivipelto L, Lehecka M, et al. Microneurosurgical management of proximal middle cerebral artery aneurysms. Surg Neurol. 2007;67(1):6–14.
5. Hernesniemi J, Ishii K, Niemela M, Smrcka M, Kivipelto L, Fujiki M, Shen H. Lateral supraorbital approach as an alternative to the classical pterional approach. Acta Neurochir Suppl. 2005;94:17–21.
6. Kivisaari RP, Salonen O, Ohman J. Basal brain injury in aneurysm surgery. Neurosurgery. 2000;46(5):1070–4; discussion 1074–6.
7. Kivisaari RP, Salonen O, Servo A, Autti T, Hernesniemi J, Ohman J. MR imaging after aneurysmal subarachnoid hemorrhage and surgery: a long-term follow-up study. AJNR Am J Neuroradiol. 2001;22(6):1143–8.
8. Molyneux A. International Subarachnoid Aneurysm Trial (ISAT) of neurosurgical clipping versus endovascular coiling in 2143 patients with ruptured intracranial aneurysms: a randomised trial. Lancet. 2002;360(9342):1267–74.
9. Nagy L, Ishii K, Karatas A, Shen H, Vajda J, Niemela M, et al. Water dissection technique of Toth for opening neurosurgical cleavage planes. Surg Neurol. 2006;65(1):38–41.
10. Spetzler RF, McDougall CG, Albuquerque FC, Zabramski JM, Hills NK, Partovi S, et al. The barrow ruptured aneurysm trial: 3-year results. J Neurosurg. 2013;119(1):146–57.

31 FLOW 800 for Vascular Surgery

Yoko Kato, Ittichai Sakarunchai, and Mohsen Nouri

31.1 Introduction

Neurovascular surgeries are sophisticated procedures, and a thorough knowledge of the vessels before and during the operation is a necessity to prevent inadvertent damage and catastrophic results. Comprehensive monitoring especially real-time evaluation of cerebral blood flow is very helpful for surgery of cerebral aneurysms, cerebral arteriovenous malformations (AVMs), and extracranial-intracranial (EC-IC) bypass.

It has been shown that addition of intraoperative angiography improves the outcome of aneurysm and AVM surgeries by approving complete obliteration of the pathology and preventing inadvertent occlusion of the adjacent vessels. Until a decade ago, there was only intraoperative conventional angiography for this purpose, but recently near-infrared fluorescence module that integrated to microscope for neurosurgery was introduced to picture blood vessels during surgical exposure. Most commonly used fluorescent dye is indocyanine green (ICG) which was first used for assessment of hepatic function in severe chronic liver diseases for which it was approved by FDA in 1959 and later for retinal and choroidal circulation, liver and renal blood flow, and cardiac output. Microscopic-integrated near-infrared ICG videoangiography (VA) has been used in several cerebrovascular surgeries since 2003. Intraoperative ICG-VA is done by using the commercially available microscopes (e.g., OPMI Pentero, Carl Zeiss, Oberkochen, Germany). This allows the surgeon to obtain an intraoperative angiography in less than 5 min (in contrast with conventional DSA which usually takes about 20 min) without the need to introduce any new device (i.e., angiography unit) into the surgical field. The main shortcoming of ICG-VA is that its images are limited to the surgical field and identifying arteries from veins is not readily possible. Also, it provides the surgeon with only anatomical data without any information about the physiology and dynamics of the blood flow. To overcome these limitations, a new image analysis software package was released later to distinguish physical properties of the flow in the vessels and demonstrate semi-quantitative data.

Y. Kato (✉)
Department of Neurosurgery, Fujita Health University, Toyoake, Aichi, Japan
e-mail: kyoko@fujita-hu.ac.jp

I. Sakarunchai
Division of Neurosurgery, Department of Surgery, Faculty of Medicine, Prince of Songkhla University, Songkhla, Thailand

M. Nouri
Gundishapour Academy of Neuroscience, Ahvaz, Iran
e-mail: nouri@gan-ac.ir

J. July, E. J. Wahjoepramono (eds.), *Neurovascular Surgery*,
https://doi.org/10.1007/978-981-10-8950-3_31

31.2 FLOW 800 Software

New image analysis software, namely, FLOW 800 (Carl Zeiss, Oberkochen, Germany) was presented in 2010 that produces intensity diagrams and color mapping. This software works on the assumption that the earlier-arriving ICG in the field belongs to the arteries and those disappearing at last belong to the veins and so depicts the vascular field in a color-coded mode [1]. The operator (e.g., the surgeon or assistants) can determine some region of interest (ROI) for the software which can be further analyzed to draw the intensity diagram. This diagram shows the intensity of fluorescence over time in the ROI. More information can be deduced from this diagram after manual analysis by an image analysis software. The combination of these two processed images in accumulation to the ICG-VA helps the surgeon to judge the anatomy and physiology of the vessels in different situations (see below).

31.2.1 Color-Coded Images

These images convert the black and white images of conventional ICG-VA into a gradient where red and blue colors represent arteries and veins, respectively (Fig. 31.1). This can be helpful especially in AVM surgeries to identify feeding arteries. Also, if the color of a distal artery changes after clipping of an aneurysm, this might imply blood flow impairment. However, one should be cautious about interpretation of these images. As mentioned earlier, the basis of this software to color a vessel in red or blue is their chronological ICG fluorescence not the real direction of blood flow. This may result in misdiagnosis in some occasions such as when one type of vessel (artery or vein) is not in the field of view (e.g., a deep feeding artery). A good knowledge of anatomy and reviewing details of the vascular pathology before the surgery are mandatory for the surgeon to compensate for these shortcomings.

31.2.2 Intensity Diagram

To draw an intensity diagram, we usually use circular or rectangular marks to define the vascular area of interest (ROI), and then the curve and some primary parameters are calculated and depicted by the software. Parameters calculated directly by the software include average intensity (shown in arbitrary intensity [AI] units), delay time (i.e., the time interval from 0 to 50% of maximum fluorescence intensities [MFI]), and the slope of the curve. On the other hand, there are some other indices presented in the literature known to be correlated with perfusion characteristics of tissues which simply can be calculated with an image analysis software such as Image J (version 1.46, National Institute of Health, USA) after delivering the data from the microscope station (Fig. 31.2). Transit time is the time difference between MFI in artery and brain tissue, and rise time is defined as time during which fluorescence intensity rises from 10 to 90% of its peak. Other variables that can be measured manually include MFI, time to peak (i.e., from the appearance of fluorescence to MFI), and cerebral blood flow index (CBFI) which is defined as ratio of MFI to rise time. These parameters can be calculated for each vessel, and their changes should be tracked throughout the procedure [2].

31.3 Special Application of FLOW 800

31.3.1 Cerebral AVMs Surgeries

During AVM surgeries, ICG-VA can detect vessels as small as 0.5 mm in diameter and is very practical for in superficial AVMs. However, the field of angiography is limited to the field of microscopic view. As the surgeon cannot see the deep vessels and the whole structure of the AVM, sometimes it gets difficult to identify arteries and veins. FLOW 800 software can help the surgeon with identification of AVM vessels by producing a color-coded map where red represents feeding arteries and blue stands for drainers (Fig. 31.1). Also, after selecting some ROIs for the software, the intensity analysis curves help to understand the hemodynamics of the vessels and the surrounding brain parenchyma. For example, both image types can be used before and after temporary clipping of the arterial feeders to evaluate its effect on the AVM nidal blood flow and as a guide

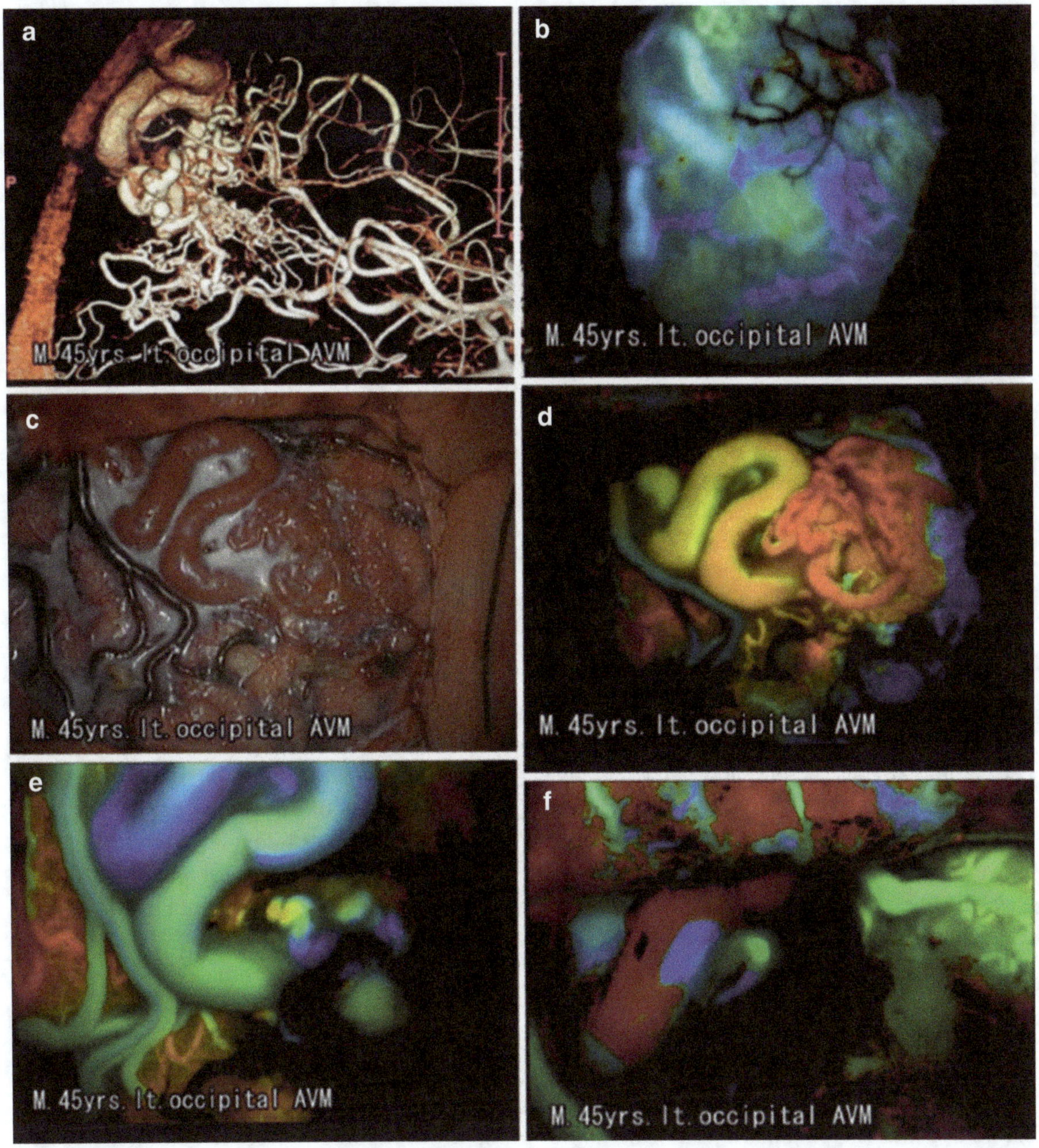

Fig. 31.1 Left occipital arteriovenous malformation (AVM) in a 45-year-old man. (**a**) Reconstructed computed tomography angiogram shows the location, feeding artery, and draining vein of the AVM. (**b**) Before opening the dura, color-coded imaging by FLOW 800 delineated vessels and helped us tailor durotomy. (**c**) The superficial presentation of the AVM after opening the dura. (**d**) Color-coded angiography immediately after opening the dura. (**e**) Color-coded imaging after partial occlusion of the feeders. Note that color changes in the vessels may indicate hemodynamic changes of the AVM. (**f**) Color-coded angiography after confirming total resection of the malformation

for the next step of the operation. Also, changes in the cerebral parenchymal blood flow can be calculated to evaluate the effect of AVM removal on cerebral perfusion and predict postoperative autoregulation disturbances (e.g., breakthrough phenomenon). However, more data are required to externally validate these data to better define their normal range and predictive capacity.

The main limitations of ICG-VA in AVM surgeries also extend to the FLOW 800 as deeply located vessels are not visualized and complementary DSA is required in such cases [3]. Also,

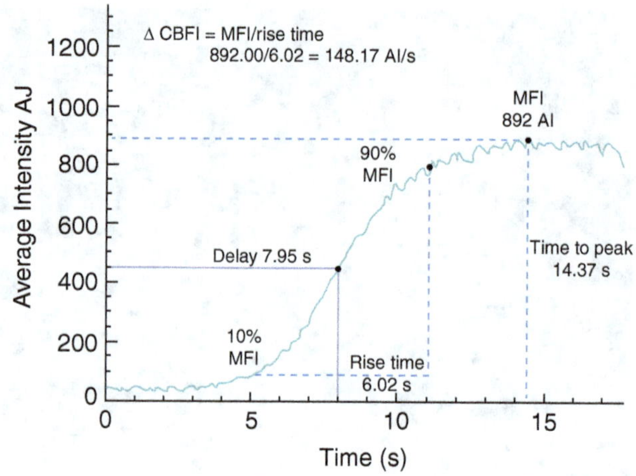

Fig. 31.2 Intensity diagram of a vessel after manual image analysis with Image J software. Maximum fluorescence intensity (MFI) is the highest intensity of fluorescence for a defined area, and time to peak is the time interval from the appearance of fluorescence until its peak. Rise time is the time interval when fluorescence intensity rises from 10 to 90% of MFI. Cerebral blood flow index (CBFI) is the ratio of MFI to rise time

in cases in which the main vessels are covered with blood clot, brain tissue, cottonoid patties, etc., the software may not be accurate in differentiating arteries from veins.

31.3.2 Cerebral Aneurysm Surgeries

In aneurysm surgeries, ICG-VA can demonstrate perforating arteries before and after clipping, check for patency of the distal vessels after clipping, and confirm complete aneurysm obliteration. However, there are certain circumstances where checking the anatomy with ICG-VA is not all enough for a safe surgery. Sometimes, despite having the distal blood flow depicted on angiograms, subtle decrease in flow presents which may compromise perfusion of the cerebral parenchyma leading to disturbed function of the brain. FLOW 800 may assist the surgeon to calculate the CBFI before and after clipping and by showing him or her the color-coded images where any change in color after clipping regarded as an alarming sign.

When ICG-VA is repeated at surgery after clipping, the dome of the aneurysm may show some residual ICG illumination from previous injections. This results in confusion as the surgeon cannot be assured of the total obliteration of the neck. In this occasion, FLOW 800 can differentiate a residual ICG from incomplete clipping: in case of clip shortage, the aneurysm dome appears red in color-coded images, and if the dome is selected as a ROI, a curve that follows an arterial diagram is produced (Fig. 31.3).

In a recent study, 2 of 12 cases needed adjustment of the clip after finding an occlusion of perforating vessels [4]. Also, after ICG-VA they found 4 cases of incomplete clipping out of 45 (8.9%) who required appropriate readjustment to complete the obliteration.

In some cases, atherosclerotic plaque in the aneurysm may make interpretation of ICG-VA very difficult if not impossible. In these cases when there is any doubt in the result of an ICG-VA, we should use other monitoring techniques such as micro-doppler or endoscope that can be used to check for residual blood flow in aneurysm sac or incomplete obliteration of the aneurysm neck.

One of the advantages of ICG-VA over DSA in aneurysm surgery is its real-time nature where the surgeon can manipulate the vessels and adjust the clip just during the angiography, if required. Also, FLOW 800 allows physiological monitoring of the clipping procedure both in the vessels and in the surrounding brain tissue. ICG-VA has largely replaced conventional DSA during aneurysm surgery in most centers, and attempts to further clarify the role of FLOW 800 in these procedures are underway.

31.3.3 Bypass Surgeries

Different stages of EC-IC bypass surgery such as to identify the recipient artery, to evaluate patency of the graft, and to detect any possible stenosis are facilitated by ICG-VA. Januszewski

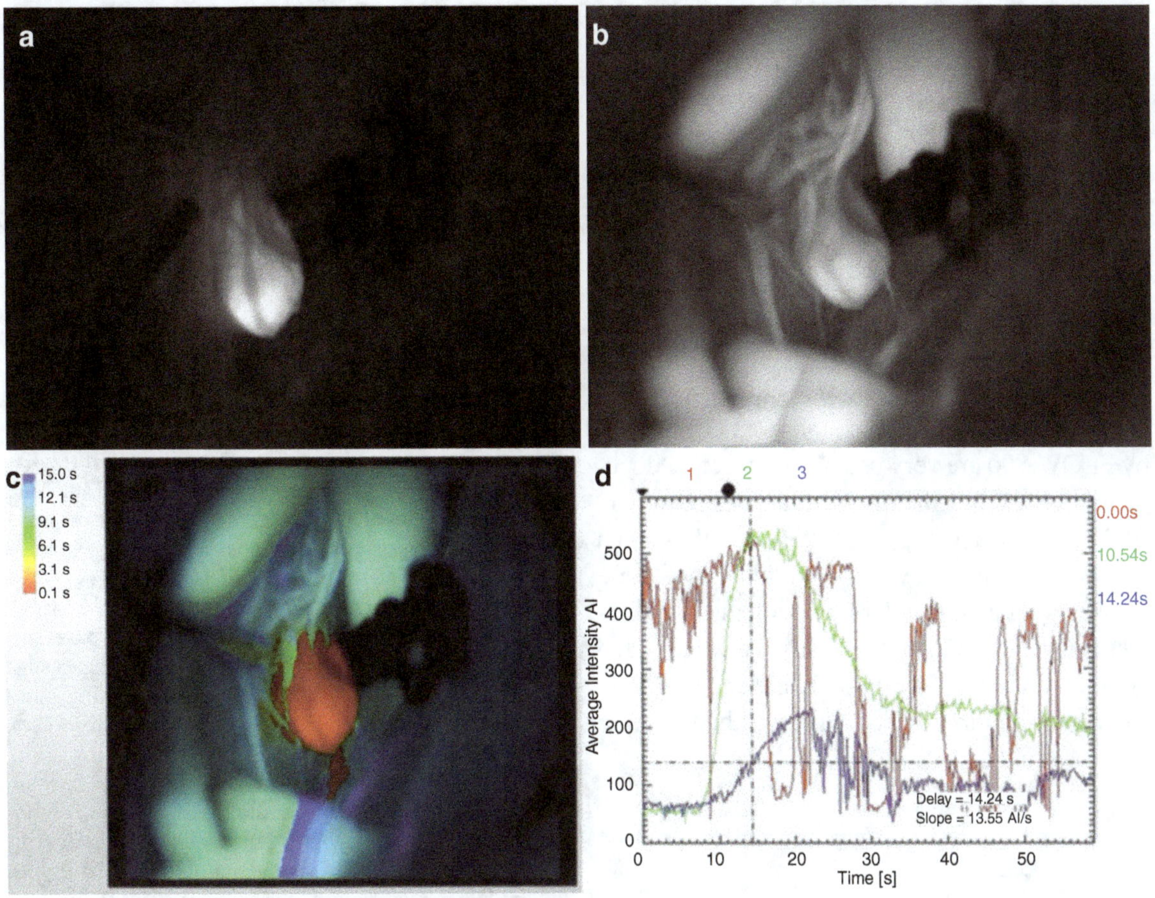

Fig. 31.3 (**a**) Surgical view under infrared camera after aneurysm clipping and before indocyanine green (ICG) injection. Note that the aneurysm glows due to previous ICG accumulated in the aneurysm sac. (**b**) The same view after ICG injection. It is difficult if not impossible to differentiate previously accumulated ICG in the aneurysm from newly injected in the vessels. This view is consistent with incomplete aneurysm obliteration. (**c**) Color-coded image by FLOW 800 software demonstrate the aneurysm in red. This is the shortcoming of the software that cannot differentiate a previously injected dye from early arrival of blood flow. (**d**) The red curve shows the intensity changes inside the aneurysm sac. Constant curve confirms absence of blood flow in the aneurysm. Some sudden changes in intensity are observed which are due to manipulation of the aneurysm with suction tip to see behind the aneurysm. Please note that delay and slope of the curve are calculated by the software

et al. used ICG-VA to analyze the blood flow type after anastomosis which can predict early postoperative graft occlusion [5]. Also, Esposto et al. used ICG-VA to identify arterial territory in temporary or permanent occlusion of the vessels [6]. Although the application of the ICG-VA in bypass evaluation is well established and widely accepted, the role of FLOW 800 is still unclear. In spite of some available limited data [7], whether pre- to post-bypass, ratio of measures such as CBFI or MFI correlates with the outcome and requires further comparative studies.

31.4 Expert Opinion

Additional hemodynamic analysis with the help of FLOW 800 to the conventional angiographies (e.g., ICG-VA) allows a real-time physiological and anatomical assessment of blood flow during cerebrovascular procedures such as aneurysms, AVMs, and bypass surgeries. Intraoperative imaging of the vessels in vascular surgeries decreases postoperative morbidities and is an inseparable adjunct in almost all centers dealing with such pathologies. This along with other intraoperative monitoring modalities such as neuroendoscopy and motor-evoked potentials results in superb outcome of the patients in the modern era of cerebrovascular surgeries [8]. Intraoperative DSA is still considered the gold standard procedure especially for AVMs where the deep vessels pose certain concerns during the surgery. However, in most aneurysm and selected AVM surgeries, ICG-VA can replace conventional DSA as it is a cheaper technique, requires less time for the procedure, and eliminates exposure to radiation. Also, physiological evaluations by FLOW 800 are very useful for objective documentation of the blood flow in aneurysm sac, AVM vessels, and bypass graft. Yet, as these data are semiquantitative, external validation of these measures against standard physiological assessments is required to better clarify the value of the numbers calculated by the software and how they can be applied in practice. This will be the topic of future studies.

References

1. Oda J, Kato Y, Chen SF, Sodhiya P, Watabe T, Imizu S, Oguri D, Sano H, Hirose Y. Intraoperative near-infrared indocyanine green–videoangiography (ICG–VA) and graphic analysis of fluorescence intensity in cerebral aneurysm surgery. J Clin Neurosci. 2011;18:1097–100.
2. Son YJ, Kim JE, Park SB, Lee SH, Chung YS, Yang HJ. Quantitative analysis of intraoperative indocyanine green video angiography in aneurysm surgery. J Cerebrovasc Endovasc Neurosurg. 2013;15(2):76–84.
3. Ye X, Liu XJ, Ma L, Liu LT, Wang WL, Wang S, Cao Y, Zhang D, Wang R, Zhao JZ, Zhao YL. Clinical value of intraoperative indocyanine green fluorescence video angiography with Flow 800 software in cerebrovascular surgery. Chin Med J. 2013;126(22):4232–7.
4. Chen SF, Kato Y, Oda J, Kumar A, Watabe T, Imizu S, Oguri D, Sano H, Hirose Y. The application of intraoperative near-infrared indocyanine green videoangiography and analysis of fluorescence intensity in cerebrovascular surgery. Surg Neurol Int. 2011;2:42.
5. Januszewski J, Beecher JS, Chalif DJ, Dehdashti AR. Flow-based evaluation of cerebral revascularization using near-infrared indocyanine green videoangiography. Neurosurg Focus. 2014;36(2):1–11.
6. Esposito G, Durand A, Doormaal TV, Regli L. Selective-targeted extra-intracranial bypass surgery in complex middle cerebral artery aneurysms: correctly identifying the recipientartery using indocyanine green videoangiography. Neurosurgery. 2012;71(ONS Suppl 2):274–85.
7. Uchino H, Nakamura T, Houkin K, Murata J, Saito H, Kuroda S. Semiquantitative analysis of indocyanine green videoangiography for cortical perfusion assessment in superficial temporal artery to middle cerebral artery anastomosis. Acta Neurochir. 2013;155(4):599–605.
8. Yamada Y, Kato Y, Nouri M. No overtaking! Take a safe trip to aneurysm. Austin J Cerebrovasc Dis Stroke. 2014;1(2):1.

32 Gamma Knife Surgery for AVM

Lutfi Hendriansyah

32.1 Symptoms and Signs

Arteriovenous malformations (AVM) are an abnormal connection between arteries and veins lacking intervening capillary network characterized by a complex, tangled web of abnormal vessels and believed to be congenital although not hereditary. This abnormal tangled web of vessels is called nidus (Latin word for nest), which has abnormally high blood flow resulting from the absence of dampening effect of capillary and has high tendency to rupture resulting in stroke. Lack of capillary network also induces enlargement of especially venous side with subsequent "growth" of AVM resulting in mass effect to surrounding brain parenchyma. AVM also disrupts normal metabolism of surrounding brain tissue by depriving them of adequate circulation (steal phenomena) causing neurological symptoms depending on its location whether superficial in cortex or deep within thalamus, basal ganglia, corpus callosum, insula/sylvian fissure, brainstem, or cerebellum. These mechanisms stated above underlie pathogenesis of symptoms and signs including hemorrhage as the most common presenting symptom in 50–52% of cases, followed by seizure in 27–30%, headache in 5–14%, and progressive neurological deficit in less than 5% [1, 2]. Hemorrhage is associated with high morbidity and mortality as much as 35% and 29%, respectively, that it becomes a primary concern in AVM management. Overall annual risk of hemorrhage on untreated AVM ranges between 2 and 4%, and although multiple studies implicated factors such as nidus size, complexity of AVM morphology, deep brain location or draining vein, associated aneurysm, and younger age to be related to hemorrhagic events, multivariate analysis indicated that only hemorrhage in initial presentation, deep AVM location or deep draining vein, and large nidus size is to be consistently predictive of higher risk of subsequent rupture up to 15% of annual rates [1, 2]. Figure 32.1 shows presentation of AVM hemorrhage on brain computed tomography (CT) scan and angiogram.

AVM management includes treatment such as microsurgical resection, Gamma Knife surgery, and embolization either individually or in combination, or just simple clinical observation. The option between doing treatment and observation or among any treatment modality has to be carefully weighed according to risk-benefit ratio and must be balanced against the risk from natural course of the disease. This chapter focuses on Gamma Knife surgery as treatment modality for AVM, which has to be considered as treatment for selected patients.

L. Hendriansyah
Gamma Knife Center Indonesia, Siloam Hospitals
Lippo Village, Tangerang, Indonesia

J. July, E. J. Wahjoepramono (eds.), *Neurovascular Surgery*,
https://doi.org/10.1007/978-981-10-8950-3_32

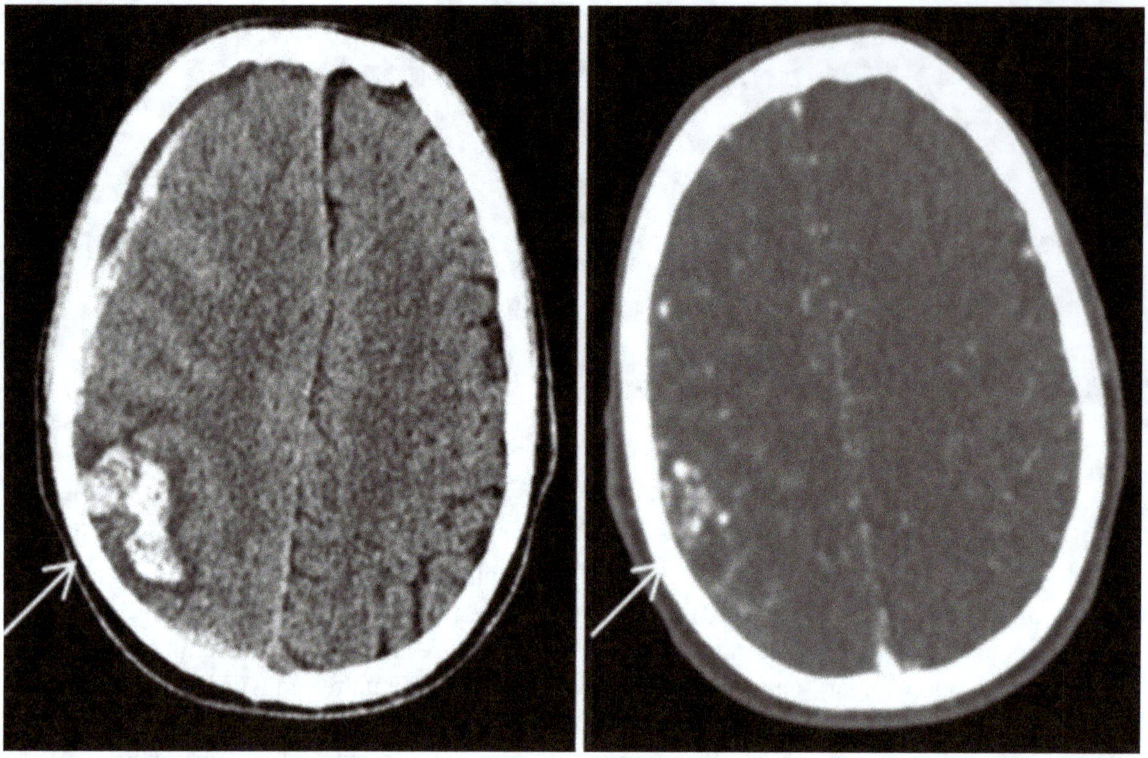

Fig. 32.1 Hemorrhage as AVM initial presentation. Spontaneous intracerebral hemorrhage in children or young adolescent, without history of hypertension and in uncommon location for hypertensive hemorrhage, should raise suspicion of AVM as the primary cause. CT scan (left, *white arrow*) showing hemorrhage and CT angiogram (right, *white arrow*) demonstrating nidus anterior to bleeding site are two investigations that reveal hemorrhage as the most common initial presentation of AVM

32.2 Gamma Knife Surgery

Gamma Knife surgery is commonly used to treat AVM that carry high risk of morbidity for microsurgical resection such as Spetzler-Martin grade III or above because it has the advantage of accurately treating small and deep-seated lesions with minimal risk of injury to surrounding structures. It delivers multiple fine beams of gamma rays radiation in such a highly focused manner that it can induce changes in AVM structure over time resulting in cessation of blood flow through the abnormal vessels leading to occlusion. The pathological changes following Gamma Knife surgery for AVM includes endothelial cell damage, proliferation of smooth muscle cells, and elaboration of extracellular collagen that subsequently lead to luminal stenosis and obliteration of nidus. Once complete obliteration of nidus happens, there will be no more blood flow through abnormal vessels. Overall total obliteration rates of AVM following Gamma Knife surgery ranges between 72 and 85% in a typical single-session treatment, and this process usually takes 2–3 years to yield in result. High chance of cure together with low risk of morbidity makes this treatment modality an interesting option for AVM.

The aim of treatment is to accomplish total obliteration of AVM in which situation the risk of hemorrhage is alleviated and the patient is cured. In other situation where partial or subtotal obliteration occur, the risk of hemorrhage still persists and hence subsequent Gamma Knife treatment has to be considered. In predicting outcome after Gamma Knife surgery for AVM, several grading scales were developed such as Virginia Radiosurgery AVM Scale (VRAS) and radiosurgery-based grading AVM Score (RBAS), which includes into consideration history of hemorrhage and patient age, respectively, beside nidus volume and location. These grading scales are considered better in predicting favorable outcome after Gamma Knife surgery, compared to previously and more commonly used Spetzler-Martin Scale [3].

32.3 Investigation

If brain AVM is suspected, magnetic resonance imaging (MRI) can much better visualize AVM structure than CT scan. High-resolution MRI not only demonstrates AVM structures mainly nidus and draining veins, but it also shows the AVM location and its relation to surrounding cortical structures that are highly essential in setting up treatment planning. Digital subtraction angiography (DSA) is still the gold standard in visualizing AVM because this imaging can best demonstrate flow through every part of AVM in addition to structure. Combination of both imaging is important in defining the lesion for treatment and subsequently influencing optimal result in Gamma Knife surgery for AVM (Fig. 32.2).

32.4 Preoperative Preparation

In our institution, we use Leksell Gamma Knife® Perfexion™ machine (Fig. 32.3, left) that is consisted of two main units; one is in radiation side and the other is in patient side. The radiation unit contains cobalt^{60} source that constantly emits gamma rays which is delivered to lesions during treatment through channel opening of 4, 8, or 16 mm collimators. Gamma rays are focused and accurately beamed to lesions through 192 collimator channels in which the opening and closing are controlled automatically according to treatment plan (Fig. 32.3, right). The patient side contains automated patient positioning system (PPS) that consists of a treatment couch where the patient lies down and of which movement is controlled according to treatment plan in such a way that lesion to be treated is positioned at the center of gamma rays cross-firing.

Leksell® Coordinate System utilizing titanium Leksell® G Frame as stereotactic frame is used to accurately localize lesion for treatment planning and to fixate the head as well as lesion in desired

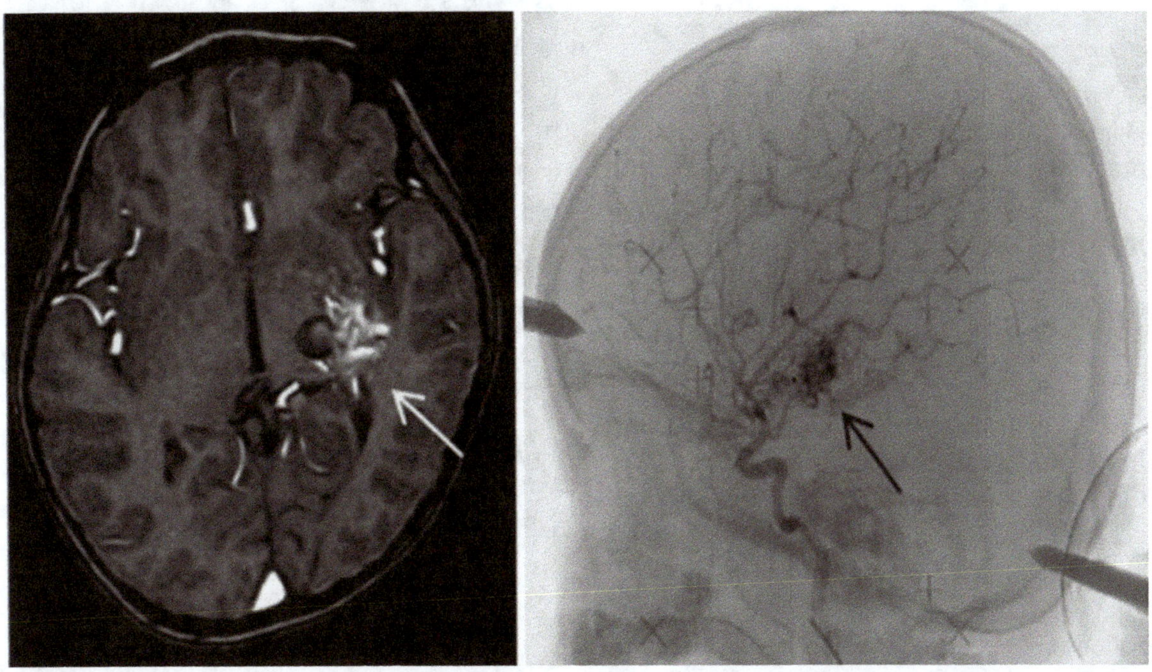

Fig. 32.2 MRI and DSA of AVM. T1 Fast Field Echo (FFE) MR images (left, *white arrow*) and DSA (right, *black arrow*) visualizing AVM nidus on posterior limb of left internal capsule. Arterial feeder comes from medial branch of lenticulostriate artery and drains into Sylvian veins

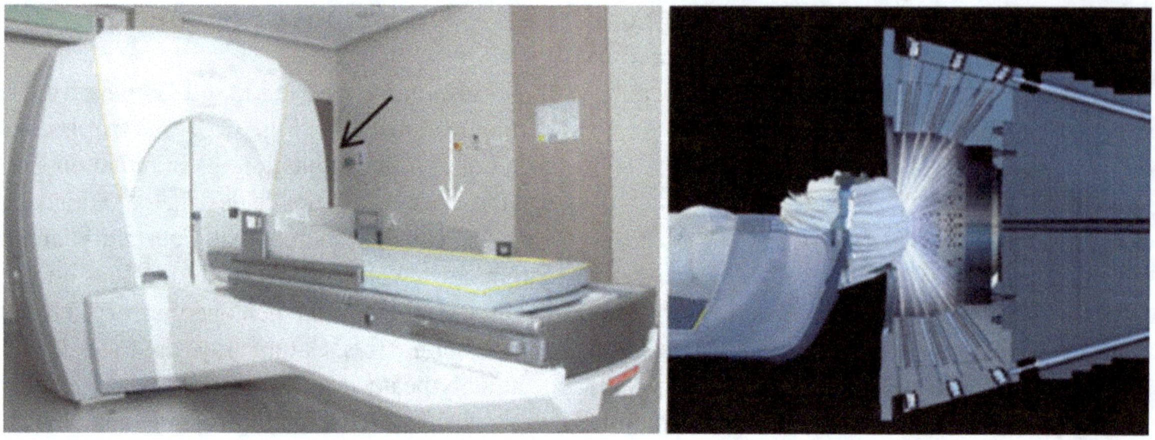

Fig. 32.3 Gamma Knife unit. Leksell Gamma Knife® Perfexion™ unit. *Left*: radiation unit on the left half part of the machine (*black arrow*) and treatment couch on the right half part (*white arrow*). *Right*: Gamma ray delivery during treatment (courtesy of Elekta Co)

position during treatment delivery. It mainly consists of rectangular frame base, front piece, and a set of fixation posts and screws. Straight or curved fixation posts and screws measuring 20–110 mm are selected accordingly to fit different patient cranial shapes and sizes and hence to optimize operative field (Fig. 32.4). Frame is assembled during treatment preparation just before fixation to patient.

32.5 Approach

Gamma knife treatment plan uses several terminologies that every neurosurgeon needs to be familiar with in order to comprehend the treatment process. They are summarized in Table 32.1.

32.6 Steps of the Surgery

Treatment process begins with stereotactic frame fixation under local anesthesia (Fig. 32.5, left). General anesthesia is rarely used and only needed for children or those who are really uncooperative during treatment procedure. Leksell® G Frame is assembled and adjusted according to patients' head size and lesion location; two assistants help in positioning the frame, while the surgeon infiltrates local anesthesia into four

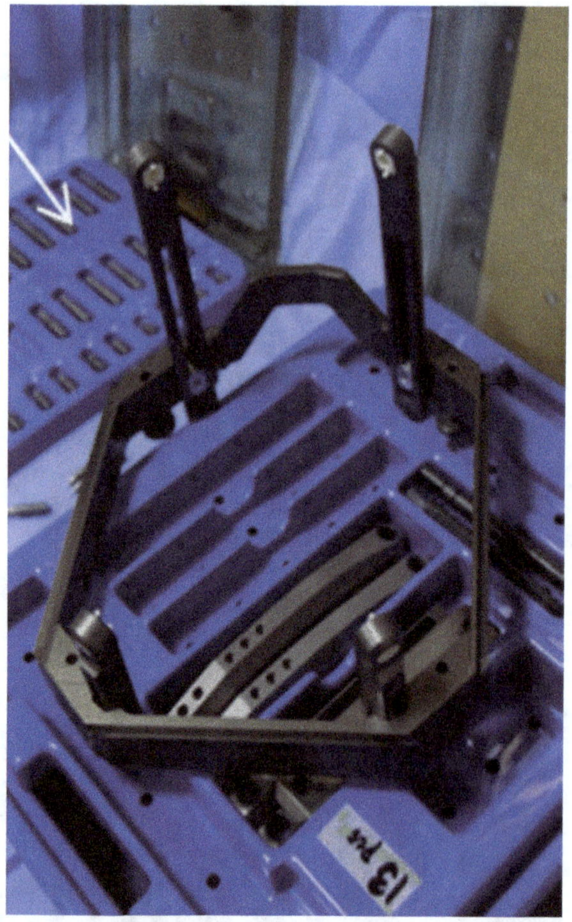

Fig. 32.4 Leksell® G stereotactic frame. Frame consisting of rectangular frame base, curved front piece, and four fixation posts has been assembled and ready for placement. A set of fixation screws of different lengths is selected from tray (upper left, *white arrow*)

Table 32.1 Terminology in Gamma Knife surgery

Terminology	Description
Target volume	Volume of lesion that is defined as target. In AVM it represents nidus volume
Isocenter	Point where radiation beams are converged by using combination of different collimators. Isocenters are placed inside target volume
Isodose line	A line indicating distribution volume of same radiation dose. It is three-dimensional and is composed by combination of isocenters. For example, 12 gray (Gy) isodose line demonstrates nidus volume receiving 12 Gy
Prescription isodose	Isodose line of prescribed effective radiation dose that covers target volume. It is stated in margin or peripheral dose. For example, margin dose of 12 Gy in 50% isodose means that nidus margin is covered by 12 Gy, which is 50% of maximum dose
Conformity index	An index that compare isodose volume (prescription) inside target with total target volume. It demonstrates degree to which target is covered by prescription dose and greater index reflects more prescription dose inside the nidus
Selectivity index	An index that compare isodose volume (prescription) inside target with total isodose volume. It demonstrates degree to which prescription dose is specific to target and do not spill to the adjacent neurovascular structure. Greater index reflects less prescription dose outside the nidus
Gradient index	An index comparing prescription isodose with half value of this isodose. It reflects the sharpness of radiation dose falloff around target margin, and smaller index demonstrates steeper dose falloff outside the nidus

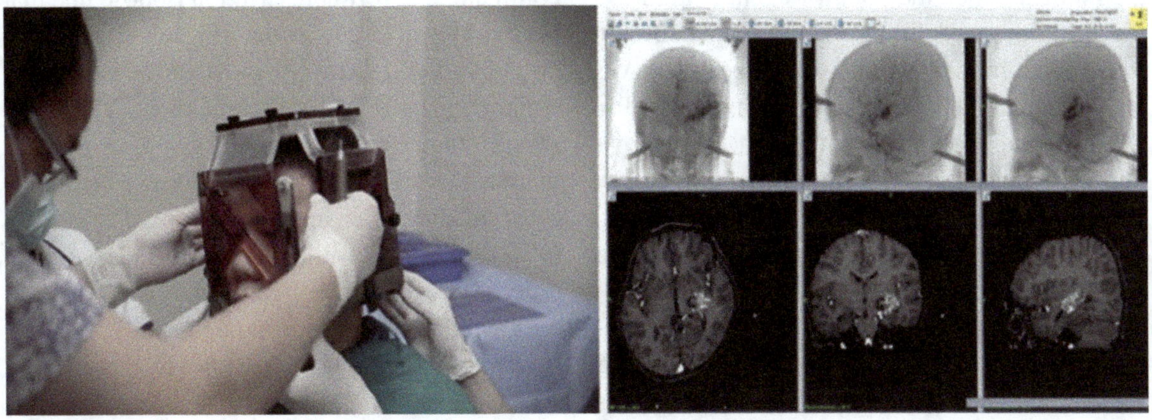

Fig. 32.5 Frame fixation and image acquisition. Sometimes MR indicator box is used during frame fixation to ensure adequate frame placement that covers optimal operative field (*left*). A combination of images from biplanar DSA and three-dimensional MR images is used for optimal nidus visualization (*right*)

points of pin insertion. A combination of lidocaine and adrenaline diluted with sterile water for injection is used for local anesthesia. As soon as anesthesia works, pins are tightened against the cranium, and frame position is checked to see whether it has fit the cranium properly or whether there is distortion caused by unequal pin pressure or excessive bending of titanium posts. Frame needs to be properly fit to cranium in order for treatment to reach lesions optimally, especially those with extremely eccentric location, and to avoid collision to collimator channel wall during treatment delivery.

When the frame is fixed, patients are ready for image acquisition (Fig. 32.5, right). Stereotactic DSA and MRI images are used for target localization. DSA is performed under local anesthesia; anteroposterior (AP) and lateral projections of feeding arteries, nidus, and draining veins are always sought for through both carotid and vertebrobasilar system bilaterally.

This way, every part of nidus can be visualized optimally and unlikely to be missed. It is essential to have optimal nidus visualization for maximum nidus coverage in treatment planning. The best images are then picked out for nidus delinea-

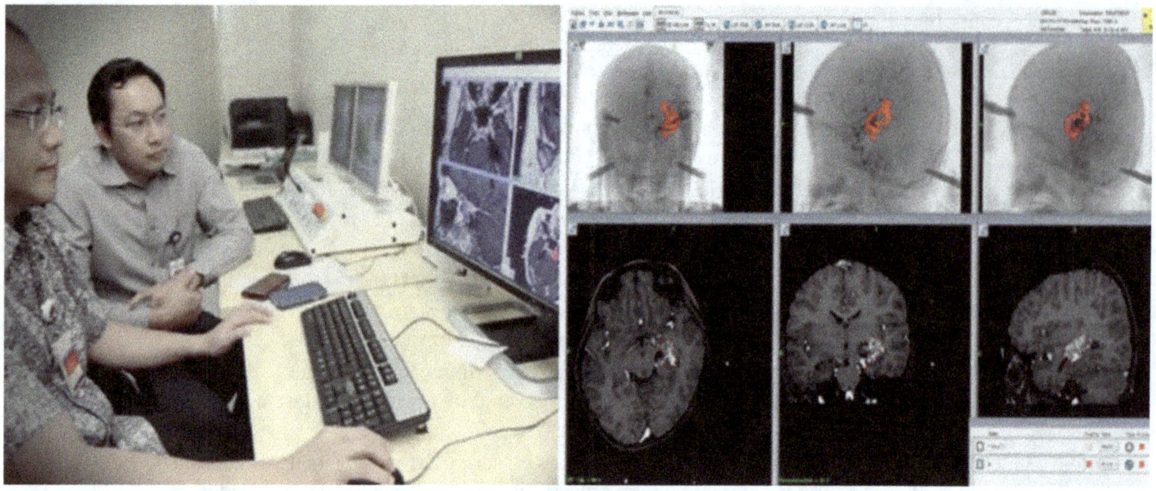

Fig. 32.6 Treatment planning and target delineation. Treatment is meticulously programmed on treatment planning system (TPS) using Gamma Plan® software. The whole nidus is defined as target volume and delineated (*red line*)

tion in order to define target volume, usually at the moment when the contrast agent starts leaving the nidus and filling up draining veins. In order not to miss this particular moment, DSA is set at minimum six frames per second (fps). Too late in taking images may result in overestimation of nidus size while too early may result otherwise. Since DSA images are made in two dimensions, they alone are not adequate to define stereotactic coordinates for accurate target localization in treatment planning that three-dimensional MRI images are needed. We use 1.5 Tesla MRI with thin slice of 1 mm-thickness without gap or overlap and usually without contrast injection. T2-weighted images together with T1 Fast Field Echo (FFE) technique are used to visualize the malformed vessels. Some patients cannot undergo MRI for many clinical reasons including severe claustrophobia and implantation of cardiac pacemakers. In these situations, three-dimensional CT angiogram is used in defining stereotactic coordinates for lesion.

As soon as images are ready, they are then exported to the Gamma Knife treatment planning system (TPS). Gamma Plan® software in TPS is used to incorporate stereotactic DSA and MRI or CT images for target volume definition and delineation (Fig. 32.6).

After nidus is defined and well delineated, isocenter placement of prescribed treatment dose is initialized using a combination of 4, 8, or 16 mm collimators, to form prescription isodose line that best conform target lesion (Fig. 32.7). Margin dose ranging 18–25 Gy in 40–50% isodose is commonly used for AVM treatment. There are several indices used to indicate how optimal treatment plan is. Conformity index, which indicates treatment coverage, is kept above 0.95 (95% coverage), while selectivity index, which reflects how selective treatment is to target and thus avoid injuring surrounding healthy tissue, is kept above 0.92 (92% selective to target), and gradient index, which reflects radiation spill outside target, is kept minimum below 3.

As soon as treatment plan is finalized, the protocol is approved and exported from TPS into control system, which will control the whole operation of Gamma Knife unit during treatment delivery. Patient is then prepared for treatment.

Patient is positioned as comfortable as possible in treatment couch; frame is fixated to its dockings, and vital sign monitors are attached; treatment plan is rechecked and confirmed during time-out period before procedure (Fig. 32.8, left). Treatment plan has been approved in control system and ready for implementation (Fig. 32.8, right). Treatment then can be initialized by pressing start button in control system. We use closed-circuit TV (CCTV) camera with speakers and microphones inside treatment

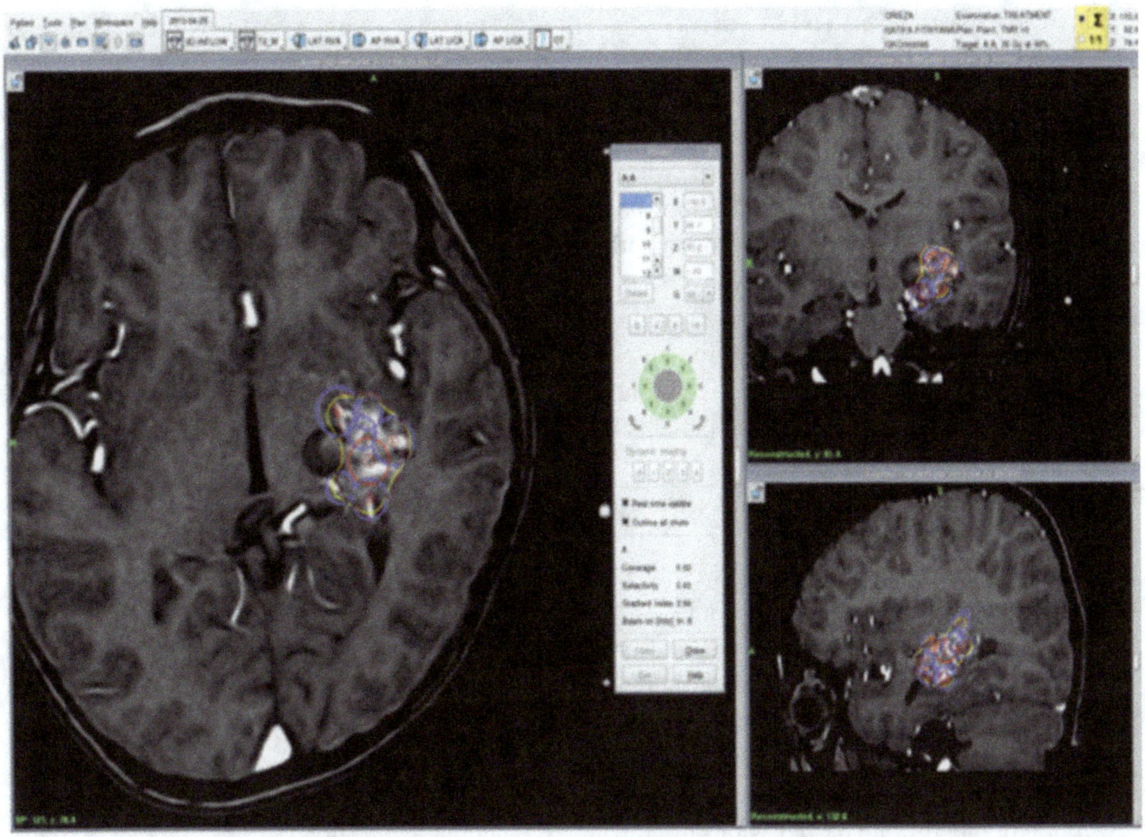

Fig. 32.7 Isocenter placement. Multiple isocenters (*circles in blue line*) are placed and arranged to form an isodose line (*yellow line*) conforming target lesion (*red line*) that has been previously delineated

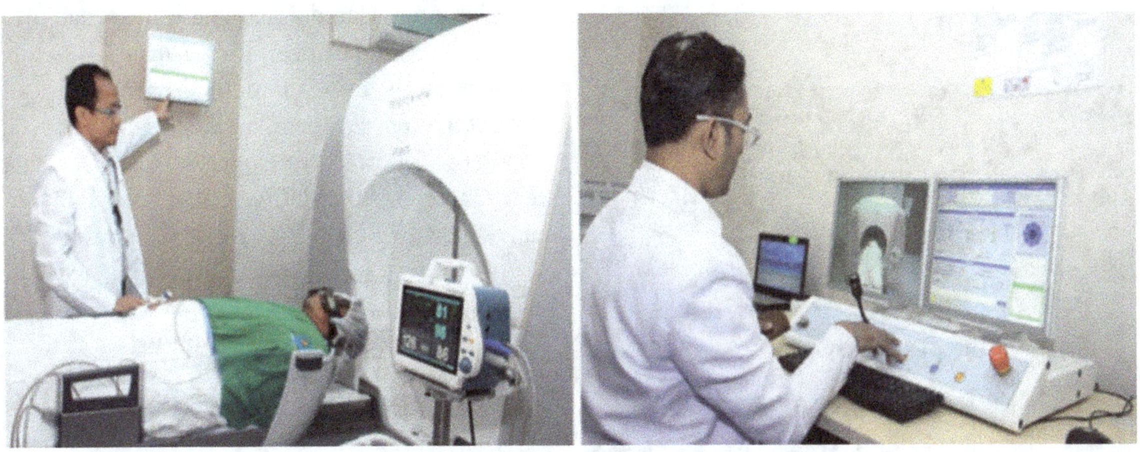

Fig. 32.8 Patient positioning and treatment delivery. Patient has been positioned, and frame is fixated; monitors for vital signs are attached, and treatment plan is rechecked and ready (*left*). Treatment then can be initiated, and patient is monitored during the whole procedure through CCTV camera (*right*)

room, which is connected to control room as intercom, to monitor and to communicate with patients during treatment delivery.

When treatment is completed, patient is removed from treatment couch, and pins are unscrewed during frame removal. Some patients may experience temporary headache after frame removal that dexamethasone and painkiller are routinely given. Finally, patients are observed for 1–2 h before discharge from hospital.

32.7 Surgeon Plan to Handle the Complication

Complications after Gamma Knife surgery includes radiation-induced changes whether symptomatic or not, cyst formation, hemorrhage, and radiation-induced neoplasm. Postradiation image change, commonly known as adverse radiation effects (ARE), are the most common adverse effects following Gamma Knife surgery occurring in 33.8% of cases within 3–12 months. They can be symptomatic in 8.6% of patients but fortunately reversible in most, and only a small number of 1.8% is associated with permanent neurological deficit [4]. These changes are demonstrated by increased signal on T2-weighted or FLAIR MRI around nidus as shown in Fig. 32.9. Several mechanisms are proposed to be responsible for these changes including radiation injury to glial cells especially oligodendroglia resulting in demyelination, damage to endothelial cells with cytokine, and antigen release causing the disruption of blood-brain barrier with subsequent edema, generation of free radicals, auto immune response, and indirect effects through vascular insults with subsequent ischemia.

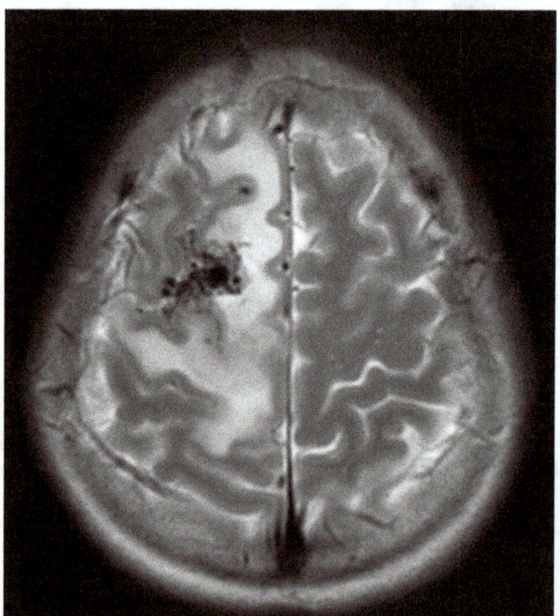

Fig. 32.9 Adverse radiation effects. Increased signal intensity on T2-weighted MRI around nidus

Many factors are related to these complications risk including larger nidus size, higher marginal dose, superficial and eloquent location, as well as less number of draining veins. Special care and considerations in treatment planning must be taken when factors related to increased risks such as larger nidus volume and eloquent locations are encountered. Lower marginal dose is typically given in these situations, and we would consider volume staging in large AVMs (nidus size above 4 cm or volume above 30 cm^3).

Surprisingly, ARE is also considered a prognostic factor to complete obliteration. Those who have complete obliteration on long-term follow-up are more common to experience ARE starting earlier within 4–6 months, peaking within 7–12 months after Gamma Knife surgery, and to have more severe symptoms. Among this group of patients, ARE were evident in 74.4% and being significant in terms of symptom in 58.1% [5]. Steroids such as dexamethasone is commonly used to treat this condition.

Gamma Knife surgery doesn't increase risk of hemorrhage, compared to natural history of AVM. In fact, although debatable, it seems to reduce the risk especially when higher margin dose is administered [6, 7]. It is reasonable to have higher margin dose for small nidus, while for larger ones, dose should be lowered. Risk of cyst formation and neoplasia or malignancy on long-term follow-up is even far less. There are very few reports currently on neoplasia or malignancy induced by Gamma Knife surgery.

32.8 Things to Be Observed and Postoperative Care/Follow-Up

Rarely we find excessive bleeding from pin site that we need to put stitches on. Some patients experience temporary headache or even being nauseous right after frame removal that we recommend observation at least an hour or two before discharge.

Patients are followed up clinically within 2 weeks posttreatment and every 6-month intervals subsequently within 3-year period. MRI examinations were scheduled within 6–12-month interval and DSA within 1–2-year interval. MRI is performed regularly to follow-up change and potential complications, while DSA is to confirm obliteration of AVM. For those who develop clinically significant ARE, intravenous steroid starting 10 mg dexamethasone four times a day is initiated and soon is tapered off as clinical condition improves.

References

1. Abecassis IJ, Xu DS, Batjer HH, Bendok BR. Natural history of brain arteriovenous malformations: a systematic review. Neurosurg Focus. 2014;37(3):E7.
2. Gross BA, Du R. Natural history of cerebral arteriovenous malformations: a meta-analysis. J Neurosurg. 2013;118:437–43.
3. Starke RM, Yen C, Ding D, Sheehan JP. A practical grading scale for predicting outcome after radiosurgery for arteriovenous malformations: analysis of 1012 treated patients. J Neurosurg. 2013;119:981–7.
4. Yen C, Matsumoto JA, Wintermark M, Schwyzer L, Evans AJ, Jensen ME, et al. Radiation-induced imaging changes following gamma knife surgery for cerebral arteriovenous malformations. J Neurosurg. 2013;118:63–73.
5. Cohen-Inbar O, Lee C, Xu Z, Schlesinger D, Sheehan JP. A quantitative analysis of adverse radiation effects following gamma knife surgery for arteriovenous malformations. J Neurosurg. 2015;123:945–53.
6. Yen C, Sheehan JP, Schwyzer L, Schlesinger D. Hemorrhage risk of arteriovenous malformation before and during the latency period after gamma knife radiosurgery. Stroke. 2011;42:1691–6.
7. Pollock BE, Link MJ, Brown RD. The risk of stroke or clinical impairment after stereotactic radiosurgery for ARUBA-eligible patients. Stroke. 2013; 44:437–41.

Index

J. July, E. J. Wahjoepramono (eds.), *Neurovascular Surgery*,
https://doi.org/10.1007/978-981-10-8950-3